handbook of
OBSTETRIC ANESTHESIA

handbook of
OBSTETRIC
ANESTHESIA

Craig M. Palmer

Professor of Clinical Anesthesiology,
University of Arizona Health Sciences Center,
Tucson, AZ, USA

Robert D'Angelo

Associate Professor of Anesthesiology,
Wake Forest University,
Winston Salem, NC, USA

Michael J. Paech

Consultant Anesthesiologist,
King Edward Memorial Hospital for Women,
Perth, WA, Australia

A CIP catalogue record for this book is available from the British Library.

ISBN 1 85996 232 7

BIOS Scientific Publishers Ltd
9 Newtec Place, Magdalen Road, Oxford OX4 1RE, UK
Tel. 144 (0) 1865 726286. Fax 144 (0) 1865 246823
World Wide Web home page: http://www.bios.co.uk/

Distributed exclusively in the United States of America, its dependent territories, Canada, Mexico, Central and South America, and the Carribean by Springer-Verlag New York Inc., 175 Fifth Avenue, New York, USA, by arrangement with BIOS Scientific Publishers Ltd., 9 Newtec Place, Magdalen Road, Oxford OX4 1RE, UK

Important Note from the Publisher
The information contained within this book was obtained by BIOS Scientific Publishers Ltd from sources believed by us to be reliable. However, while every effort has been made to ensure its accuracy, no responsibility for loss or injury whatsoever occasioned to any person acting or refraining from action as a result of information contained herein can be accepted by the authors or publishers.

The reader should remember that medicine is a constantly evolving science and while the authors and publishers have ensured that all dosages, applications and practices are based on current indications, there may be specific practices which differ between communities. You should always follow the guidelines laid down by the manufacturers of specific products and the relevant authorities in the country in which you are practising.

Production Editor: Andrea Bosher
Designed and typeset by J&L Composition Ltd, Filey, North Yorkshire
Printed by Cromwell Press, Trowbridge, UK

Contents

Contents

Abbreviations

Ach	acetylcholine	IV	intravenous
AMPA	α-amino-3–hydroxy-5–4–isoxazolepropionic acid	IVC	inferior vena cava
		IVH	intraventricular hemorrhage
BP	blood pressure	LA	local anesthetic
bpm	beats per minute	LBW	low birth weight
CNS	central nervous system	LOR	loss of resistance
CPD	cephalopelvic disproportion	MAC	minimum alveolar concentration
CS	cesarean section	MLK	myosin light-chain kinase
CSEA	combined spinal-epidural anesthesia	NMDA	N-methyl-D-aspartate
CSF	cerebrospinal fluid	PCEA	patient-controlled epidural anesthesia
DIC	disseminated intravascular coagulation	PCIA	patient-controlled intravenous analgesia
EA	epidural anesthesia	PDPH	post-dural puncture headache
EBP	epidural blood patch	PIH	pregnancy-induced hypertension
ECG	electrocardiogram	p.p.m.	parts per million
ECV	external cephalic version	PPV	positive-pressure ventilation
EGA	estimated gestational age	PTL	preterm labor
FHR	fetal heart rate	PVR	pulmonary vascular resistance
FRC	functional residual capacity	RDS	respiratory distress syndrome
GA	general anesthesia	SA	spinal anesthesia
HOCM	hypertrophic obstructive cardiomyopathy	SVC	superior vena cava
		SVR	systemic vascular resistance
ICP	intracranial pressure	UPP	uterine perfusion pressure
IM	intramuscular	WDR	wide dynamic range
IUGR	intrauterine growth retardation		

Contributors

Valerie A. Arkoosh, MD
Associate Professor of Anesthesiology and Obstetrics & Gynecology, MCP Hahnemann University Philadelphia, PA, USA

Laura S. Dean, MD
Assistant Professor, Department of Anesthesiology, Wake forest University, Winston-Salem, NC, USA

Paul Fenton, MD
Associate Professor of Anaesthesia, Malawi College of Medicine, Blantyre, Malawi, Africa.

Kenneth E. Nelson, MD
Assistant Professor, Department of Anesthesiology, Wake Forest University, Winston-Salem, NC, USA

Medge D. Owen, MD
Assistant Professor, Department of Anesthesiology, Wake Forest University, Winston-Salem, NC, USA

John A. Thomas, MD
Assistant Professor, Department of Anesthesiology, Wake Forest University, Winston-Salem, NC, USA

Preface

Obstetric anesthesia is a rapidly expanding and evolving field, and this is certainly not the first book to address the subspecialty. When the idea of a completely new text was first raised, our first questions were whether there was a need for a book, and how it would differ from previous textbooks.

We saw a need for a practical guide to patient care and management, one that could be consulted quickly (and often) to outline a concrete course of clinical management: how to manage specific patients in specific situations, what drug to give, how to give it, how much to give, and when to stop and try something different. Our goal in this book has been to provide anethesiologists and anesthetists, both in training and in practice, with that practical reference.

We have worked diligently to make the information easy to use—when possible, we have tried to distill essential information down into tables, charts, diagrams, and flowcharts which can be quickly accessed and applied. We have tried to limit the discussion to the essential background, rationale, and science behind clinical decision-making. This is not intended to be an exhaustive reference textbook, though the readings and references at the end of each chapter do provide additional background and the basis for further study.

Of course, as the saying goes, ". . . there is more than one way to skin a cat." Where our experience has shown one approach works best, we have advocated it; where there are equally viable options, we have tried to present each, with the advantages and disadvantages of alternate approaches.

All three of us are full-time clinical obstetric anethesiologists, as are most of our contributors. We care for these patients and deal with these problems everyday. The *Handbook of Obstetric Anesthesia* draws on our experience and study to tell you what we do, how we do it and why.

Craig M. Palmer, M.D.
Robert D'Angelo, M.D.
Michael J. Paech, FANZA

Chapter 1

Overview of obstetric anesthesia

Craig M. Palmer, MD

Contents

1.1 Introduction

The field of obstetric anesthesia has a long and proud tradition, very nearly as long as the specialty of anesthesiology itself. The way obstetric anesthesia is practiced today has been shaped by the social pressures of the last century. Much more than other subspecialties within anesthesiology, and more than most other fields of medicine in general, the practice of obstetric anesthesia has been shaped by the desires of the patients it serves – laboring women. The demands and desires of the parturient remain the strongest influence on the field today.

1.2 A brief history of obstetric anesthesia

The year 1997 marked the 150th anniversary of the birth of obstetric anesthesia. On 19 January 1847, James Young Simpson (*Figure 1.1*) administered diethyl ether to a young woman with a deformed pelvis to aid in the vaginal delivery of her stillborn infant. Simpson was Professor and Chair of Midwifery and Diseases of Women and Children at the University of Edinburgh in Scotland. It was only 5 years earlier that Crawford Long, a physician in Georgia, was the first to use ether for a surgical procedure, the painless removal of a neck tumor.

Simpson immediately became a great advocate of the use of ether to relieve the pain accompanying labor and delivery, but most of the established institutions of the day failed to exhibit his enthusiasm. The Church of Scotland condemned its use as contrary to God's will, citing the book of Genesis in the Bible: 'In sorrow thou shalt bring forth children.' Many of the most eminent physicians of the day also opposed its use. Charles Meigs, Professor of Obstetrics at Jefferson Medical College in Philadelphia, was representative of many of the opponents of ether, arguing that pain was a necessary and useful part of childbirth, and relieving pain might interfere with the normal progress of labor. Some of this opposition was

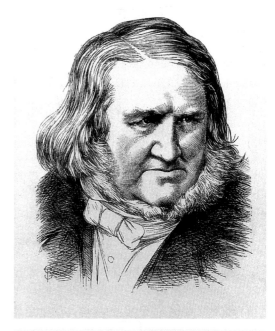

Figure 1.1 James Young Simpson. Simpson was Professor and Chair of Midwifery and Diseases of Women and Children at the University of Edinburgh in Scotland. In January of 1847 he used ether to assist a patient during a difficult delivery. He is considered the 'Father of Obstetric Anesthesia'. Courtesy of The Wood Library-Museum of Anesthesiology, Park Ridge, IL.

well founded – little or nothing was known about ether's effects on the infant, mother, or progress of labor. As neither side had much in the way of objective evidence on their side, the debate continued for years. The controversy about anesthetic effects on labor continues to this day (see Section 5.8).

The first use of ether for childbirth in the USA also occurred in 1847. Fanny Longfellow, wife of the poet Henry Wadsworth Longfellow, had heard of the use of this new drug for analgesia during labor, and enlisted the aid of a dentist, Nathan Cooley Keep, to administer it when she could not find a physician willing to do so. Also in 1847, Walter Channing, Dean of the Harvard Medical School, first used ether for a forceps delivery.

The popularity of anesthesia for labor and delivery was greatly accelerated in 1853, when John Snow (*Figure 1.2*) administered chloroform to Queen Victoria for the birth of her eighth child, Prince Leopold. This event quickly gave the use of inhaled anesthetics during labor a measure of validity in the public eye. Snow was also among the first to begin to look at the use of anesthesia during childbirth in a careful, rational way. That same year, 1853, he observed that infants born to mothers who had received chloroform during delivery were less vigorous at birth than those born without anesthesia; he concluded that the chloroform must also affect the infant, though to a lesser extent than the mother.

Use of inhaled anesthesia for labor continued to gain momentum through the latter half of the 19th century. Ether was usually the anesthetic of choice. While gaining in popularity, inhaled anesthesia for labor still presented problems – the risk of aspiration became apparent, and the potential for asphyxia of both mother and infant in untrained hands. The vast majority of births during this period occurred at home, attended by lay midwives; since only physicians could use anesthetics, they were actually available to very few women. Further, as labor was often prolonged for several hours, even in those cases where anesthesia was used, its actual administration was often left to the husband or some other untrained bystander who happened to be available.

By the turn of the century, a new approach was being developed. Morphine had first been isolated in the early 1800s, but was not used for labor analgesia until the 1900s. By 1907, Richard von Steinbuchel, an Austrian physician, described a method for labor analgesia that had been used by surgeons for several years: *Dämmerschlef*, or 'Twilight Sleep'. Twilight sleep entailed subcutaneous injections of morphine and scopolamine; used alone, neither provided a satisfactory result and could even be dangerous, but two German obstetricians, Carl Gauss and Bernhardt Krönig, believed that by combining the two in the correct amounts, the benefits of each could be gained without the drawbacks. The parturient was given an initial injection of both drugs at the beginning of labor, then intermittent injections of scopolamine throughout the duration of labor. The initial morphine given, about 10 mg, provided a modest degree of analgesia, while the scopolamine was an amnestic; pain may not have been eliminated, but it was rarely remembered. In addition to amnesia, however, scopolamine disinhibited many patients, causing them to become disoriented and thrash about; because of this, parturients required constant attendance.

Despite these drawbacks, twilight sleep gained a popular following. A popular US magazine of the pre-war period, *McClure's*, sent two journalists, Mary Boyd and Marguerite Tracy to

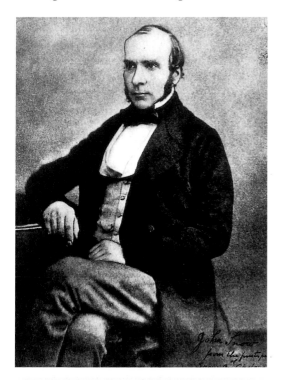

Figure 1.2 John Snow. In 1853, he administered chloroform to Queen Victoria of England for the birth of her eighth child, Prince Leopold. The event catalyzed the use of inhaled anesthetics for obstetric anesthesia. Courtesy of The Wood Library-Museum of Anesthesiology, Park Ridge, IL.

3

the Freiburg, Germany clinic of Gauss and Krönig to report on the technique firsthand. In 1914, *McClure's* published an article detailing Boyd's own experience giving birth at the clinic; the article presented the technique in a very favorable light, characterizing twilight sleep as a safe and effective method of pain relief during labor. Upon their return, the two women were instrumental in the founding of the National Twilight Sleep Association. The Association was a 'grassroots' lay organization dedicated to expanding the use of this form of analgesia in the US. It was formed as a reaction to the lack of enthusiasm the medical establishment of the day showed for the technique. The association was part of a larger social feminist movement of the time, aimed at improving the health and welfare of women and children in a wide array of areas.

Several years later, in 1927, a similar organization was founded in Great Britain, the National Birthday Trust Fund. The Fund was initiated by two upper class women, Ladies Rhys-Williams and Cholmondelay, with the aim of extending to all classes of the British public the same quality of maternal and obstetric care enjoyed at the time only by the aristocracy and royalty. While providing maternal labor analgesia was a major part of the drive, the Fund had broader goals than the Twilight Sleep Association; it aimed to improve all aspects of obstetric care, not just obstetric anesthesia. Rather than just championing a single method, they encouraged the involved professionals – obstetricians, midwives, and anesthetists – to actively innovate and develop better methods for health care delivery. The Fund provided monies to research new techniques and agents for the provision of labor analgesia. Over the succeeding 20 years, the Fund was able to dramatically improve the delivery of health care to British women and children.

Together, both these movements had an important secondary effect – moving labor and delivery from the home to hospitals and nursing homes. Because of the maternal supervision which twilight sleep entailed, it was ill suited to being administered in parturients' homes, even if individuals who understood the technique would have been available. Likewise, many of the inhalation techniques that were developed with the help of the National Birthday Trust Fund required apparatus that was not easily moved to individual homes. Movement of deliveries to nursing homes and hospitals also had the benefit of providing cleaner surroundings, and increased the use of aseptic techniques during the delivery process. From the anesthetic perspective, this movement from home to hospital had a dramatic effect – the flow of patients through these facilities allowed physicians to specialize in the provision of labor analgesia, and develop the regional anesthetic techniques that have become the mainstay of labor analgesic practice today.

Despite the ever-increasing enthusiasm of the lay public for labor analgesia, not all professionals were convinced of its merits. Grantly Dick-Read published his first book, *Natural Childbirth*, in 1933, though he had written his first draft over 10 years earlier while still in training to be an obstetrician (*Figure 1.3*). Based partly on his observations of childbirth in 'primitive' societies, Dick-Read believed that it was society that was responsible for labor pain, by propagating misconceptions, superstitions, and misinformation about childbirth which caused women to fear childbirth. Fear produces tension, which in turn produces pain; eliminate the fear, and the pain of labor will be eliminated also. The key to the elimination of fear, according to Dick-Read, is education about the delivery process, and training in breathing exercises to attain a state of relaxation.

A second vocal opponent of the use of medication to relieve labor pain was Fernand Lamaze of France (*Figure 1.4*). Lamaze ran a clinic in Paris, and built upon the work of the Russian physiologist Velvoski who used 'psychoprophylaxis' for pain relief during labor. Lamaze and Velvoski believed that positive conditioned reflexes could be used to eliminate labor pain, and pregnant women could learn to use this method with training in

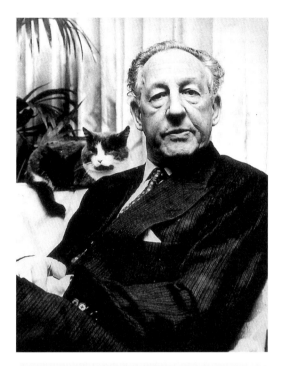

Figure 1.3 Grantly Dick-Read. In 1933 he published his first book, *Natural Childbirth*. Dick-Read, a British obstetrician, did not believe labor and delivery were inherently painful; he believed society was responsible for labor pain, causing women to fear childbirth. This fear produced tension, which in turn produced pain. Courtesy of The Wellcome Trust, London, UK.

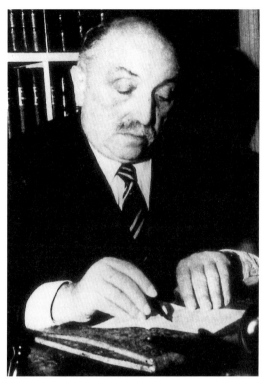

Figure 1.4 Fernand Lamaze. Lamaze was a French obstetrician who popularized the use of 'psychoprophylaxis' for pain relief during labor. Lamaze believed that positive conditioned reflexes, based on breathing exercises and relaxation techniques, could be used to eliminate labor pain. Lamaze's book, *Painless Childbirth*, has become the basis of most 'natural childbirth' classes today. Courtesy of The Wood Library-Museum of Anesthesiology, Park Ridge, IL.

breathing exercises and relaxation techniques. Such psychoprophylactic techniques are the direct application of Pavlovian conditioning to labor. Lamaze wrote a book, *Painless Childbirth*, that was widely read and has become the basis of most 'natural childbirth' classes today.

Regional anesthesia for labor and delivery was slowly advancing during this period. In 1900, Oskar Kreis first described the use of spinal anesthesia in parturients. He injected 10 mg of cocaine into the lumbar spine of six parturients, and observed pain relief that lasted about 2 hours. Despite such early successes, regional anesthesia took many years to gain momentum. Part of the reason for this slow development was the relative paucity of equipment and medication, but part was also due to the fact that obstetricians, who were providing the vast majority of anesthesia during labor, reserved spinal anesthesia for delivery.

In the early 1930s, a Romanian anesthesiologist, Eugene Aburel, described the sensory innervation of the uterus and perineum. He also pioneered early sacral epidural techniques and caudal analgesia for the second stage of labor. Unfortunately, due to the fact that he published his findings in the German and French literature, the disruption of scientific literature that surrounded World War II prevented his work from appearing in the West for almost 40 years.

About the same time, in 1933, John Cleland published a report on the use of paravertebral block for labor analgesia and also outlined the relevant nerve pathways associated with sensation and pain during labor. In 1942, Robert Hingson and Waldo Edwards published a report detailing the use of caudal anesthesia for labor and delivery, in which they used a small malleable needle that remained taped in place during labor. Later, the development of flexible catheters that could be threaded into the epidural space sparked a shift to lumbar epidural anesthesia that remains the dominant method of regional anesthesia for labor today.

It took more than just the development of regional techniques to supplant the use of twilight sleep and inhalational anesthesia for labor, however. Though pain was reduced with these systemic techniques, the amnesia induced often left the mother feeling disconnected from the birth experience, and somehow 'unfulfilled'. By the 1960s, the desire to be actively involved in the birth process was overtaking the desire for analgesia in the minds of parturients, and enhanced the popularity of Dick-Read's and Lamaze's 'natural childbirth' methods. The rapid development in the last two decades of regional anesthetic techniques that lack significant motor block, and even allow ambulation, has eliminated most of the concerns associated with systemic analgesics, and (much to their surprise) has fulfilled the expectations of 'natural childbirth' advocates.

It is interesting to note that the goals of both the natural childbirth movement and the obstetric anesthesia community have been the same: an awake, fully-functional, and participating mother during delivery, without neonatal side effects or interference with the natural course of labor. Despite occasional tensions between the two camps, only the paths they have taken to this common goal differ.

Further reading

Caton, D. (1970) Obstetric anesthesia – the first ten years. *Anesthesiology* **33**: 102–109.

Caton, D. (1994) The history of obstetric anesthesia. In: *Obstetric Anesthesia: Principles and Practice* (ed. Chestnut, D.H.), pp. 3–13. Mosby-Yearbook, Inc., St Louis, MO.

Caton, D. (1999) What a blessing she had chloroform. Yale University Press, New Haven.

Cleland, J.G.P. (1933) Paravertebral anaesthesia in obstetrics. *Surg. Gynecol. Obstet.* **57**: 51–62.

Curelaru, I. and Sandu, L. (1982) Eugene Bogdan Aburel (1899–1975). The pioneer of regional anesthesia for pain relief in childbirth. *Anaesthesia* **37**: 663–669.

Dick-Read, G. (1944) Childbirth without fear. Harper and Row, New York.

Eisenach, J.C. and Dewan, D.M. (2000) Evolution in analgesia in obstetrics over the last 30 years. *Am. J. Anesthesiol.* **27**: 26–28.

Farr, A.D. (1980) Early opposition to obstetric anesthesia. *Anaesthesia* **35**: 896–907.

Hingson, R.A. and Edwards, W.B. (1943) Continuous caudal anesthesia: an analysis of the first ten thousand confinements thus managed with the report of the authors' first thousand cases. *JAMA* **123**: 538–546.

Lamaze, F. (1956) Painless childbirth: psychoprophylactic method. Burke, London.

Stampone, D. (1990) The history of obstetric anesthesia. *J. Perinat. Neonatal Nurs.* **4**: 1–13.

Chapter 2

Anatomic and physiologic changes of pregnancy

Laura S. Dean, MD and
Robert D'Angelo, MD

Contents

2.1 Introduction

Profound physiologic and mechanical changes occur during pregnancy. Unique alterations allow for the development of a growing fetus and prepare the parturient for the demands of labor and delivery. Anesthesia providers must recognize the anesthetic implications of this altered physiology in order to care for patients throughout the puerperium as well as during non-obstetric surgery. Many of the physiologic adaptations occur during the first trimester making recognition of pregnancy in women of childbearing age imperative.

2.2 Cardiovascular

2.2.1 Hemodynamics

Cardiovascular parameters are altered progressively throughout pregnancy and are accentuated in pregnancies subsequent to the first (*Table 2.1*). Beginning as early as 4–8 weeks gestation and plateauing between 16 and 24 weeks, these alterations become further dependent on changes in the parturient's position as aortocaval compression worsens during the third trimester. In general, these alterations return to pre-pregnancy baseline during the first 6 months to 1 year postpartum.

Initially, systemic vascular resistance decreases as a result of increased circulating estrogen and progesterone. This decrease in systemic tone results in reduced afterload and preload triggering a reflex increase in heart rate. Volume restoring mechanisms including angiotensin and aldosterone are activated to elevate blood volume. Cardiac output elevation thus results from an increase in both stroke volume and heart rate. Increased left ventricular wall thickness and ventricular cavity accommodate the elevated cardiac output. Despite this remodeling, contractility is probably unchanged. It is crucial to recognize the normal changes in the cardiac exam that occur during pregnancy (*Table 2.2*). While diastolic murmurs and S4 heart sounds are not uncommon, both should be further evaluated for underlying heart disease. The increased blood flow is redistributed to meet the demands of the growing fetus and altered maternal physiology (*Table 2.3*).

Table 2.1 Cardiovascular adaptations during pregnancy

Parameter	Change
Cardiac output	↑ 20–40%
Stroke volume	↑ 30%
Heart rate*	↑ 16%
Systemic vascular resistance	↑ 30%
Mean arterial pressure**	↑ 8%
Plasma volume	↑ 11–50%
Oxygen consumption †	↑ 20%

*At 4 weeks gestation there is a 20 bpm increase in heart rate. **Mean arterial blood pressure will fall as a result of a decrease in systemic vascular resistance despite an increase in cardiac output. † Cardiac oxygen consumption increases in conjunction with resting tachycardia.

Table 2.2 Cardiac exam findings during pregnancy*

Accentuated and split S$_1$

Normal S$_2$

Systolic ejection murmur (90%)

Diastolic flow murmur (20%)

S$_3$ heart sound (80%)

Occasional S$_4$

*Flow murmurs correlate with the increase in blood volume rather than the alteration in the cardiac output. A pericardial effusion (9%) may cause isoelectric T waves and ST changes on the electrocardiogram.

Table 2.3 Redistribution of cardiac output during pregnancy

Organ	Increase in blood flow
Uterus	500 ml/min
Skin	300–400 ml/min
Renal	400 ml/min
Breasts	200 ml/min
Overall increase during pregnancy	1.5–2 l/min

2.2.2 Blood volumes

A 40–50% increase in blood volume during pregnancy meets the metabolic demands of the enlarging uterus and growing fetus. This relative hypervolemia is crucial for protecting the mother and fetus from hemorrhage at delivery and from the deleterious effects of decreased venous return in the supine position. The mechanisms accounting for the increase in blood volume are multifactorial. Progesterone relaxes venous smooth muscle thus increasing venous capacitance. The increase in blood volume may be a response to fill this increased vascular capacity. Estrogen and progesterone are also thought to directly mediate an increase in hepatic renin production which triggers enhanced secretion of aldosterone. The resultant retention of sodium allows for the increase in total body water. As early as the first trimester, increased renin and angiotensin diminish the pressor response to angiotensin during pregnancy. In contrast, response to norepinephrine infusions is unchanged. Enhanced renal erythropoietin production simultaneously increases red blood cell volume. However, the plasma volume increase is proportionately greater than the red cell volume increase resulting in a hemodilutional anemia (*Table 2.4*).

2.2.3 Aortocaval compression

A symptomatic reduction in cardiac output in the supine position occurs in 5–10% of parturients and is referred to as the supine hypotensive syndrome. Manifestations include dizziness, nausea, maternal hypotension, shortness of breath, tachycardia and possibly fetal distress. Compression of the inferior vena cava by the enlarged uterus reduces venous return and can result in profound hypotension. Abdominal aortic compression further compromises uterine blood flow. Neuraxial or general anesthesia may exaggerate these hemodynamic effects. It is important to recognize that the standard 15 degree lateral tilt that is vital for the obstetric patient may not be adequate to relieve aortocaval compression in all parturients. The lateral decubitus position or even the knee chest position may be necessary to alleviate maternal hypotension or fetal heart rate changes. Although supine hypotension is classically described beyond 20 weeks gestation, partial or complete compression can occur before this time. Anesthesia providers should consider left uterine displacement in pregnant women beyond 12–16 weeks gestation.

If aortocaval compression is suspected in a hypotensive patient, the compressed inferior vena cava may act like two pieces of wet glass that resist separation. Alleviating the compression and restoring adequate venous return are paramount. Treatment consists of ensuring left uterine displacement, ephedrine administration, and elevation of the legs, rather than placing the patient in the Trendelenburg's position.

2.3 Pulmonary

As summarized in *Table 2.5*, there are numerous mechanical and physiologic pulmonary adaptations that occur during pregnancy.

2.3.1 Mechanical effects

Venous engorgement and edema of the upper airway involves the pharynx, glottis, trachea and vocal cords making visualization during endotracheal intubation more challenging than in the nonpregnant patient. Enlarged breasts and redundant soft tissue in the neck and chest may inhibit placement of the laryngoscope. Chest circumference increases 5–7 cm as a result of both increased anterior posterior and transverse diameters. The anesthetic implications of these anatomic changes are shown in *Table 2.6*.

Table 2.4 Physiologic anemia of pregnancy

Parameter	Level during pregnancy
Blood volume	↑ 45%
Plasma volume	↑ 55%
Red cell volume	↑ 30%
Hemoglobin (average)	11.6 mg/dl
Hematocrit (average)	33.5 mg/dl

Table 2.5 Pulmonary alterations during pregnancy

Parameter	Change during pregnancy
Respiratory rate	↑ 9%*
Tidal volume	↑ 19–28%
Expiratory reserve volume	↓ 17%
Residual volume	No change–↓ 20%
Functional residual capacity	↓ 12–25%**
Vital capacity	No change–↑ 6%***
Total lung capacity	No change–↓ 5%
O_2 consumption	↑ 20–40%†
Minute ventilation	↑ 20–50%
FEV_1	No change‡
Basal metabolic rate	↑ 14%

*Early in the first trimester, hyperventilation is stimulated by a progesterone-mediated hypersensitivity of respiratory centers to CO_2. ** The decrease in FRC may result in airway closure during tidal breathing in as many as 50% of term parturients in the supine position. *** Despite elevation of the diaphragm by the enlarging uterus there is no change in vital capacity because of the simultaneous increase in chest wall diameter. † The increase in cardiac output is greater than the increase in oxygen consumption so the AVO_2 difference in early pregnancy is decreased. As cardiac output plateaus and the metabolism of the fetus and growing uterus further increases O_2 consumption the AVO_2 difference approaches pre-pregnancy levels. ‡ There are no documented changes in airway flow or diffusion capacity.

2.3.2 Acid-base physiology in pregnancy

Hyperventilation induces a slight respiratory alkalosis. Renal compensation decreases plasma HCO_3 allowing for a near normal pH. Although respiratory alkalosis shifts the oxyhemoglobin dissociation curve to the left, 2,3-DPG production rises 30% above nonpregnant levels and shifts the curve back to the right. P_{50} is increased from 26.7 to 30.4 aiding delivery of oxygen to the fetus. The increase in minute ventilation, cardiac output and blood volume along with a fall in alveolar dead space contribute to a negligible arterial to end tidal CO_2 difference at term. Arterial blood gas values seen in nonpregnant and pregnant patients are listed in *Table 2.7*.

2.4 Gastrointestinal

Controversy exists over the effects of pregnancy on the rate of gastric emptying. Some investigators have suggested that motility decreases early in pregnancy, some not until the third trimester and others contend there is never any alteration in gastric emptying. This issue is important clinically during pregnancy but also in the days post delivery. *Table 2.8* reviews studies that have examined the changes in gastric physiology. The placenta and fetus produce gastrin which increases the volume and acidity of gastric contents. Progesterone slows gastric motility by inhibiting motilin and diminishes the lower esophageal sphincter tone by relaxing smooth muscle. The gravid uterus increases gastric pressure and elevates the lower esophagus into the thorax in many women. Consequently, 80% of term parturients experience pyrosis. Opioids administered during labor or for non-obstetric surgery will further impair gastric motility. All pregnant women should be considered to have full stomachs regardless of NPO status. Obstetrics provides a unique anesthetic setting during which the likelihood of difficult mask ventilation and failed intubation is higher than normal at a time when aspiration is also more likely to occur. Aspiration prophylaxis to reduce the chance of pneumonitis should be routinely followed. Recommendations are noted in *Table 2.9*.

2.5 Renal

The renal system undergoes anatomical and physiologic changes during pregnancy. Increased vascular and interstitial volumes result in slightly enlarged kidneys. The pelvis, calyces and ureters are dilated by the effects of progesterone and probably by the mechanical effects of the gravid uterus. Renal plasma flow and glomerular filtration increase early in the first trimester. These changes precede the

Table 2.6 Anesthetic implications of pulmonary manifestations of pregnancy*

Anatomic/physiologic change	Anesthetic implication/recommendations
Redundant soft tissue: neck, chest, breasts	May obstruct laryngoscope placement: Have short handle available.
Mucosal venous engorgement/edema Increased Mallampati scores throughout labor	May result in impaired visualization and a friable bleeding airway with intubation. Avoid nasal instrumentation. Have smaller ETT available. Important to have experienced personnel available.
↓ FRC, ↑ O_2 consumption	Prone to hypoxia during general anesthesia induction. Maximal preoxygenation is crucial. Rapid sequence induction with cricoid pressure indicated.
Normal $paCO_2$ – 32 mmHg There is little to no arterial/end-tidal CO_2 gradient.	Maintain normocarbia during general anesthesia. Avoid hyperventilation (↓$paCO_2$ will cause uterine vasoconstriction and ↓placental blood flow. Alkalosis will shift $HgbO_2$ curve to the left decreasing release of O_2 to the fetus).

*The leading causes of anesthesia related morbidity and mortality in pregnancy are failure to intubate or ventilate and aspiration.

Table 2.7 Arterial blood gas results in normal pregnancy

Parameter	Pregnant	Nonpregnant
$PaCO_2$	30–32 mmHg	40 mmHg
PaO_2	92–106 mmHg	100 mmHg
Supine paO_2	101–94 mmHg	100 mmHg
HCO_3	16–21 meq/l	24 meq/l
PH	7.405–7.44	7.40

increase in plasma volume suggesting hormonal mechanisms. BUN and creatinine are lowered as GFR and renal plasma flow increase. (*Table 2.10*) Even mild elevations in plasma levels should be investigated for evidence of renal disease.

Glucosuria, independent of blood sugar concentration, is noted soon after conception. The renal tubules are likely unable to accept the

Table 2.8 Summary of studies investigating gastric emptying during pregnancy

Study	Findings
1. Davison JS *et al.*	Positive delayed emptying
2. O'Sullivan GM *et al.*	No difference in rate of emptying during pregnancy
3. Simpson KH *et al.*	Positive delay at 12–14 weeks gestation compared to controls
4. Macfie AG *et al.*	No delay during pregnancy compared to controls
5. Sandhar BK *et al.*	No statistically significant change in gastric emptying as a result of pregnancy.
6. Carp H *et al.*	Emptying of the stomach is delayed for many hours after the onset of labor.
7. Whitehead EM *et al.*	Significant delay in gastric emptying 2 hours post partum, but no differences in emptying times during three trimesters of pregnancy when compared to 18 hours after delivery.
8. Levy DM *et al.*	Positive delay at 8–12 wks
9. Gin T	Rapid emptying post-partum

1. *J. Obst. Gyn. Br. Com.* 1970; **77**:37. 2. *Anaesth. Analg.* 1987; **66**:505. 3. *Br. J. Anaesth.* 1988; **60**: 24. 4. *Br. J. Anaesth.* 1991; **67**: 54. 5. *Anaesthesia* 1992; **47**: 196. 6. *Anesth. Analg.* 1992; **74**: 683. 7. *Anaesthesia* 1993; **48**: 53. 8. *Br. J. Anaesth.* 1994; **73**: 237. 9. *Anaesthesia.* 1993; **48**: 821.

Table 2.9 Recommended aspiration precautions

- Nonparticulate antacid – 30 ml, 30–45 minutes before surgery
- Metoclopramide – Consider in high risk patients 30–90 minutes before surgery
- Consider all pregnant patients to have full stomachs
- Use rapid sequence induction with cricoid pressure
- Avoid positive pressure mask ventilation if possible
- Extubate patients when fully awake

Table 2.10 Renal hemodynamics

Parameter	First trimester	Third trimester
RPF (renal plasma flow)	↑ 75– 85%	↓ 50%
GFR (glomerular filtration rate)	↑ 50%	↑ 50%
Filtration fraction – RPF/GFR	↓	↔
Creatinine	WNL	↓ 0.4–0.6 mg/dl
BUN	8 – 9 mg/dl	↓ 6–8 mg/dl

increased filtered load of glucose accompanying the increase in GFR. Uric acid tubular reabsorption declines so that plasma uric acid concentration increases in the third trimester. Plasma osmolality decreases early in pregnancy as water is retained in excess of sodium. The osmotic threshold for thirst declines further increasing fluid intake to contribute to the decline in osmolality.

2.6 Hepatic

The diagnosis of liver disease in pregnancy is confounded by the normal changes that occur in liver function studies during gestation (*Table 2.11*). Plasma cholinesterase levels decline 20–30% by term pregnancy. However, the simultaneous increase in volume of distribution likely counters any clinically significant prolongation of neuromuscular blockade from succinylcholine.

Table 2.11 Diagnostic signs of liver disease vs. normal pregnancy

Parameter	Liver disease	Pregnancy
Clinical signs	Spider angiomata/ palmar erythema	Spider angiomata/ palmar erythema
Protein synthesis	Normal ↓↓↓	↓ 20–30%
Alkaline phosphatase	Normal to ↑↑↑ secondary to obstructive disease	↑ 200–400% by placental production
GGT, LDH, AST, ALT	Normal to ↑↑↑	High normal to ↑

2.7 Gallbladder

Decreased cholecystokinin release and a reduced contractile response of the gallbladder to cholecystokinin is mediated by increased progesterone levels. This combined effect yields a sluggish milieu with propensity for gallstone formation.

2.8 Glucose metabolism

Although insulin secretion rises during gestation, pregnancy is considered to be a 'diabetogenic' state. There is a relative insulin resistance mediated by decreased peripheral sensitivity to insulin evoked by circulating placental hormones (particularly human placental lactogen (HPL)). Carbohydrate loads result in higher plasma glucose levels than in nonpregnant patients allowing for placental transfer of glucose to the fetus. These alterations in glucose metabolism likely contribute to the propensity for gestational diabetes. Shortly after delivery of the fetus and placenta, insulin sensitivity returns to baseline. Insulin should be administered cautiously prior to delivery because of the possibility of hypoglycemia immediately postpartum. Insulin does not cross the placenta so the fetus is responsible for secreting its own insulin in response to glucose loads. The fetus of a hyperglycemic mother may become profoundly hypoglycemic after delivery when it no longer receives a glucose load but still has elevated circulating levels of insulin.

2.9 Thyroid

Although there is an elevation of total serum thyroxin during gestation and the thyroid gland is noted to be enlarged, a euthyroid clinical state is maintained throughout pregnancy.

2.10 Hematologic

The hemodilutional anemia of pregnancy was discussed earlier in this chapter. Platelets remain unchanged or fall slightly with no apparent clinical effect. Clotting mechanisms are activated with an elevated serum concentration of fibrinogen and all clotting factors except XI and XIII. Although this hypercoagulable state may be a protective mechanism to allow hemostasis after delivery, embolic complications remain a leading cause of morbidity and mortality during pregnancy. Leukocytosis peaks postpartum complicating the clinical diagnosis of infection and response to antibiotics (*Figure 2.1*).

2.11 Neurologic

Pregnant patients require approximately one third less local anesthetic for regional anesthesia. Theoretical explanations for this increased sensitivity to local anesthetics are listed in *Table 2.12*. Although there may be some contribution of mechanical effects, most experts favor the elevated progesterone theory. Pregnant women have elevated CSF progesterone levels that are speculated to alter neuronal structure and allow for increased local anesthetic effect.

2.12 Uterus

The uterus undergoes massive change during pregnancy. An organ that is 5 cm × 6 cm

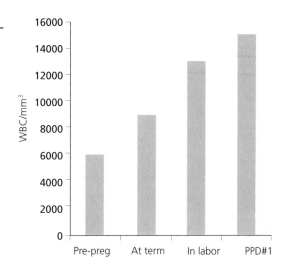

Figure 2.1 WBC count during pregnancy. WBC count increases slightly during pregnancy, acutely increases during labor, and remains elevated for at least the first week postpartum.

Table 2.12 Theories for increased local anesthetic sensitivity during pregnancy

1. A decreased epidural space secondary to epidural venous engorgement

2. Increased abdominal pressure enhancing transdural spread of local anesthetics

3. Exaggerated lumbar lordosis allowing increased cephalad spread of local anesthetic.

4. Progesterone enhanced sensitivity of nerves to local anesthetics.

increases in size to 25 cm × 30 cm at term. Uterine blood flow in nonpregnant females increases from 50 ml/min to 500–800 ml/min. The uterine vessels are maximally vasodilated. The fraction of cardiac output to the uterus increases from 3–4% up to 12% at term. Perfusion is not autoregulated so that a decrease in systemic blood pressure will result in impaired uteroplacental blood flow. Uterine contractions result in decreased placental perfusion and can lead to fetal compromise. Indirect acting agents, such as ephedrine, are preferred over peripheral α-1 agonists for maintaining arterial pressure and uterine blood flow.

2.13 Skeletal

<u>Corpus luteal production of relaxin increases</u> joint laxity. Exaggerated lumbar lordosis may contribute to the back and joint pain seen in some parturients.

2.14 Summary

The anatomic and physiologic changes that occur during pregnancy place the parturient at greater risk for complications during anesthesia than the nonpregnant patient. In particular, pregnant women are at an increased risk of complications during general anesthesia. A thorough understanding of these changes allows the anesthesia care provider to alter their anesthetic management to maximize benefits while minimizing risks.

Further reading

Blechner, J.N. (1993) Maternal–fetal acid-base physiology. *Clin. Obstet. Gynecol.* **36:** 3–12.

Clapp, J.F. (1988) Maternal heart rate in pregnancy. *Am. J. Obstet. Gynecol.* **152:** 659–660.

Clapp, J.F. 3rd, Seaward, B.L., Sleamaker, R.H. and Hiser, J. (1988) Maternal physiologic adaptations to early human pregnancy. *Am. J. Obstet. Gynecol.* **159:** 1456–1460.

Clapp, J.F. 3rd and Capeless, E. (1997) Cardiovascular function before, during and after the first and subsequent pregnancies. *Am. J. Cardiology.* **80:** 1469–1473.

Cutforth, R. and MacDonald, C.B. (1966) Heart sounds and murmurs in pregnancy. *Am. Heart J.* **71:** 741–747.

Dafnis, E and Sabatini, S. (1992) Effect of pregnancy on renal function. Physiology and pathophysiology. *Am. J. Med. Sci.* **303:** 184–205.

Datta, S., Lambert, D.H., Gregus, J., Gissen, A.J. and Covino, B.J. (1983) Differential sensitivity of mammalian nerve fibers during pregnancy. *Anesth. Analg.* **62:** 1070–1072.

Datta, S., Hurley, R.J., Naulty, J.S. et al. (1986) Plasma and cerebrospinal fluid progesterone concentration in pregnant and nonpregnant women. *Anesth. Analg.* **65:** 950–954.

Duvekot, J.J., Cheriex, E.C., Pieters, F.A. et al. (1993) Early pregnancy changes in hemodynamics and volume homeostasis are consecutive adjustments triggered by a primary fall in systemic vascular tone. *Am. J. Obstet. Gynecol.* **169:** 1382–1392.

Lund, C.J. and Donovan, J.C. (1967) Blood volume during pregnancy. Significance of plasma and red cell volumes. *Am. J. Obstet. Gynecol.* **98:** 394–403.

Mendelson, C.L. (1946) The aspiration of stomach contents into the lungs during obstetric anesthesia. *Am. J. Obstet. Gynecol.* **53:** 191–205.

Metcalf, J., McAnulty, J.H. and Ueland, K. (1981) CV physiology. *Clin. Obstet. Gynecol.* **24:** 693–710.

NcNair, R.D. and Jaynes, R.V. (1960) Alterations in liver function during normal pregnancy. *Am. J. Obstet. Gynecol.* **80:** 500.

Weinberger, S.E., Weiss, S.T., Cohen, W.R. et al. (1980) Pregnancy and the lung. *Am. Rev. Respir. Dis.* **121:** 559–581.

Chapter 3

Fetal assessment

Craig M. Palmer, MD

Contents

3.1 Introduction

Obstetric anesthesia is unique among the anesthetic subspecialties in its responsibility to not one, but two patients: the parturient and the fetus. Not only must anesthetic interventions be in the best interests of the mother, but they must also, as far as possible, be in the best interests of the unborn infant. Often, the 'best' interests of these two patients are at odds with each other, and there is no single 'best' course of action. The appropriate anesthetic interventions will depend upon the clinical circumstances and the judgment and experience of the individual anesthesiologist.

Obstetric anesthesiologists need to be familiar with available means of fetal assessment for two reasons. First, all maternal anesthetic interventions have at least the potential to impact fetal well being. Second, in many (most?) emergent situations, anesthetic interventions are undertaken on the mother because of the fetus: understanding the role and limitations of fetal assessment is the knowledge that allows the anesthesiologist to exercise appropriate judgment.

3.2 Normal fetal growth and development

Estimated gestational age (EGA) is defined by obstetricians as the time from the first day of the last menstrual period. The actual time of fertilization is about two weeks later. On average, delivery occurs about 280 days from the first day of the last menstrual period, amounting to 40 weeks, or roughly 9 months. This 9-month gestation period is often divided into trimesters of 3 months each, corresponding to various obstetrical milestones.

About 1 week after ovulation and fertilization (which are closely related temporally) the blastocyst implants in the uterine lining. Development of the placenta and chorionic villi begin almost immediately; once this development begins, the products of conception are termed an 'embryo'. By 3 weeks after fertilization, a true intervillous space has developed, and maternal blood supply to the placenta is established.

Most major structures of the embryo have been formed by 8 weeks after fertilization. By 12 weeks EGA (10 weeks after fertilization), the uterus has enlarged enough to be palpable above the pubic symphysis. At midpoint of the pregnancy, 20 weeks EGA, the fetus weighs roughly 300 g. Over the next 4 weeks, weight more than doubles to over 600 g and passes 1000 g (2.2 lbs) by an EGA of 28 weeks. While the fetus is small, survival after delivery at this gestational age is almost 100% with skilled neonatal care. At term, 40 weeks EGA, average fetal weight is about 3400 g (*Table 3.1*).

3.3 Utero–placental physiology

The placenta is the organ of interface and communication between the mother and the

Table 3.1 Fetal developmental milestones

Estimated gestational age (weeks)	Average fetal weight (g)	Characteristics
2	—	Fertilization
3	<1	Implantation
12	14	Intestines in abdomen; Eyes closed
14	45	Identifiable external genitalia
18	200	Prominent ears; Lower limbs well-developed
22	460	Lanugo (hair) visible; Vernix present
26	820	Fingernails present; Little adipose tissue
28	1000	Eyelashes present
32	1700	Toenails present; Testes descending
40	3400	Fingernails beyond fingertips; Testes in scrotum

After Cunningham, F.G., MacDonald, P.C., Gant, N.F. *et al.* (eds) (1993) The morphological and functional development of the fetus. In: *Williams Obstetrics*, 19th edn, pp.165–207. Appleton & Lange, Norwalk, CT.

fetus. Through the placenta, oxygen and nutrients pass from the maternal circulation to the fetus, and carbon dioxide and waste products pass from the fetal circulation to the mother. There is no direct communication between maternal and fetal circulations. Fetal blood stays within the fetal capillaries of the chorionic villi, and maternal blood stays within the intervillous space of the placenta.

In order for a substance to pass from the maternal to the fetal circulation, it must traverse the trophoblast (the cells which form the boundary between the intervillous space and the chorionic villi), the stroma of the intravillous space, and the fetal capillary wall, or endothelium. Transfer across this barrier is not strictly passive; the trophoblast can actively speed or slow the transfer of many substances, particularly those of high molecular weight. Other important factors that impact placental transport include concentration gradients, the degree of protein binding, the rate of both maternal and fetal blood flow, and total surface area.

Molecules with a molecular weight of under 500 d move primarily by simple diffusion; this is the mechanism for transport of oxygen, carbon dioxide, water and electrolytes. Anesthetic gases, being relatively small molecules, also traverse the placenta via passive diffusion.

The rate of oxygen transfer across the placenta is limited by maternal and fetal blood flow. The placenta supplies approximately 8 ml min^{-1} kg^{-1} fetal body weight of oxygen to the developing fetus. Because of mixing of blood within the intervillous space, oxygen saturation of maternal blood in the intervillous space is lower than maternal arterial oxygen saturation (about 70%) with a pO$_2$ of 30 to 35 mmHg. Oxygen saturation of fetal blood in the umbilical vein is about the same, but the pO$_2$ is lower (*Table 3.2*). Despite this low pO$_2$, the fetus has several adaptations allowing it to grow and thrive *in utero*. These include a higher cardiac output per body weight than adults, increased oxygen affinity of fetal hemoglobin, and a higher hemoglobin concentration than adults. All these factors increase oxygen delivery at the tissue level.

Carbon dioxide transfer is by simple passive diffusion. Carbon dioxide crosses the placenta faster and more readily than oxygen. The pCO$_2$ in fetal blood returning to the placenta via the umbilical arteries is slightly higher than maternal venous pCO$_2$, which facilitates diffusion, as does the mild maternal hyperventilation and resulting respiratory alkalosis in the third trimester.

3.4 Fetal circulation

The fetal circulation is highly adapted to this metabolic environment (*Figure 3.1*). Oxygenated fetal blood returns from the placenta

Table 3.2 Normal values for oxygen, carbon dioxide, and pH in human maternal and fetal blood

	Uterine		Umbilical	
	Artery	Vein	Vein *from placenta* (O$_2$)	Artery
pO$_2$ (mmHg)	95	40	27	15
SaO$_2$ (percent saturation)	98	76	68	30
O$_2$ content (ml/dl)	15.8	12.2	14.5	6.4
Hemoglobin (g/dl)	12.0	12.0	16.0	16.0
O$_2$ capacity (ml O$_2$/dl)	16.1	16.1	21.4	21.4
Pco$_2$ (mmHg)	32	40	43	48
CO$_2$ content (mM/l)	19.6	21.8	25.2	26.3
HCO$_3$ (mM/l)	18.8	20.7	24.0	25.0
pH	7.40	7.34	7.38	7.35

After Cunningham, F.G., MacDonald, P.C., Gant, N.F. *et al.* (eds) (1993) The morphological and functional development of the fetus. In: *Williams Obstetrics*, 19th edn, pp.165–207. Appleton & Lange, Norwalk, CT.

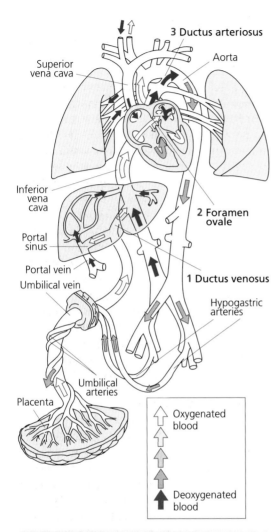

Figure 3.1 Fetal circulation. See text for complete explanation. Well-oxygenated blood returning from the placenta is selectively shunted to the heart and brain via the ascending aorta. The three major shunts of the fetal circulation are the ductus venosus (1), the foramen ovale (2) and the ductus arteriosus (3). After Cunningham, F.G., MacDonald, P.C., Gant, N.F., et al. (eds) (1993) The morphological and functional development of the fetus. In: *Williams Obstetrics*, 19th edn, pp. 165–207. Appleton & Lange, Norwalk, CT.

via the umbilical vein; the umbilical vein enters the abdomen and follows the abdominal wall to the liver, where it divides. The smaller division carries blood to the portal sinus and hepatic veins, while the major division joins the inferior vena cava (IVC). In the IVC, the oxygenated placental blood mixes with deoxygenated blood returning to the heart from the lower half of the fetal body. While mixing results in a lower pO_2, the oxygen content of blood returning to the fetal heart from the IVC is still considerably higher than that returning from the superior vena cava (SVC).

Upon entering the heart, blood from the IVC is shunted primarily through the foramen ovale; this has the effect of delivering the better-oxygenated blood to the left ventricle, and thence to the heart and brain. Blood from the SVC enters the right ventricle and pulmonary artery before being shunted via the ductus arteriosus to the descending aorta. A portion of this blood flows through the umbilical arteries to return to the placenta.

This pattern of shunts allows the fetal ventricles to pump in series while *in utero*, rather than in parallel as in adults. This series arrangement contributes to a higher cardiac output per weight (as much as three times that of an adult at rest), and helps compensate for the lower O_2 content of fetal blood.

3.5 Prepartum fetal assessment

The primary goal of intrauterine fetal surveillance is to prevent fetal demise, or stillbirth, and to decrease neonatal morbidity. An ideal prepartum test would be quick and simple to perform, inexpensive, accurate, and would produce objective results. There is no single test that meets these criteria. Despite this, a number of prepartum tests are used by obstetricians, often in selected populations, to improve the outcome of pregnancy. The results of these tests may have implications for the anesthesiologist in the timing and urgency of delivery and are reviewed below.

3.5.1 Fetal movement

Quantification of fetal activity perceived by the mother was one of the earliest prepartum fetal assessment tests devised. It has the advantage of being simple and cheap to perform, and can therefore be applied to large numbers of patients. The underlying premise is that fetal movement is decreased by hypoxia. During uterine contractions associated with late decelerations (see Section 3.6), fetal movements decrease significantly; during uterine contractions not associated with decelerations, no change in fetal activity is seen.

In the simplest form of fetal activity monitoring, the mother is instructed to count the number of times she feels the fetus kick, turn, or otherwise move during a set time period. The average time it takes to feel 10 fetal movements in the third trimester is about 18 minutes; a 1-hour time period for 10 movements is greater than three standard deviations beyond the mean. To perform the test, the mother records the amount of time it takes for her to feel 10 movements; if she fails to feel 10 movements within 1 hour, further fetal evaluation is indicated.

3.5.2 Contraction stress test

Contraction stress testing combines the use of continuous fetal heart rate and uterine contraction monitoring. It was a direct outgrowth of the use of intrapartum fetal heart monitoring which linked fetal hypoxia and asphyxia with certain fetal heart rate patterns, particularly late decelerations. Uterine contractions can be induced in the non laboring patient during the third trimester by either nipple stimulation or intravenous oxytocin administration. A satisfactory test requires three contractions within 10 minutes while the fetal heart rate is continuously recorded. In a confusing twist of terminology, a negative test is reassuring, with no decelerations associated with contractions; a positive test indicates the presence of decelerations and the need for further evaluation. Disadvantages of the test include the time, effort, and equipment necessary; further, it is contraindicated in conditions such as placenta previa and premature rupture of membranes, where labor must be avoided.

3.5.3 Nonstress test

The nonstress test was derived from the contraction stress test when it was observed that contraction stress tests were rarely abnormal as long as fetal heart rate accelerations were associated with fetal movement. This simplifies the test and eliminates the need for uterine contractions. The fetal heart rate (and usually uterine activity) is monitored for 20 – 40 minutes, while the mother simultaneously notes fetal movement. A normal, or reactive, test exhibits a normal baseline fetal heart rate, adequate variability, and at least two fetal heart rate accelerations of 15 beats per minute or more lasting 15 seconds associated with fetal movement.

Due to its simplicity, the nonstress test is currently the mainstay of prepartum fetal surveillance. There are both maternal (diabetes, collagen vascular disorders, chronic disease) and fetal (intrauterine growth retardation, multiple gestation, decreased movement) indications for its use. Typically, the test is performed twice weekly when indicated for on-going evaluation.

3.5.4 Ultrasonography

The widespread availability and accuracy of ultrasonography has made it an essential tool in the pre- and intrapartum evaluation of fetal well being. Among the most valuable information that ultrasonography can provide is an estimate of gestational age. Particularly in the late first and early second trimesters, fetal measurements obtained with ultrasound are the most accurate means available of determining gestational age. Accurate dating is especially useful for determining options when pregnancy is threatened before fetal viability, or when viability is marginal.

Ultrasonography is also highly useful in identifying fetal anomalies. As with accurate dating, identification of lethal fetal anomalies permits rational choices to be made regarding route of delivery. Identification of serious but nonlethal anomalies prior to delivery allows planning for appropriate postpartum care of the neonate, to optimize outcome; on occasion, such anomalies may be amenable to improvement with *in utero* therapy.

Table 3.3 Elements of the biophysical profile

Nonstress test
  Reactive test = 2 points

Fetal breathing movements
  At least one episode of fetal breathing of 60 sec
  duration = 2 points

Gross fetal body movements
  At least three discrete episodes of fetal movement
  = 2 points

Fetal tone
  At least one episode of extension and return to
  flexion of extremities or spine or hand open/close
  = 2 points

Amniotic fluid volume
  At least one amniotic fluid pocket of at least 1 cm
  in depth = 2 points

Total available
  10 points

3.5.5 Biophysical profile

The biophysical profile utilizes ultrasonography to measure several parameters in conjunction with a nonstress test to provide an assessment of the fetus' overall development and well being. There are five elements that are assessed for the biophysical profile (*Table 3.3*); each is assigned a score of either 0 or 2. A score of 8 – 10 is generally associated with a favorable outcome, while a score of 2 – 4 indicates a high perinatal mortality rate that usually requires intervention. The amniotic fluid volume tends to receive greater weight in determining a course of action with intermediate values (*Table 3.4*). Testing is usually performed at 34 – 36 weeks gestation, but may be performed as early as 28 weeks.

Table 3.4 Interpretation and management of biophysical profile score

Score	Comment	Perinatal mortality within 1 wk without intervention	Management
10 of 10	Risk of fetal asphyxia extremely rare	<1/1000	Intervention only for obstetric and maternal factors
8 of 10 (normal fluid)	No indication for intervention for fetal disease		
8 of 10 (abnormal fluid)	Probable chronic fetal compromise	89/1000	Determine that there is functioning renal tissue and intact membranes: if so, deliver for fetal indications
6 of 10 (normal fluid)	Equivocal test, possible fetal asphyxia	Variable	If the fetus is mature, deliver. In the immature fetus, repeat test within 24 h; if <6/10 deliver
6 of 10 (abnormal fluid)	Probable fetal asphyxia	89/1000	Deliver for fetal indications
4 of 10	High probability of fetal asphyxia	91/1000	Deliver for fetal indications
2 of 10	Fetal asphyxia almost certain	125/1000	Deliver for fetal indications
0 of 10	Fetal asphyxia certain	600/1000	Deliver for fetal indications

From: Manning FA, Morrison I, Harman CR, et al. Fetal assessment based on fetal biophysical profile scoring: Experience in 19,221 referred high-risk pregnancies. *Am J Obstet Gynecol* **157**:880, 1987.

3.6 **Intrapartum fetal heart monitoring**

To understand the fetal response to labor, it is necessary to understand the hemodynamics of utero-placental blood flow. Uterine perfusion pressure (UPP) is approximated as mean maternal uterine arterial pressure minus mean uterine venous pressure; the maternal mean arterial pressure minus the maternal central venous pressure is a slightly higher approximation. In a healthy parturient, UPP is approximately 60 mmHg or less (due to the vascular resistance of intraplacental vessels, it is slightly lower than the equation indicates) (*Figure 3.2*). During a normal uterine contraction, intrauterine pressure can easily exceed 60 mmHg. As the pressure increases during a contraction, first the uterine venous pressure will be exceeded, which constricts uterine outflow, and eventually uterine arterial pressure will be exceeded, preventing perfusion. The fetal circulation through the placenta continues throughout the contraction; therefore, at the peak of most contractions, there is a period where uterine blood flow is essentially cut off, and no exchange occurs. The analogy can be made that the fetus is required to 'hold its breath' for a few moments every few minutes during labor. A healthy, term fetus has sufficient metabolic reserve to tolerate this stress without problems.

Monitoring the fetal heart rate (FHR) is the primary means of assessing fetal status during labor, specifically the response of the fetus to the added stress of uterine contractions. While, ultimately, interpretation of the fetal heart trace is the responsibility of the obstetrician, it is important that the anesthesiologist be familiar with the basics of FHR monitoring, as he or she is often the first physician in the position to identify potentially ominous signs and take corrective action. Elements of the FHR to be considered in interpretation include the baseline fetal heart rate, variability of the FHR, and the presence or absence of decelerations and accelerations.

3.6.1 Baseline FHR

The normal baseline FHR is between 110 and 160 beats per minute (bpm). Fetal tachycardia is a persistent FHR above 160 bpm and can be the result of maternal fever or infection (particularly chorioamnionitis). Medications administered to the mother can also cause fetal tachycardia – atropine and β-sympathomimetics (terbutaline or ritodrine, often used for tocolysis). Fetal tachycardia does not usually require urgent intervention as long as variability is maintained.

Fetal bradycardia is defined as a FHR below 110 bpm. In contrast to adults, cardiac output of the fetus is highly rate dependent; the fetus has a very limited ability to compensate for decreased heart rates by increasing stroke volume. At a FHR below 90 bpm, cardiac output falls, resulting in the shunting of blood to the brain, heart, and vital organs; other tissue will become progressively anaerobic, and pO_2 and pH will decrease. While a healthy fetus can probably tolerate a heart rate of 90 – 100 bpm for a prolonged period due to its metabolic reserve, a stressed infant will experience progressive hypoxemia unless the heart rate is increased. Due to the episodic interruptions of uterine blood flow during labor described above, even a healthy infant cannot tolerate such a low heart rate during active labor. Bradycardia may be associated with some congenital heart lesions and maternal medications (beta-blockers and high levels of local anesthetics). More significantly, fetal bradycardia is often a response to a hypoxic insult (see below).

UPP = (M.M.U.A.P – M.M.U.V.P.)
    = 70 mmHg – 10 mmHg
    = 60 mmHg

UPP – Uterine Perfusion Pressure
MMUAP – Mean Maternal Uterine Arterial Pressure
MMUVP – Mean Maternal Uterine Venous Pressure

Figure 3.2 Derivation of uterine perfusion pressure

3.6.2 Variability

Variability in the FHR refers to the minute fluctuations between the R-waves of the fetal ECG. The SA node sets the intrinsic FHR; in the absence of any other influences, the R–R interval would be constant, and the FHR trace would appear as a straight, flat line. A constantly changing balance of autonomic influences affects the SA node, however, with the result that the R–R interval is constantly changing slightly. This results in the jagged, 'saw-tooth' pattern seen in normal FHR monitor strips (*Figure 3.3*). Normal variability is defined as fluctuation of 6–10 bpm. The presence of variability in the FHR is taken as evidence of an intact, functional neuraxis: appropriate CNS traffic between aortic arch and carotid chemo- and baroreceptors, through the cerebral cortex and brainstem, and out through the vagus nerve and cardiac sympathetics. Diminished or absent variability is taken as a sign of central nervous system (CNS) hypoxia.

3.6.3 Decelerations

Decelerations are periodic FHR changes that occur in response to fetal insults and may be related to the uterine contraction pattern. They are defined as early, variable and late.

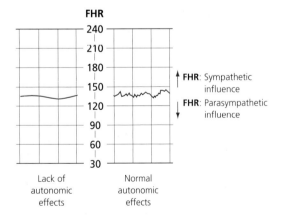

FHR

FHR: Sympathetic influence

FHR: Parasympathetic influence

Lack of autonomic effects

Normal autonomic effects

Figure 3.3 Autonomic influences and the fetal heart rate. Sympathetic influences tend to increase the baseline heart rate, while parasympathetic influences tend to decrease it.

Early decelerations are considered to be a vagal response to fetal head compression during contractions. They begin with the onset of the contraction, with a gradual decrease in the FHR and a gradual return to baseline before the end of the contraction; they are sometimes said to 'mirror' the contraction (*Figure 3.4*). They are generally considered benign.

Variable decelerations are considered to be a vagal reflex to umbilical cord compression. Their temporal relation to uterine contractions is appropriately 'variable'. They are characterized by an abrupt onset and abrupt return to baseline and are irregular in shape (*Figure 3.5*). They are considered 'severe' when the FHR drops 60 or more bpm below baseline for 60 seconds or more. If repetitive and severe, variable decelerations may lead to progressive fetal acidosis, and efforts to eliminate them should be undertaken (see Section 3.7).

Late decelerations are considered ominous because they are assumed to indicate uteroplacental insufficiency. As noted above, uterine blood flow ceases at the peak of normal uterine contractions; this leads to a brief period during each contraction when oxygen exchange is markedly reduced and fetal pO_2 falls slightly (*Figure 3.6*). A healthy fetus has sufficient reserve to tolerate this short interruption, but a stressed fetus may not be able to tolerate even these brief interruptions in oxygen supply. The result is that blood is shunted to the brain and heart and away from peripheral tissues. This activates a vagal reflex due to transient fetal hypertension activating baroreceptors of the aortic arch and carotids. Late decelerations are characterized by a smooth decrease in FHR baseline after the start of the contraction, and a smooth return to baseline after the end of the contraction (*Figure 3.7*). If repetitive, late decelerations can lead to progressive fetal acidosis and deterioration. Aggressive efforts to eliminate the decelerations or to deliver the fetus should be made.

Late decelerations with absent variability are a particularly ominous sign, indicating severe fetal hypoxemia. Every effort should be made to deliver the infant as quickly as possible.

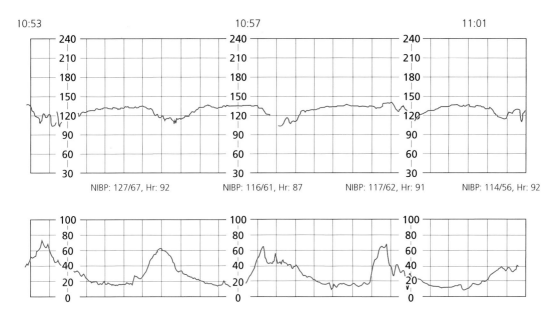

Figure 3.4 Early decelerations in a 23-year-old parturient in early labor. The decelerations tend to 'mirror' the uterine contraction pattern, and the FHR returns to baseline before the end of the contraction. (Note: The uterine contraction pressure scale is not accurate.)

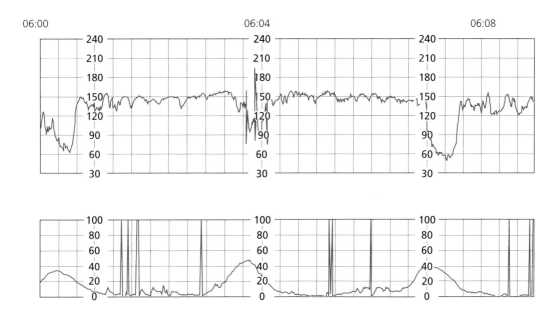

Figure 3.5 Severe variable decelerations in a 30-year-old parturient in active labor. The decelerations begin after the start of the uterine contraction, and the fetal heart rate has returned to baseline before the end of the contraction. Note that FHR variability is well maintained between the decelerations.

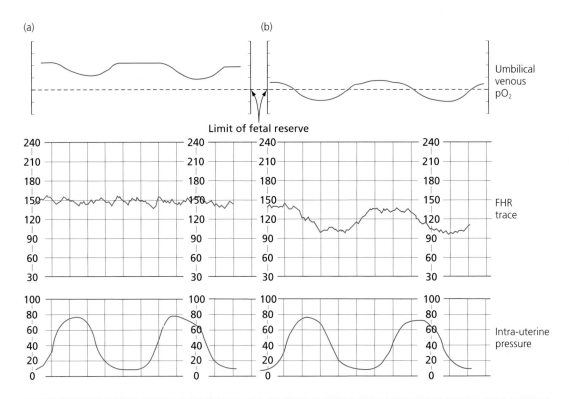

Figure 3.6 Mechanism of late FHR decelerations. As uterine blood flow decreases during a uterine contraction, placental oxygen exchange is briefly disrupted, resulting in a transient drop in fetal pO_2. A healthy fetus has sufficient reserve to tolerate this brief interruption, but in a stressed fetus the fetal pO_2 drops below a critical level causing a vagally mediated decrease in fetal heart rate.

3.7 *In-utero* resuscitation

In-utero resuscitation, or fetal resuscitation, is the first intervention that should be attempted when fetal compromise or distress is suspected. It may prevent the need for urgent interventions or delivery, or at least may improve fetal status during the period before delivery can be affected. *In-utero* resuscitation consists of several distinct interventions that should all be applied at the same time, as it is rarely possible to determine exactly which step will alleviate the fetal insult.

3.7.1 Interventions

Position change

The rationale for maternal position change is to eliminate aorto-caval compression that may be impeding uterine blood flow. Avoidance of supine positioning, and use of the left uterine displacement position should be routine during all phases of labor, but the mass of the gravid uterus may still impinge on the abdominal aorta in certain situations in some patients. This can restrict uterine blood flow to the placenta. The 'supine hypotension syndrome' results from similar compression of the abdominal vena cava; in this instance, however, the decrease in venous return because of caval compression results in maternal hypotension. With either situation, the mother should be turned to the full lateral position, either left or right; if one side does not relieve the problem, the other should be tried. In extreme situations, the mother should be placed in the 'knee-chest' position (i.e.

11:31   11:35   11:39

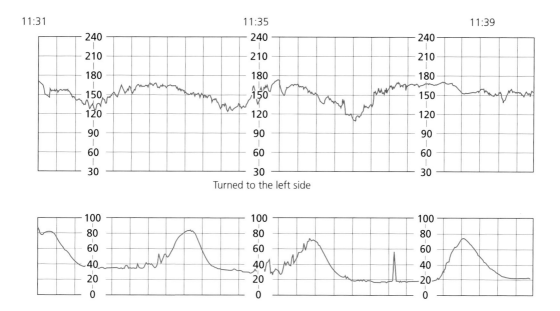

Turned to the left side

Figure 3.7 Repetitive late decelerations in a 31-year-old parturient in active labor. The decelerations in the FHR lag behind the uterine contraction pattern: the drop in FHR begins after the start of the contraction, and persists after the contraction has resolved. (Note: the uterine contraction pressure scale is not accurate.)

turned prone and positioned with her knees and upper chest or anterior shoulders on the bed). This tends to move the fetus' weight cephalad, and can decrease umbilical cord compression or fetal head compression at the pelvic brim.

Oxygen administration. Despite large increases in maternal pO_2 with increasing FiO_2, maternal blood oxygen content does not increase significantly because even on room air ($FiO_2 = 0.21$) maternal hemoglobin is nearly saturated with oxygen. Fetal hemoglobin has a different affinity for oxygen, however, and available evidence indicates that fetal pO_2 and oxygen saturation do increase significantly with increases in maternal FiO_2. If fetal oxygen delivery decreases for any reason (decreased uterine blood flow, increased uterine tone, or umbilical cord compression), increasing fetal blood oxygen content may improve fetal status (*Table 3.5*).

Unfortunately, it is not usually possible to increase maternal FiO_2 to 1.0 in the standard labor suite (though this can be accomplished with an anesthesia machine). Administering oxygen via simple face mask at high flows (15 l/min or more) can significantly increase maternal FiO_2, and it is reasonable to assume a corresponding improvement in fetal blood oxygen content.

Table 3.5 Relation between maternal FiO_2 and umbilical artery and vein oxygen gradient

Maternal FiO_2	Umbilical venous blood oxygen content (ml O_2/100 ml blood)	Umbilical arterial blood oxygen content (ml O_2/100 ml blood)
0.21	13.2 ± 0.5	5.3 ± 0.6
0.47	15.9 ± 0.8	7.9 ± 0.4
1.0	17.7 ± 0.1	11.8 ± 0.8

Adapted from Ramanathan, S., Gandhi, S., Arismandy, J. *et al.* (1982) Oxygen transfer from mother to fetus during cesarean section under epidural anesthesia. *Anesth. Analg.* **61**: 576–581.

Blood pressure support. Since decreases in maternal blood pressure can clearly result in decreases in uterine blood flow, increasing maternal blood pressure may improve uterine and placental perfusion. Except in those unusual circumstances where maternal blood pressure is known to be excessive (as in severe preeclampsia), empirically increasing maternal blood pressure in the face of fetal compromise is indicated.

The most rapid means of elevating maternal blood pressure is with intravenous ephedrine, 5–10 mg; this should be accompanied by vigorous intravenous fluid administration, with nonglucose-containing fluids (normal saline, lactated Ringer's solution, or Plasmalyte®). The blood pressure response should be closely monitored during and following these interventions.

Decreasing uterine tone. As described above, increases in uterine tone or an increase in the intensity and frequency of uterine contractions can decrease placental perfusion by impeding uterine blood flow. A very rapid contraction pattern may not allow a fetus sufficient time to recover between contractions from the episodic decrease in oxygen delivery.

The most widely used method of decreasing uterine tone or stopping uterine contractions is probably terbutaline, either subcutaneous or intravenous, 0.25 mg. Nitroglycerin, either intravenous or sublingual, is another agent for rapidly producing uterine relaxation that has proven effective. Intravenous nitroglycerin should be administered beginning at a dose of 50 µg: the dose can be increased to as high as 500 µg until the desired relaxant effect is seen. Intravenous nitroglycerin has a rapid speed of onset (30–45 s) and a short duration of action (1–2 min), so it should be viewed as a temporizing measure. Sublingual nitroglycerin, either tablets or spray, has also been shown to be effective. Careful maternal blood pressure monitoring is necessary, as both terbutaline and nitroglycerin can cause significant decreases in maternal blood pressure.

Further reading

American College of Obstetricians and Gynecologists (1995) Fetal heart rate patterns: Monitoring, interpretation, and management. ACOG Technical Bulletin No. 207.

Bekedam, M.D. and Visser, G.H.A. (1985) Effects of hypoxemic events on breathing, body movements, and heart rate variation: a study in growth-retarded human fetuses. *Am. J. Obstet. Gynecol.* **153**: 52–56.

Evertson, L.R., Gauthier, R.J., Schifrin, B.S. *et al.* (1979) Antepartum fetal heart rate testing: I. Evolution of the nonstress test. *Am. J. Obstet. Gynecol.* **133**: 29–33.

Huddleston, J.F. (1984) Management of acute fetal distress in the intrapartum period. *Clin. Obstet. Gynecol.* **27**: 84–94.

Longo, L.D. (1991) Respiration in the fetal-placental unit. In: *Principles of Perinatal-Neonatal Metabolism* (ed. Cowett, R.M.), pp. 304–315. Springer-Verlag, New York.

Manning, F.A., Morrison, I., Harman, C.R. *et al.* (1987) Fetal assessment based on fetal biophysical profile scoring: experience in 19,221 referred high-risk pregnancies. *Am. J. Obstet. Gynecol.* **157**: 880–884.

Moore, K.L. (1988) *The Developing Human: Clinically Oriented Embryology*, 4th edn. WB Saunders Company, Philadelphia.

Moore T.R., and Piacquadio, K. (1990) A prospective evaluation of fetal movement screening to reduce the incidence of antepartum fetal death. *Am. J. Obstet. Gynecol.* **162**: 1168–1173.

Parer, J.T. (1999) Fetal heart rate. In: *Maternal-Fetal Medicine*, 4th edn (eds Creasy, R.K. and Resnik, R.), pp. 270–299. WB Saunders Company., Philadelphia.

Platt, L.D., Paul, R.H., Phelan, J. *et al.* (1987) Fifteen years experience with antepartum fetal testing. *Am. J. Obstet. Gynecol.* **156**: 1509–1515.

Ramanathan, S., Gandhi, S., Arismandy, J. *et al.* (1982) Oxygen transfer from mother to fetus during cesarean section under epidural anesthesia. *Anesth. Analg.* **61**: 576–581.

Rochard, F., Schifrin, B.S., Goupil, F. *et al.* (1976) Nonstressed fetal heart rate monitoring in the antepartum period. *Am. J. Obstet. Gynecol.* **126**: 699–706.

Vintzileos, A.M. and Knuppel, R.A. (1994) Multiple parameter biophysical testing in the prediction of fetal acid-base status. *Clin. Perinatol.* **21**: 823–848.

Chapter 4

Neuroanatomy and neuropharmacology

Craig M. Palmer, MD

Contents

4.1 Introduction

Even with the development of regional techniques such as subarachnoid and epidural blocks, and their application to obstetric patients in the middle of this century, what anesthesiologists usually provided their laboring patients was more appropriately termed anesthesia, rather than analgesia. Dense sensory and motor block from high concentrations of local anesthetics has, until recent years, been the norm when it came to regional techniques for labor analgesia. While effective at alleviating pain, the motor block inherent in such techniques interfered with the mother's participation in the process of labor, and may have contributed to problems such as malpresentation and a decrease in spontaneous vaginal deliveries.

Within the past 2 decades, and even the past few years, our understanding of the structure and function of the nervous system, particularly at the cellular and molecular level, has been advancing at a truly astounding rate. Applying this new knowledge to laboring patients brings us closer to the ideal of true analgesia without bothersome side effects, and avoids any impact upon the natural processes inherent in parturition.

4.2 Neuroanatomy

4.2.1 Afferent neural pathways

Peripheral pathways

The peripheral neural pathways associated with labor sensation were first described by Head in 1893. More recent work, notably by Cleland and Bonica, has clarified our understanding. Sensation from the first stage of labor (i.e. the onset of contractions through complete cervical dilation) travels with the lumbar sympathetics and enters the spinal cord between the T_{10} and L_1 levels. Sensation from the second stage of labor (from complete cervical dilatation through delivery of the infant) travels peripherally *via* the pudendal nerve and enters the spinal cord at the S_2 through S_4 levels (*Figure 4.1*).

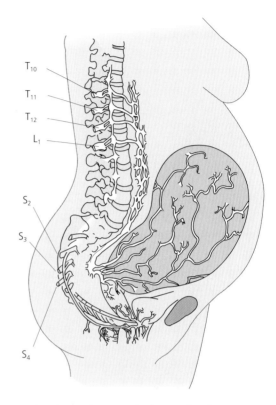

Figure 4.1 Peripheral neural pathways associated with labor sensation. Sensation from the first stage of labor is carried by neurons that travel with the lumbar sympathetic plexus and enter the spinal cord between levels T_{10} to L_1. Sensation from distention of the perineum (largely during the second stage of labor) enters the spinal cord between S_2 through S_4, traveling peripherally *via* the pudendal nerve. From: Brown, D.L. (1994) Spinal, epidural and caudal anesthesia: anatomy, physiology, and technique. In: *Obstetric Anesthesia, Principles and Practice* (ed. Chestnut, D.H.) pp. 181–201. Mosby-Year Book, Inc., St. Louis, MO.

Central pathways

The pathways labor sensation travels after entry into the central nervous system are less widely known. The cell bodies of the primary afferent neurons lie in the dorsal root ganglion and send their projections into the spinal cord through the dorsal root entry zone. The first synapse in the pathway occurs in the dorsal gray matter of the spinal cord. Histologically, several (10) distinct zones are found in the

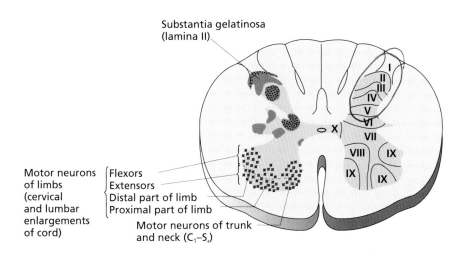

Figure 4.2 Diagrammatic cross section of the spinal cord illustrating Rexed's lamina of the gray matter. Most primary afferent neurons associated with labor sensation synapse initially between laminas II through V. Lamina II is also referred to as the *substantia gelatinosa*, and is the primary synaptic site of most sensory afferent fibers entering at the T10 to L1 levels (i.e., the first stage of labor). The ventral lamina are associated primarily with motor neurons. After: Watson C. (1995) *Basic Human Neuroanatomy*. Little, Brown and Co., Boston, MA.

gray matter, commonly referred to as Rexed's lamina. These zones are distinct because of variations in the cell type and neuronal connections within each, reflecting differences in information processing and function. Lamina I is the most superficial and dorsal of these laminae in the spinal cord. Laminae I through V are most important in discussion of afferent sensory information associated with labor (*Figure 4.2*).

The initial synapse may be located in any of the laminae between I and V, but current understanding of these pathways focuses on laminae II and V. Lamina II is also referred to as the substantia gelatinosa, and is the primary synaptic site of most sensory afferent fibers entering at the T_{10} to L_1 levels. In order for primary afferent input to reach the level of conscious sensation, second or higher order neurons must project cephalad to the primary sensory cortex. Neurons within lamina V known as 'wide dynamic range' (WDR) neurons play an important role in the initial processing of afferent input. These WDR neurons receive afferent projections from large numbers of other neurons at the same and nearby

levels of the cord. These afferent projections may be from primary afferent neurons, but can also be from local 'interneurons', which extend short distances between a few laminae or levels within the gray matter. As noted above, most of the primary afferent neurons synapse initially in the more superficial laminae (I and II); locally projecting interneurons in turn synapse on the more deeply located WDR neurons.

The WDR neurons process the input they receive from these multiple synapses; their name derives from the wide range of responses characteristic of these neurons. With minimal input, their rate of firing is very low; with greater input, they are capable of firing action potentials in great bursts (*Figure 4.3*). Through this variability in firing rate, these spinal WDR neurons modulate input to higher levels of the CNS.

Projections from the dorsal gray matter cross to the contralateral ventral white matter of the cord and then the cephalad via the spinothalamic tract (*Figure 4.4*). The next synapse occurs, appropriately enough, in the thalamus. Neurons located in the thalamus project at last to the primary sensory cortex, and the

afferent sensory → dorsal gray matter → contralateral ventral white matter → spinothalamic tract → thalamus → 1° sensory cortex

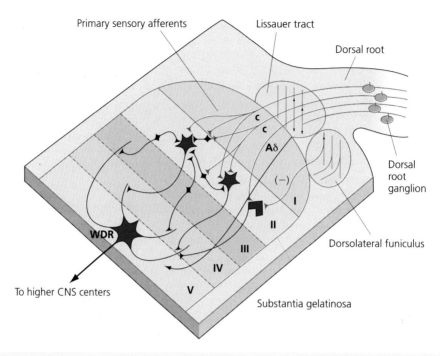

Figure 4.3 Diagrammatic cross section of the dorsal nerve root entry zone of the spinal cord. Wide dynamic range (WDR) neurons are located in deeper levels of the gray matter, receiving synaptic connections and input from many other neurons and projecting centrally. The dorsolateral funiculus carries a descending pathway (see 4.2.2). Primary afferent neurons may send branches to spinal levels above and below their level of entry to the cord via Lissauer's tract (see 4.2.3). Interneurons project between lamina and levels of the gray matter (see 4.2.4). A wide variety of both excitatory and inhibitory synaptic connections are possible.

parturient finally becomes aware she is having a contraction.

4.2.2 Descending pathways

In addition to the afferent pathways described above, descending pathways within the central nervous system play an active role in the processing of nociceptive information (*Figure 4.5*). These descending pathways originate in the primary sensory cortex and project caudally to the midbrain, synapsing on neurons in the periaquaductal gray matter. These neurons in turn project to the medulla, to the rostral ventral nuclei. Neurons with cell bodies lying in these nuclei project to the spinal cord via the dorsilateral funiculus to synapse within the dorsal gray matter of the spinal cord. It is not clear at present exactly what activates this descending pathway *in vivo*, but it is clearly effective. Studies in ani-

mals have shown that electrical stimulation of the periaquaductal gray matter and the rostral ventral nuclei not only produces analgesia in animals (by behavioral criteria), but also inhibits output of lamina V (WDR) neurons in the afferent (ascending) pathway.

4.2.3 Neuronal morphology

In addition to the anatomic separation of the pathways of the first and second stages of labor, the neurons of these pathways are also morphologically distinct. Peripheral neurons can be characterized on the basis of their size and degree of myelination (*Table 4.1*). Type C fibers predominate in the first stage of labor; these small fibers are poorly myelinated (if myelinated at all), and their conduction velocity is quite slow. It is important to recognize that these primary afferents synapse not at one

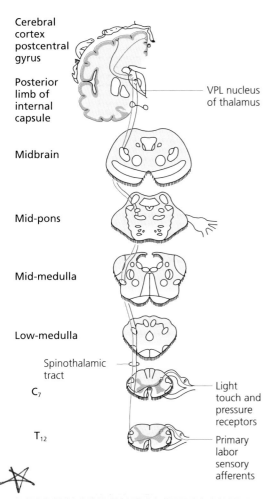

Cerebral cortex postcentral gyrus

Posterior limb of internal capsule

VPL nucleus of thalamus

Midbrain

Mid-pons

Mid-medulla

Low-medulla

Spinothalamic tract

C_7

T_{12}

Light touch and pressure receptors

Primary labor sensory afferents

Figure 4.4 Cephalad extension of labor sensory pathways. Secondary neurons whose cell bodies lie in the dorsal gray matter of the spinal cord project via the spinothalamic tract to the thalamus. Another synapse occurs in the pathway before projection to the primary sensory cortex. After: Palmer C. (2000). Spinal neuroanatomy and neuropharmacology. In: *Seminars in Anesthesia, Perioperative Medicine and Pain*. Vol. 19 No. 1. WB Saunders, Philadelphia, PA.

single point or on a single secondary neuron, but branch widely with multiple synaptic connections not only at the level of entry to the cord, but also one or two levels above and below the level of entry. The wide 'arborization' of these primary afferents contributes to the diffuse, poorly localized nature of sensation associated with the first stage (*Figure 4.6*).

During the second stage of labor (distention of the perineum), type Aδ fibers dominate. These neurons are significantly larger in diameter and better myelinated, with more rapid conduction velocities.

The anatomic and morphologic distinctions between the first and second stage pathways have clear clinical correlates. First stage labor pain results from uterine contractions and cervical stretching; it is cramping and visceral in nature, diffuse and poorly localized. Second stage pain is well localized and somatic, due mainly to less arborization and the faster conduction velocity in the sacral pathways. Parturients feel this sensation between their legs rather than in their abdomen. This more discrete sensation is the reason parturients will feel 'the urge to push' and know 'the baby's coming!'

Finally, it is important to realize that these two types of sensation are not mutually exclusive: pain associated with the first stage of labor does not stop miraculously with the entry into the second stage of labor, but it is often superseded by pain resulting from distention of the perineum due to descent of the fetal head. Dependent on the progression of a woman's labor, sensation typically ascribed to the second stage may be significant during the first stage of labor if the fetal station (the level of the fetal head within the maternal pelvis) is changing rapidly. Generally speaking, however, sensations traveling via the sacral nerve roots do not become significant until labor is well advanced.

4.2.4 Endogenous neurotransmitters

In order for information to be passed between neurons, neurotransmitters are necessary (*Table 4.2*). Understanding which neurotransmitters are released by which cells in response to which stimuli can be invaluable information if we want to alter perception of painful or nociceptive stimuli. Due to the incredible complexity of the CNS, researchers are only beginning to shed light on many of these compounds.

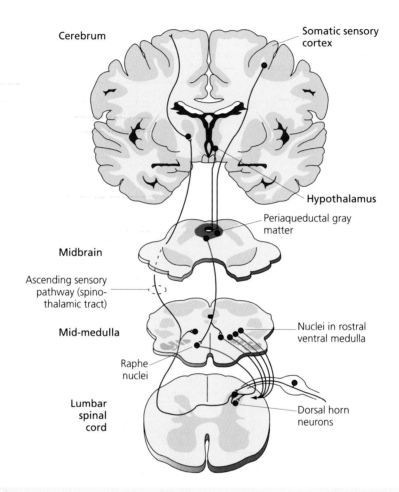

Figure 4.5 Descending inhibitory pathway. Neurons with cell bodies in the sensory cortex project caudally, synapsing in the periaqueductal gray matter of the midbrain. Another synapse occurs in the medulla before the pathway terminates in the gray matter of the dorsal lumbar spinal cord. After: Palmer C. (2000). Spinal neuroanatomy and neuropharmacology. In: *Seminars in Anesthesia, Perioperative Medicine and Pain*. Vol. 19 No. 1. WB Saunders, Philadelphia, PA.

The primary neurotransmitter between first order type C afferent neurons and second order neurons appears to be glutamate, an excitatory amino acid neurotransmitter. Substance P is also released synaptically by these neurons as a facilitative neurotransmitter, but it appears to function only to augment the post-synaptic response. Glutamate acts primarily at non-NMDA (α-amino-3-hydroxy-5-4-isoxazolepropionic acid, or AMPA) receptors on the post-synaptic membrane (aspartate, another excitatory amino acid neurotransmitter, acts primarily at N-methyl-D-aspartate

(NMDA) receptors, but does not appear to be the significant neurotransmitter in these pathways). Substance P acts on neurokinin receptors (*Figure 4.7*).

A second major neurotransmitter is norepinephrine, a catecholamine (monoamine) with an affinity for α_2 adrenergic receptors. As noted above, a descending inhibitory pathway terminates in lamina II of the dorsal gray matter, the substantia gelatinosa. Norepinephrine release from these descending neurons inhibits transmission in the primary afferent pathway. Receptors for norepinephrine are located both

Table 4.1 Classification of peripheral nerve fibers

Fiber	Myelinated	Fiber diameter (microns)	Conduction velocity (m/sec)	Function	Resistance to local anesthetic blockade
A-alpha	Yes	12–20	70–120	Innervation of skeletal muscles Proprioception	++++
-beta	Yes	5–12	30–70	Tactile sensory receptors (touch, pressure)	+++
-gamma	Yes	3–6	15–30	Skeleton muscle tone	+++
-delta	Yes	2–5	12–30	Stabbing pain Touch Temperature	++
B	Yes	<3	3–15	Preganglionic autonomic fibers	+
C	No	0.3–1.3	0.5–2	Burning and aching pain Touch Temperature Pruritus	+

Adapted from: Voulgaropoulos, D. and Palmer, C.M. (1996) Local Anesthetic Pharmacology. In: Prys-Roberts C, Brown BR Jr. and Nunn JF (eds). *International Practice of Anaesthesia*. Butterworth-Heinemann, Oxford.

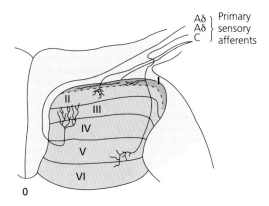

Figure 4.6 Synaptic connections of primary sensory afferents in the dorsal gray matter. The wide branching of the primary sensory fibers, both within and between spinal levels (see *Figure 4.3*) contributes to the diffuse, poorly-localized nature of labor sensation. After: Palmer C. (2000). Spinal neuroanatomy and neuropharmacology. In: Seminars in Anesthesia, Perioperative Medicine and Pain. Vol. 19 No. 1. WB Saunders, Philadelphia, PA.

pre- and post-synaptically on primary afferent neurons and secondary neurons, respectively. Significant α_2 agonist binding occurs on dorsal root ganglion cells, which suggests the presynaptic action, but the most profound inhibitory effect occurs within the substantia gelatinosa in response to excitatory amino acid (glutamate) discharge, indicating a postsynaptic effect. The result is selective inhibition of C and Aδ fiber-evoked activity in the WDR neurons of lamina V (*Figure 4.8*).

Acetylcholine is another important neurotransmitter, also apparently in the descending inhibitory pathway. Muscarinic (cholinergic) receptors are found in the gray matter of the dorsal horn of the spinal cord. Application or release of norepinephrine at this level of the spinal cord increases the level of acetylcholine (Ach) in spinal cord interstitial fluid at the same time as it produces analgesia. Applying an anticholinergic along with norepinephrine significantly *decreases* the analgesic response; applying an anticholinesterase (to inhibit

Table 4.2 Major neurotransmitters in labor sensation pathways

Neurotransmitter	Class	Released by	Site of action	Comments
Glutamate	Excitatory amino acid	Primary sensory afferents	Secondary afferent nerons	Primary neurotransmitter labor sensory pathways
Norepinephrine	Monoamine	Descending inhibitory neurons	Primary and secondary afferent neurons	Both pre- and post-synaptic effects
Acetylcholine	Monoamine	Interneurons of dorsal gray matter	Secondary afferent neurons	A major inhibitory interneuronal neurotransmitter
Substance P	Neurokinin	Primary sensory afferents	Secondary afferent neurons	A facilitative neurotransmitter

Table 4.3 Pharmacological options in neuraxial labor analgesia

Class	Agents	Target neurons	Mechanism/site of action	Comments
Local anesthetics	Bupivacaine Lidocaine Ropivacaine 2-Chloroprocaine Other	Primary sensory afferents	Na$^+$ channel blockade	Effective in very low concentrations
Opioids	Fentanyl Sufentanil Morphine Meperidine	Primary and secondary sensory afferents	Opioid receptors (primarily μ receptors)	Receptors found pre-synaptically on type C fibres and post-synaptic membranes
Adrenergic agonists	Epinephrine Clonidine	Primary and secondary sensory afferents	α_2 adrenergic receptors	Post-synaptic effects dominate
Anticholinesterases	Neostigmine	Secondary sensory afferents	Increase interstitial acetylcholine concentration	Side effects limit clinical utility

breakdown of Ach) along with the α-adrenergic agonist significantly *increases* the analgesic response. This evidence indicates that acetylcholine is most likely released by locally projecting interneurons to act on second or higher order (WDR) neurons in the primary afferent pathway.

4.3 Neuropharmacology (Table 4.3)

4.3.1 Practical membrane channel pharmacology

Local anesthetics
Local anesthetics have been the mainstay of regional anesthesia in obstetrics for decades,

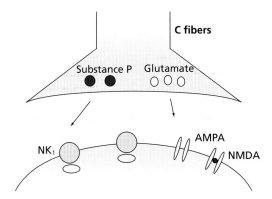

Figure 4.7 C-fiber synaptic terminal. Glutamate, the primary neurotransmitter is released by C-fibers, and interacts with AMPA (non-NMDA) receptors on the post-synaptic membrane. Substance P may also be released, interacting with post-synaptic neurokinin receptors (NK₁), but it is merely a facilitative neurotransmitter. Aspartate acts primarily at NMDA receptors but does not appear important in these pathways.

and will likely continue in this role for decades to come. All local anesthetics share a similar molecular structure: all have an aromatic ring at one end, a hydrocarbon chain of varying length and composition in the middle, and an amine group ($-NH_2$) at the other end. The aromatic ring and hydrocarbon chain are nonpolar, but the amine group may reversibly bind a free proton (H^+) to acquire a positive charge, and allow the molecule to become polar (*Figure 4.9*). This is a physical characteristic that can be described in terms of pK_a. When placed in solution, the pK_a is the pH at which the molecules are evenly split between their charged (polar) and uncharged (nonpolar forms). Decreasing the pH (increasing the free H^+ concentration) will increase the proportion of molecules in the charged or polar state; increasing the pH (decreasing the free H^+ concentration) will have the opposite effect. Both the charged and uncharged forms of the

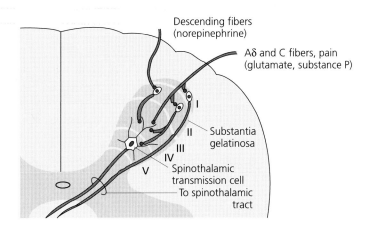

Figure 4.8 Neurotransmitters in the dorsal horn. Descending inhibitory pathways release norepinephrine, which is excitatory and acts primarily on locally projecting neurons in the gray matter. These neurons in turn release acetylcholine, which is inhibitory, at synapses with neurons of the afferent sensory pathway projecting cephalad via the spinothalamic tract. Neurotransmitters released by primary afferent neurons include glutamate and substance P. After: Palmer C. (2000). Spinal neuroanatomy and neuropharmacology. In: *Seminars in Anesthesia, Perioperative Medicine and Pain*. Vol. 19 No. 1. WB Saunders, Philadelphia, PA.

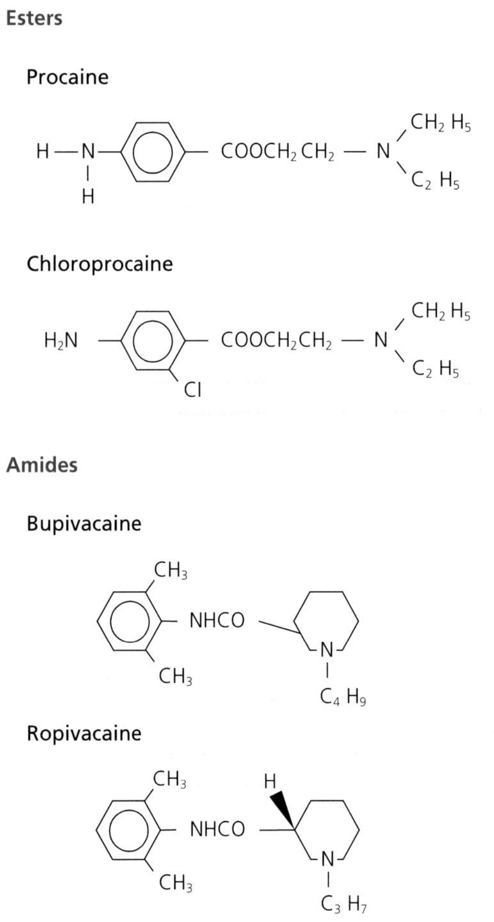

Esters

Procaine

Chloroprocaine

Amides

Bupivacaine

Ropivacaine

Figure 4.9 Representative chemical structures of commonly used local anesthetics. All local anesthetics have an aromatic ring at one end, an intermediate hydrocarbon chain linkage, and an amine group at the other end. The intermediate linkage may be either an ester (-COO) or an amide (-NH).

molecule are necessary for the clinical effects of local anesthetics.

The site of action of local anesthetics is the sodium channel of the neuronal cell membrane. The sodium channel is a large transmembrane protein with four repeating 'domains'. *In vivo*, the channel forms a donut-shaped ring with a central pore. In the resting state, the pore is closed and the channel is inactive; in response to depolarization of the neuronal membrane, the channel undergoes a conformational change that opens the pore and allows the passage of sodium ions. Local anesthetics reversibly bind to the intracellular surface of the sodium channel in its resting state and prevent the conformational change. It is the polar, protonated form of the local anesthetic molecule that is able to bind to the channel.

Unfortunately, we cannot apply local anesthetics directly to the intracellular surface of the sodium channel. Whether placed in the epidural space or directly into the cerebrospinal fluid, the local anesthetic must diffuse across at least two barriers to reach its site of action (*Figure 4.10*). Both the lipid bilayer of the neuronal membrane and the overlying epineurium are nonpolar environments, difficult for the local anesthetic to traverse in its active, charged state. The molecules diffuse across these membranes much more readily in the nonpolar, uncharged form. Unfortunately, the pK_as of all the clinically used local anesthetics are above the physiological pH of 7.4; upon injection, equilibrium favors the protonated, charged form of the molecule, slowing penetration to the site of action. By raising the pH, the equilibrium can be shifted to favor the uncharged state and speed the clinical onset of the block. This is the physiochemical basis for the addition of bicarbonate to epidural local anesthetics to speed their action.

Neuronal morphology also has important clinical implications for local anesthetic blockade. The smaller and more poorly myelinated the neuron, the more susceptible it is to local anesthetic block. The type C fibers transmitting first stage sensation are readily blocked with very low concentrations of local anesthetic. The Aδ fibers innervating the perineum require a higher local anesthetic concentration for effective blockade, but both types can be readily blocked with concentrations of local anesthetics that should have a minimal effect on large motor fibers to not only the lower extremities, but also to the musculature of the pelvic floor. Maintaining muscular tone of the pelvic muscles may play an important role in the progress of labor by guiding the descent

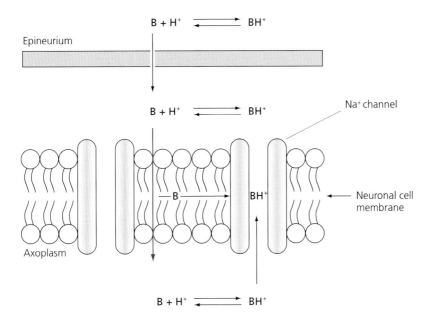

Figure 4.10 Local anesthetic action. The site of action of the local anesthetic (B) is the intracellular portion of the transmembrane Na^+ channel of the neuron. In order to reach this site of action, the anesthetic molecule must traverse several non-polar barriers (the lipid bi-layer of the cell membrane, the epineurium, the dura mater, etc.). These are most readily traversed in the uncharged state, but it is the protonated, charged form of the molecule which ultimately interacts with the Na^+ channel. From: Santos, A.C., Pederson, H. and Finster, M. (1994) Local anesthetics. In: *Obstetric Anesthesia, Principles and Practice* (ed. Chestnut, D.H.) pp. 202–228. Mosby-Year Book, Inc., St. Louis, MO.

and rotation of the fetal head as it traverses the pelvic outlet. Finally, this 'differential block-ade' explains our ability to eliminate nociception (pain) without completely eliminating awareness of labor; the sensation of 'pressure' associated with contractions is carried mainly via larger Aδ fibers, which are relatively resistant to blockade.

4.3.2 Practical applied pharmacology

Opioid receptors and agonists

Though the idea that cell membrane receptors can mediate drug effects was first postulated in the 1800s, only recently has substantial progress been made in the area of receptor pharmacology. With regard to opioid receptors, by the mid-1970s, Martin had described and characterized two opioid receptors, the mu and kappa receptors. A third opioid receptor type, the delta receptor, was described by others shortly thereafter. In 1975, enkephalins, a form of endogenous opioid, were isolated and characterized. By the late 1970s, autoradiographic mapping had revealed opioid receptor distribution within the central nervous system – notably, high concentrations of opioid receptors are found in the substantia gelatinosa of the spinal cord and periaqueductal gray matter of the midbrain.

The initial synapses of many of the primary afferents associated with labor occur in the substantia gelatinosa (lamina II), particularly for the first stage of labor. Here, opioid receptors are concentrated on the terminals of type C, but not Aδ neurons (*Figure 4.11*). To a lesser extent, they are also found on the surface of post-synaptic second order neurons (about 75% of opioid receptors are on the presynaptic C fiber terminals). Presynaptically, opioid agonists result in decreased release of neurotransmitter by the primary afferent. Postsynaptically, receptor activation decreases excitability of the postsynaptic membrane. Both effects are mediated by membrane-bound G protein and result from an increase in K+ permeability.

Once again, this understanding of cellular anatomy correlates with clinical results. Spinal or epidural opioids are much more effective analgesics during the first stage of labor where C fiber input predominates. Though not completely ineffective during the second stage, the lack of presynaptic inhibition on the Aδ fibers which dominate the second stage significantly reduces opioid efficacy. Like the substantia gelatinosa, the periacqueductal gray matter of the midbrain has a very high concentration of opiate receptors and is an important synaptic junction of the descending inhibitory pathway discussed above. In animals, injection of an opioid such as morphine in the midbrain substantially inhibits spinal nociceptive reflexes. This action is inhibited by α-adrenergic

antagonists applied locally at the spinal level, implying that the analgesic effects of *systemic* opioids are at least partly due to activation of the descending inhibitory pathway mentioned above.

α₂ adrenergic agonists

The discovery of α₂ adrenergic receptors in the superficial lamina of the spinal cord has opened new options for provision of spinal analgesia. For most of this century, the analgesic effects of spinal epinephrine have been known, and for decades epinephrine has been used with local anesthetics for surgical anesthesia to prolong the duration of the block. Almost invariably, the reason advanced for this prolongation was epinephrine's action as a local vasoconstrictor, slowing the uptake (and therefore metabolism) of the local anesthetic. The same mechanism was offered for the prolongation of epidural local anesthetics by added epinephrine. A more plausible explanation of epinephrine's action is probably its ability to activate spinal α₂ adrenergic receptors on afferent neurons.

Epinephrine added to both intrathecal and epidural local anesthetics augments the resulting block, not only in terms of duration but also intensity, as evidenced by reports of increased motor block associated with epinephrine-containing mixtures. Among other α-2 adrenergics, only clonidine has been systematically investigated and used as a labor analgesic in humans. Like norepinephrine, neuraxial clonidine results in significant analgesia; however, it also causes major dose-related side effects, such as decreased blood pressure and heart rate, and sedation. While the effectiveness of intrathecal and epidural clonidine for labor analgesia is apparent, these side effects have so far prevented widespread clinical utilization (see Chapter 5). It may eventually prove to be a useful agent for post-operative (post-cesarean) analgesia. It may be necessary to await the development of novel adrenergic agonists to fully apply adrenergic pharmacology to neuraxial analgesia in parturients.

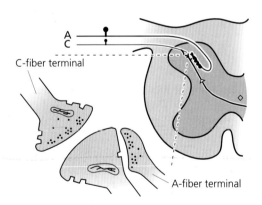

Figure 4.11 Location of opioid receptors in the dorsal horn of the spinal cord. Opioid receptors (the dots in the cell membranes) are located both pre- and post-synaptically. Pre-synaptically, they are found on C, but not Aδ fibers. About 75% of opioid receptors are presynaptic, while about 25% are postsynaptic. After: Palmer C. (2000). Spinal neuroanatomy and neuropharmacology. In: *Seminars in Anesthesia, Perioperative Medicine and Pain.* Vol. 19 No. 1. WB Saunders, Philadelphia, PA.

Cholinergic agents

At present, the only agents available that can be used to exploit the cholinergic receptors of the spinal cord are the anticholinesterases. By preventing the breakdown of acetylcholine released by inhibitory interneurons in the dorsal gray matter, anticholinesterases can provide significant analgesia. Neostigmine is the only anticholinesterase that has been systematically investigated as a neuraxial labor analgesic in humans to date, but, like clonidine, its effectiveness as an analgesic has been overshadowed by an unacceptable side effect profile. In the case of neostigmine, even when used in very low doses in combination with opioids and local anesthetics, the incidence of nausea and vomiting has proven unacceptable. It is not clear whether other anticholinesterases will eventually prove to have fewer side effects and be safe for use in humans. Direct muscarinic agonists may also eventually be clinically useful as neuraxial analgesics.

4.4 Conclusion

As our understanding of the complexity of the human nervous system has increased, so has our ability to selectively use interventions to achieve the goal of providing analgesia during labor without side effects or impact on the progress of labor. Concepts such as 'walking epidurals' and the use of ultra-low dose local anesthetics, which were unheard of ten years ago, have been proven not only possible, but also practical for routine use. While clonidine and neostigmine have not had the impact on labor analgesia practice that opioids such as fentanyl and sufentanil have, it is quite probable that other adrenergic and cholinergic agents will have an impact in the future.

Further reading

Bouaziz, H., Hewitt, C. and Eisenach, J.C. (1995) Subarachnoid neostigmine potentiation of alpha2-adrenergic agonist analgesia. Dexmedetomidine versus clonidine. *Reg. Anesth.* **20**: 121–127.

Butterworth, J.F. and Strichartz, G.R. (1990) Molecular mechanisms of local anesthesia: a review. *Anesthesiology* **72**: 711–734.

Carr, D.B. and Cousins, M.J. (1998) Spinal route of analgesia: opioids and future options. In: *Neural Blockade in Clinical Anesthesia and Management of Pain* (eds. Cousins, M.J. and Bridenbaugh, P.O.), pp. 915–941. Lippincott-Raven Publishers, Philadelphia.

Collins, J.G., Kitahata, L.M., Matsumoto, M. *et al.* (1984) Spinally administered epinephrine suppresses noxiously evoked activity of WDR neurons in the dorsal horn of the spinal cord. *Anesthesiology* **60**: 269–275.

Cleland, J.G.P. (1933) Paravertebral anesthesia in obstetrics. *Surg. Gynecol. Obstet.* **57**: 51–62.

Detweiler, D.J., Eisenach, J.C., Tong, C. and Jackson, C. (1993) A cholinergic interaction in alpha 2 adrenoreceptor mediated antinociception in sheep. *J. Pharmacol. Exp. Ther.* **265**: 536–542.

Dougherty, P.M. and Staats, P.S. (1999) Intrathecal drug therapy for chronic pain. *Anesthesiology* **91**: 1891–1918.

Eisenach, J.C., Detweiler, D. and Hood, D.D. (1993) Hemodynamic and analgesic actions of epidurally administered clonidine. *Anesthesiology* **78**: 277–287.

Gordh, T. Jr., Jansson, I., Hartvig, P. *et al.* (1989) Interactions between noradrenergic and cholinergic mechanisms involved in spinal nociceptive processing. *Acta Anaesthiol. Scand.* **33**: 39–47.

Klimscha, W., Tong, C. and Eisenach, J.C. (1997) Intrathecal α2-adrenergic agonists stimulate acetylcholine and norepinephrine release from the spinal cord dorsal horn in sheep. An *in vivo* microdialysis study. *Anesthesiology* **87**: 110–116.

Naguib, M. and Yaksh, T.L. (1994) Antinociceptive effects of spinal cholinesterase inhibition and isobolographic analysis of the interaction with μ and α2 receptor systems. *Anesthesiology* **80**: 1338–1348.

Paech, M.J., Pavy, T.J.G., Orlikowski, C.E.P. and Evans, S.F. (2000) Patient-controlled epidural analgesia in labor: the addition of clonidine to bupivacaine-fentanyl. *Reg. Anesth. Pain Med.* **25**: 34–40.

Palmer, C.M. (2000) Spinal neuroanatomy and neuropharmacology. In: *Seminars in Anesthesia, Perioperative Medicine, and Pain,* (ed. Katz R.L), Vol 19, No. 1, pp. 10–17. W.B. Saunders Company, Philadelphia.

Purves, D., Augustine, G.J., Fitzpatrick, D., Katz, L.C., LaMantia, A. and McNamara, J.O. (eds) (1997) *Neuroscience.* Sinauer Associates, Inc., Sunderland, MA.

Sabbe, M.B. and Yaksh, T.L. (1990) Pharmacology of spinal opioids. *J. Pain Symptom Manage.* **5**: 191–203.

Stamford, J.A. (1995) Descending control of pain. *Br. J. Anaesth.* **75**: 217–227.

Sukara, S., Sumi, M., Morimoto, N. and Saito, Y. (1999) The addition of epinephrine increases the intensity of sensory block during epidural anesthesia with lidocaine. *Reg. Anesth. Pain Med.* **24**: 541–546.

Voulgaropoulos, D. and Palmer, C.M. (1996) Local anesthetic pharmacology. In: *International Practice of Anaesthesia* (eds Prys-Roberts, C. and Brown, B.R.). Butterworth-Heinemann, Oxford.

Chapter 5

Regional analgesia in obstetrics

Robert D'Angelo, MD and
John A. Thomas, MD

Contents

5.1 Introduction

The use of regional analgesic techniques has revolutionized pain relief in obstetrics. The utilization of epidural analgesia in obstetrics within the US has increased from < 20% of parturients in 1981 to > 50% in 1997. Contemporary regional analgesic techniques provide rapid, almost complete analgesia while minimizing risk to the mother and fetus. It is no coincidence that as the use of regional anesthesia has increased during the past two decades the incidence of anesthesia-related maternal mortality has dramatically decreased. Since the majority of maternal deaths occur during general anesthesia from either failed intubation or aspiration, the use of regional analgesia avoids the need for general anesthesia and its related complications. Statistics indicate that the use of general anesthesia in the United States has fallen from 35% to 8% since 1981. Additionally, administration techniques have been refined over the past two decades to reduce local anesthetic toxicity (see Section 15.7). Prior to 1984, large boluses of concentrated local anesthetic were routinely administered through the epidural needle. This practice resulted in approximately 20 maternal deaths from bupivacaine-induced cardiac arrest. Following these deaths, 0.75% bupivacaine was withdrawn from obstetrics and recommendations were made that epidural catheters be inserted and tested for proper location rather than dosing through the epidural needle, that all local anesthetics be administered incrementally, and that dilute concentrations of local anesthetic solutions be used for maintenance. These recommendations significantly increased the safety of regional anesthesia and decreased the incidence of undesirable side effects such as motor block. As a result, there have been no reported local anesthetic-induced maternal deaths during labor in the US since 1984.

5.2 Epidural analgesia

5.2.1 Advantages
The advantages of continuous epidural techniques include the ability to produce analgesia over a prolonged period of time that can be altered in intensity throughout labor, and to provide anesthesia for instrumental or operative delivery if necessary. In addition, epidural analgesia has a low incidence of side effects and reduces the need for general anesthesia in high-risk patients.

5.2.2 Disadvantages
The disadvantages of epidural analgesia are primarily related to increased manpower requirements. Providing epidural analgesia in obstetrics is relatively labor intensive since it takes approximately 20 minutes to induce each anesthetic; as many as 30% of epidural catheters require manipulation for intravenous cannulation or inadequate analgesia at some point during labor; nearly 10% require replacement; and most labor suites are not situated near the main operating suite. With approximately 2 million parturients requesting epidural analgesia in the United States each year, many anesthesia practices are struggling to provide coverage for both the operating room and the labor suite. To survive, these practices must maximize the efficiency of their obstetric epidural services, without compromising patient safety. This chapter focuses on an evidence-based approach to providing labor analgesia while accomplishing both of these goals. In addition, Section 5.7 of this chapter specifically addresses efficiency.

5.2.3 Indications
As noted in a joint statement by the ASA and ACOG, 'There is no other circumstance when it is considered acceptable for a person to experience severe pain, amenable to safe intervention, while under a physician's care.'

Contemporary obstetric anesthesia practice dictates that any parturient requesting pain relief during any phase of labor and irrespective of cervical dilatation is a candidate for epidural or regional analgesia. This assumes an epidural service exists at that institution and that the patient has no contraindications to regional anesthesia.

5.2.4 Contraindications

Although absolute contraindications to neuraxial blockade are rare, a number of relative contraindications occur that may preclude the use of regional anesthesia *(Table 5.1)*. When relative contraindications exist, the risk of a complication occurring must be weighed against the benefits of the regional anesthetic on a case-by-case basis.

5.2.5 Preparation

All patients should have a brief history and physical exam and the risks of the procedure explained prior to epidural catheter placement. Laboratory tests are not routinely recommended unless the history warrants them, such as a platelet count in a patient with a history of preeclampsia (see Chapter 9). Prior to inducing any regional anesthetic, the anesthesia care provider must be prepared to treat any side effects that may be encountered, including, but not limited to hypotension, seizures and cardiopulmonary arrest. Drugs and equipment for resuscitation should be immediately available, intravenous access should be established, and the patient's obstetrician should be notified prior to induction of epidural analgesia. These recommendations are based on the Guidelines for Regional Anesthesia in Obstetrics established by the ASA *(Table 5.2)*. If time allows, it is also advisable to administer 250–500 ml of a nondextrose containing balanced salt solution before epidural placement. If not, waiting until the fluid bolus is administered to begin the procedure is not routinely necessary since hypotension induced by epidural labor analgesia is usually easily treated with small intravenous boluses of ephedrine.

5.2.6 Equipment

Key essentials of a disposable epidural kit include sterile skin preparation solutions, anesthetic and needles for local infiltration, a sterile drape, an epidural needle, a syringe for loss of resistance, saline, and an epidural catheter. Although there are many types of epidural needles, each with advantages and disadvantages, a winged needle with a 9 cm barrel marked into 1 cm increments to assist with insertion and with determining the depth from the patient's skin to the epidural space is widely used and probably optimal. Likewise, an epidural catheter that is clearly marked along the distal 20 cm into 1 cm increments to assist with determining the amount of catheter that remains within the epidural space after

Table 5.1 Contraindications to regional anesthesia

Absolute	Relative[a]
Patient refusal or the inability to cooperate	Mild coagulopathy (i.e. isolated decreased platelet count)
Localized infection at the insertion site	
Sepsis	Severe maternal cardiac disease such as Eisenmenger's syndrome or aortic stenosis (see Chapter 13)
Severe coagulopathy	
Uncorrected hypovolemia	Neurological disease (spina bifida) (see Chapter 13)
	Severe fetal depression

[a]The risk of a complication occurring must be weighed against the benefits of the regional anesthetic on a case-by-case basis.

Table 5.2 Guidelines for regional anesthesia in obstetrics[a]
1. Appropriate resuscitation equipment and drugs must be immediately available, including: oxygen, suction, equipment to maintain an airway and perform endotracheal intubation, ability to provide positive pressure ventilation, and ability to perform advanced cardiac life support.
2. Regional anesthesia should be initiated by or under the medical direction of a physician with appropriate privileges.
3. Regional anesthesia should not be initiated until the patient is examined by a qualified individual and the obstetrician with the knowledge of maternal and fetal status and the progress of labor approves of the labor anesthetic and is readily available to supervise labor and manage any complications that may arise.
4. An intravenous infusion should be established and maintained throughout the regional anesthetic.
5. The parturient's vital signs and fetal heart rate should be monitored.
6. Regional anesthesia for cesarean section requires that the Standards for Basic Anesthetic Monitoring be applied and that the obstetrician be immediately available.
7. Qualified personnel, other than the attending anesthesiologist, should be immediately available for newborn resuscitation.
8. The anesthesia care provider should remain readily available during the regional anesthetic to manage anesthetic complications until the post anesthesia condition is stable.
9. The Standards for Post Anesthesia Care should be applied.
10. A physician should be available to manage complications and provide CPR for patients receiving post anesthesia care.

[a]Adapted from the guidelines approved by the ASA House of Delegates on October 12, 1988 and last amended on October 18, 2000.

removal of the epidural needle is recommended. Multiport catheters (closed tip and with three lateral holes at 0.5, 1.0 and 1.5 cm from the distal tip) are recommended since they reduce the incidence of inadequate analgesia, require less manipulation and make identification of an intravenous catheter easier than do uniport (open-end, distal port) epidural catheters. Finally, a clear sterile drape may assist with interspace and midline identification, especially during difficult epidural placement.

5.2.7 Technique

For quick reference, a recommended technique for continuous lumbar epidural analgesia is outlined in *Table 5.3*.

Positioning and choice of interspace

The patient may be positioned in either the lateral decubitus or sitting position during epidural catheter placement. Although both positions have advantages, the sitting position theoretically makes identification of the mid-line easier, especially in obese patients. On the other hand, many patients may be more comfortable in the lateral decubitus position, especially if the procedure occurs when the patient is in the late phases of labor. Occasional clinical scenarios, such as a prolapsed cord, will necessitate the lateral position should a regional anesthetic be required. Therefore, regardless of personal preference the anesthesia care provider must be adept at epidural catheter insertion with the patient in either the lateral or sitting position. With either position, it is helpful to have the patient place her elbows on her knees. To do so she must reach around her abdomen, which in turn reduces the amount of lumbar lordosis. To facilitate the elbow on knee position, having the patient sit cross-legged, with the ankles crossed and the knees fully abducted is recommended. If the patient cannot assume this position, have them place their feet on a stool so that their knees are raised and flexed rather than dangling off the bed. Once the patient has been positioned, the midline should be identified

Table 5.3 Technique for lumbar epidural analgesia

- Sitting position
- Sterile prep and drape, any interspace between L_2 and S_1
- LOR for identification of epidural space, cephalad-directed bevel
- Midline approach
- Once the epidural space is identified, insert a multiport epidural catheter 5–6 cm
- If aspiration negative, test catheter for IT or IV placement
- *See text for details of test-dosing*
- Initiate catheter dosing with divided (5 ml) doses of:
  - ➤ 0.9%–2.0% lidocaine (10–12 ml total)
  - ➤ 0.0625%–0.25% bupivacaine (10–12 ml total)
  - ➤ 0.1%–0.2% ropivacaine (10–20 ml total)
  - ➤ 0.0625%–0.25% levobupivacaine (10–12 ml total)
  - ➤ Adjuncts: Fentanyl (50 µg total)
      Epinephrine (1:200 000–400 000)
- Adequate analgesia: Begin infusion of bupivacaine (0.04%–0.125%) + fentanyl (1.5–2 µg/ml) at 12–16 ml/h
  - ➤ Consider PCEA | Settings:

	Basal rate	8–10 ml/h
	Bolus dose	5 ml
	Lockout	10 min
	Hourly limit	30 ml

- If pain persists 15 min after initial injection, pull catheter so 3–4 cm remains within the epidural space and administer additional local anesthetic
- If pain persists after 5 min, remove and replace epidural catheter

and any interspace between the L_2 spinous process and the sacrum selected. The lowest interspace that can be readily palpated is generally recommended.

Loss of resistance and needle advancement

The epidural space should be identified using a loss of resistance (LOR) technique; however, the use of air or saline for LOR remains controversial (see also Section 15.1.1). Proponents of the air technique suggest a 'better feel', easier identification of accidental dural puncture and avoiding the extra step of opening a vial of saline. In contrast, air causes an almost immediate headache if injected intrathecally and theoretically prevents diffusion of local anesthetic to all nerve roots. On the other hand, saline theoretically expands the epidural space that in turn reduces the incidence of intravenous cannulation and inadequate analgesia. Either air or saline can be used safely and

effectively for LOR to identify the epidural space; if air is used, the volume actually injected into the epidural space should be minimized. However, when learning to insert epidural catheters, saline may be preferential since it is less compressible than air.

Two common techniques for epidural needle advancement have been described: an intermittent LOR technique and a continuous LOR technique *(Figure 5.1(a) and (b))*. A winged needle is typically used for the intermittent technique. The wings are grasped between the thumbs and index fingers while the middle fingers of each hand are pressed against the needle shaft near the insertion sight to prevent excess movement. The needle is advanced a short distance (1–2 mm), then intermittent LOR is ascertained *(Figure 5.1 (a))*. With the continuous technique the back of the hand is pressed onto the patient's back to prevent excess movement and the epidural needle is held securely near the patient's back between the thumb and index finger of the non-dominant hand. Continuous pressure is then applied to the syringe with the dominant hand as the needle is slowly but continuously advanced *(Figure 5.1 (b))*. With either technique depression of the plunger will be met with resistance while the epidural needle is in either the interspinous ligament or the ligamentum flavum. When the epidural needle bevel passes through the ligamentum flavum and into the epidural space, gentle pressure will easily depress the plunger.

Bevel direction
It has been suggested that in cases of accidental dural puncture, positioning the epidural needle bevel so that it punctures the dura vertically, rather than horizontally, across the long axis of the back may reduce the incidence of post dural puncture headache. When using

the vertical needle technique, however, the epidural needle should be rotated so that the bevel is oriented in a cephalad direction once the epidural space has been identified and prior to epidural catheter insertion. This rotation theoretically facilitates midline epidural catheter insertion. However, rotation of the epidural needle may in itself increase the likelihood of dural puncture. Therefore, to avoid the extra step of rotating the epidural needle, the epidural needle should be inserted with a cephalad orientation and the epidural space entered cautiously.

Epidural catheter insertion
Inserting epidural catheters 5–6 cm within the epidural space is optimal. Catheters inserted greater than 6 cm increase the risk of intravenous cannulation and those inserted less than 5 cm are more likely to become dislodged

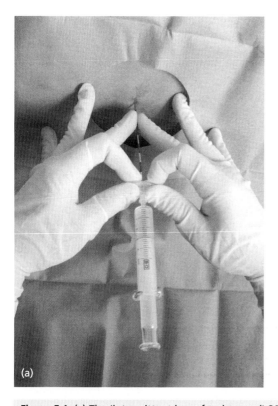 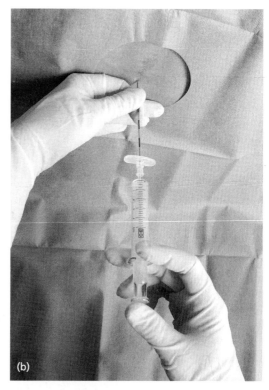

(a)   (b)

Figure 5.1 (a) The 'intermittent loss of resistance (LOR) technique' for epidural catheter placement. (b) The 'continuous LOR technique'.

during prolonged labors. Although epidural catheters can deviate from midline during insertion, it makes sense to maximize the chance of a midline insertion by holding the catheter during insertion so that the coils do not generate right or left rotational force.

Occasionally, a persistent paresthesia or blood is noted during insertion. When this occurs the epidural catheter must be removed and replaced. However, withdrawing the epidural catheter through the epidural needle can lead to a shearing of the catheter tip. To prevent this from occurring, the epidural catheter should never be pulled back through the epidural needle; remove the epidural catheter and needle as one unit. If a piece of epidural catheter is believed to have broken off in the patient's back in this fashion, the patient should be informed and a neurosurgeon consulted, although surgical removal is rarely warranted unless there are persistent neurological symptoms.

Epidural catheter testing

After securing the catheter, place the patient in the semi-lateral position to avoid aorta caval compression and carefully aspirate the epidural catheter. If negative, the catheter should be tested to rule out accidental intravenous or intrathecal placement. The goal of a test dose is to produce early signs of toxicity but not produce seizures or cardiopulmonary arrest. If a test dose containing local anesthetic is administered, the patient should be monitored for motor block to rule out intrathecal placement and signs such as tinnitus or peri-oral numbness to rule out intravenous placement. In addition, many patients will develop a 'glassy-eyed look' and will not be able to communicate effectively for 2–3 minutes after intravenous injection of a large bolus of local anesthetic.

Many epidural test solutions have been proposed (*Table 5.4*; see also Sections 15.6 and 15.7). A commonly used test dose is 1.5% lidocaine 45 mg (3 ml) plus epinephrine 15 µg administered as a single test to rule out both intrathecal and intravenous catheter placement. However, because painful labor potentially increases maternal heart rate, this test dose must be administered between contractions and the reliability of further increasing maternal heart rate has been questioned. In addition, even this small dose of epinephrine produces transient increases in uterine artery tone in sheep, which if also true in humans, may theoretically produce fetal bradycardia in patients with preexisting placental insufficiency. The double test entails administering two doses of plain 2% lidocaine: a 40 mg (2 ml) intrathecal test followed in 5 minutes by a 100 mg (5 ml) intravenous test. This test dose solution avoids the pitfalls associated with epinephrine- containing test doses and may be used in cases where it is essential the epidural catheter functions properly, such as in patients at high risk for requiring urgent operative delivery. Regardless of test dose chosen, careful observation of the patient with each injection of the epidural catheter reduces maternal and fetal risk, and is recommended.

Table 5.4 Epidural catheter test doses (see also Section 15.7)

Double test dose	2% lidocaine 40 mg (2 ml) IT test followed if negative in 3–5 minutes by 2% lidocaine 100 mg (5 ml) IV test
Single test doses	1.5% lidocaine 45 mg + Epi 15 µg (3 ml) 2% chloroprocaine 60 mg + Epi 15 µg (3 ml) 0.25% bupivacaine 7.5 mg + Epi 15 µg (3 ml)
Others	Isoproterenol 5 mg Fentanyl 100 µg Doppler detection of air 1–2 ml

If an intrathecal catheter is noted, the catheter can either be removed or left in place as a spinal catheter. Section 5.4 discusses the indications and risks of spinal catheters.

If an intravenous catheter is detected by either aspiration or from the test dose, withdrawing the catheter in 1 cm increments while gently aspirating may be effective since 50% of these catheters can be 'salvaged' to produce adequate labor analgesia. At some point during withdrawal of each intravenous catheter, blood will no longer be aspirated when either the catheter has been pulled out of the epidural vein, but remains within the epidural space or when it has been withdrawn back through the ligamentum flavum. If the catheter tip rests 3 cm or more within the epidural space, adequate analgesia will be produced in >90% of patients. If not, simply remove and replace the epidural catheter. This maneuver saves time and minimizes the need for epidural catheter replacement.

Establishing a block

Once a negative test dose is established, local anesthetic should be administered incrementally to obtain a T_8–T_{10} sensory block. If the single lidocaine plus epinephrine test dose was administered, an additional 10–15 ml of dilute local anesthetic plus opioid will be required to produce adequate labor analgesia. If the double test dose was administered, an additional 3 ml of 2% lidocaine to total 200 mg will produce a dense sensory block and some degree of motor block, both of which assist in determining how well the epidural catheter is functioning. Given the wide variety of local anesthetics (and concentrations) that can be administered, it is impossible to describe all the initial injections that can and are used to establish effective analgesia.

Management of epidural catheters

As many as 20–30% of patients may experience inadequate epidural analgesia. The most likely cause is catheter deviation from midline during insertion that then leads to a maldistribution of local anesthetic within the epidural space. Septa, the use of air for loss of resistance, and mechanical obstructions have also been postulated as causes for maldistribution of local anesthetic. Regardless of the cause, these epidural catheters should be actively managed until adequate analgesia is established. An aggressive approach to epidural catheter management should be taken so that within 20 minutes of epidural catheter insertion, the patient is either comfortable or the epidural catheter is replaced. If pain persists longer than 15 minutes after local anesthetic administration, withdrawing the catheter 1–2 cm (so that 3–4 cm remains within the epidural space) and administering additional local anesthetic is recommended. If the patient is not comfortable within 5 minutes, remove and replace the epidural catheter. This approach improves overall efficiency and increases the likelihood that epidural anesthesia will be successful should urgent cesarean section be required. Alternatively, it has been suggested that patients should be placed with their inadequate analgesia side into the dependent position and additional local anesthetic administered rather than withdrawing the epidural catheter. This technique is, however, less effective than first withdrawing the epidural catheter (91% vs 74%), and therefore wastes time if the catheter eventually requires manipulation.

Once the patient develops adequate analgesia, administering a dilute local anesthetic solution for maintenance is recommended. Using low concentrations of local anesthetic minimizes maternal motor block; the addition of an opioid (usually fentanyl) and often epinephrine as adjuncts in the solution allows lowered concentrations to be effective.

The optimal concentration of local anesthetic and mixture for epidural infusion probably varies with patient population, physician experience, available manpower, and other factors. Bupivacaine concentrations as low as 0.04% (with fentanyl and epinephrine) have been advocated, and 0.0625% is commonly used. Other anesthesiologists prefer to use concentrations as high as 0.125%, albeit at a lower infusion rate.

Fentanyl at a concentration between 1.25 and 2.0 µg/ml is commonly used as an adjunct in epidural infusion solutions. Many anesthesiologists also advocate the routine use of epinephrine at a dilution of 1:600 000 to 1:800 000.

In situations where mixing of infusion solutions may be impractical, ropivacaine 0.1% to 0.2% has been used as a plain local anesthetic infusion with some success.

Maintenance

Labor analgesia can be maintained by intermittent bolus, continuous infusion, and patient-controlled epidural analgesic techniques. Generally speaking, the intermittent bolus technique requires the most anesthetic interventions, followed by the continuous infusion technique, and lastly by the PCEA technique. Although many 'cocktails' have been described, one technique for each method is described in *Table 5.5*. Patient-controlled epidural analgesia with a background infusion may be optimal since this technique is associated with high patient satisfaction and may decrease manpower require-

ments. Although background infusions may increase total drug use without significantly enhancing analgesia, PCEA can be primarily utilized as a 'continuous infusion technique' that allows for patient-administered boluses should breakthrough pain be experienced.

Regardless of the maintenance technique utilized, analgesic requirements vary throughout labor and for delivery, and occasionally patients experience breakthrough pain or perineal pressure as labor progresses. Administering additional boluses of local anesthetic (5–10 ml of 0.1%–0.25% bupivacaine, depending on circumstances) when this occurs will be necessary; adding fentanyl to the bolus may also be helpful. If discomfort persists, manage the epidural catheter as described in the preceding section.

5.2.8 Complications

Epidural analgesia is associated with many side effects and complications *(Table 5.6)*, although the most common ones are easily treated. Risks of epidural analgesia include: backache, inadequate analgesia, hypotension, motor block, require replacement, fetal bradycardia, intravenous cannulations, dural puncture, spinal catheters, post dural puncture headache,

---

Table 5.5 Solutions for various epidural analgesia maintenance techniques

Technique	Concentration and dosing schedule
Intermittent bolus	0.1%–0.25% bupivacaine + fentanyl 3 µg/ml + Epi 1:200 000 10 ml (5 + 5 ml) Boluses as needed
Continuous infusion	0.044%–0.125% bupivacaine + fentanyl 1.5–2 µg ml^{-1} at 8–14 ml/h
PCEA with basal infusion	0.0625%–0.125% bupivacaine + fentanyl 2 µg ml^{-1} at the following settings: Basal rate: 8–12 ml/h Bolus dose: 5 ml Lockout: 10 min Hourly limit: 30 ml
PCEA without a basal infusion	0.125% bupivacaine + fentanyl 2 µg/ml at the following settings: Bolus dose: 8 ml Lockout: 15 min Hourly limit: None

Table 5.6 Complications and side effects associated with epidural analgesia[a]

Complication or side effect	Incidence
Backache at insertion site	75%
Inadequate labor analgesia	25%
Hypotension	Varies with dose
Motor block	Varies with dose
Urinary retention	Varies with dose
Require replacement	10%
Fetal bradycardia	8%
Intravenous cannulation	6%
Dural puncture	2%
Post dural puncture headache	1%
Spinal catheter	<1%
Subdural catheter	Rare (1:1000)
High spinal block	Rare (1:10 000)
Permanent neurologic injury	Extremely rare (<1:10 000)
Epidural hematoma	Extremely rare (<1:100 000)
Epidural abscess	Extremely rare (<1:100 000)
Death	Extremely rare (<1:100 000)

[a]The listed incidence for each complication or side effect is an average value obtained from numerous sources within the literature (see also Chapter 15).

urinary retention, and the very rare risks of subdural catheter placement, permanent neurological injury, epidural hematoma, epidural abscess and death (see also Chapter 15). Back pain is usually self-limited and easily treated with oral analgesics and ambulation. Hypotension results from sympathetic blockade, which may cause fetal bradycardia by reducing uterine artery blood flow and fetal oxygenation. Hypotension and/or fetal bradycardia should both be treated immediately with ephedrine 5–10 mg administered intravenously as needed and ensuring left uterine displacement, followed by intravenous fluid infusion.

5.2.9 Medications
Local anesthetics
Local anesthetics interfere with axonal sodium channels to inhibit propagation of action potentials. They are weak bases with pK_as approximating 8.0. At physiological pH most of the local anesthetic molecules exist in the ionized form; however, it is the unionized molecules that diffuse through tissues and across cell membranes. Therefore, speed of onset is generally inversely related to pKa since local anesthetics with lower pK_as will have a higher

fraction of unionized molecules (see also Section 4.3.1). A notable exception is chloroprocaine whose rapid onset is related to the high concentrations utilized rather than from a low pK_a. Local anesthetics are classified according to the alkyl chain linking the lipophilic carbon ring and the tertiary amine as either amides or esters. The esters include cocaine, tetracaine, procaine and chloroprocaine, while the amides include lidocaine, etidocaine, mepivacaine, prilocaine, bupivacaine, ropivacaine and levobupivacaine. Esters are degraded in the plasma by pseudocholinesterase and non-specific esterases, while amides are metabolized in the liver. Esters are hydrolyzed to produce para-aminobenzoic acid (PABA), which gives them greater allergic potential than the amides.

Blood levels are influenced by the dose of drug administered, physiochemical properties of the drug, the addition of vasoconstrictors, metabolism, and the vascularity of the administered site. For example, while 5 mg/kg of lidocaine administered within the epidural space is considered safe, 20 mg injected directly into the carotid artery will likely produce a seizure. Similar doses of lidocaine

Table 5.7 Commonly administered local anesthetics in obstetrics

Drug	Class	Concentration	Dose[a]	Onset	Minimum duration of labor analgesia[b]	pKa	Protein bound (%)
Chloroprocaine	Ester	2–3%	10–30 ml	Rapid	30 min	8.7	0
Lidocaine	Amide	1–2%	10–30 ml	Intermediate	45 min	7.9	70
Bupivacaine	Amide	0.04–0.5%	10–30 ml	Slow	60 min	8.1	95
Levobupivacaine	Amide	0.04–0.5%	10–30 ml	Slow	60 min	8.1	97
Ropivacaine	Amide	0.04–0.5%	10–30 ml	Slow	60 min	8.1	94

[a] Local anesthetics should be administered incrementally rather than as a bolus. [b] Duration of labor analgesia from a single 15 ml epidural dose administered incrementally.

produce varying plasma levels with different regional techniques in the following order: intercostal > caudal > epidural > brachial plexus = femoral that directly correlate with the vascularity of each site. The addition of epinephrine 1:200 000 lowers plasma concentrations and prolongs the duration of the block. The physiochemical properties such as pK$_a$, lipid solubility, and protein binding determine variables such as speed of onset, potency and duration of action, respectively.

Based on these physiochemical properties the most appropriate local anesthetics for use in obstetrics are bupivacaine, chloroprocaine, levobupivacaine, lidocaine and ropivacaine (Table 5.7). Lidocaine is best suited for testing epidural catheters for location and to establish labor analgesia, bupivacaine to maintain labor analgesia, and chloroprocaine to provide anesthesia (rapidly, if necessary) for instrumental and operative deliveries.

All local anesthetics are toxic if administered in high enough doses. As blood levels increase, local anesthetics at first cause excitatory neurological symptoms such as tinnitus and perioral numbness followed by CNS depression, respiratory arrest and eventual cardiac arrest (Table 5.8). The key to preventing local anesthetic toxicity is maintaining vigilance during administration and by administering low enough doses of local anesthetics that they may produce early signs of CNS toxicity, but not seizures or cardiopulmonary arrest. Testing epidural catheters after insertion and fractionating each dose into 5 ml aliquots

Table 5.8 Signs and symptoms of local anesthetic toxicity[a]

1. Tinnitus, perioral numbness
2. Inability to communicate appropriately (glassy-eyed look)
3. Loss of consciousness
4. Seizure
5. Respiratory arrest
6. Cardiac arrest

[a]Any local anesthetic can produce these reactions. The signs and symptoms generally occur in the listed order as blood levels increase. A test dose containing local anesthetic should produce early signs and symptoms, but not loss of consciousness or seizures. To prevent severe toxic reactions, local anesthetics should always be administered incrementally.

administered at least 30–60 seconds apart while observing the patient for signs and symptoms of CNS toxicity will reduce (or eliminate) the likelihood of a catastrophic toxic event. Large boluses of concentrated local anesthetics should never be administered as a single rapid bolus even in patients with a functioning epidural catheter since epidural catheters can migrate into epidural veins or intrathecally. When dosing for urgent cesarean section, 30 ml of concentrated local anesthetic can safely be administered in 3–4 minutes, rather than as a single bolus.

At clinically relative doses, local anesthetics have no adverse effect on the uterine vasculature or umbilical artery blood flow. However, at higher concentrations local anesthetics can result in uterine artery vasoconstriction and uterine hypertonus. Unionized local anesthetic molecules freely pass through the placenta. Since fetal pH is lower than the maternal pH, more local anesthetic becomes ionized and accumulates in the fetal circulation in a phenomenon known as 'ion trapping'. This may become clinically significant in a distressed acidotic fetus, which then 'traps' additional local anesthetic molecules.

Bupivacaine

Bupivacaine is the most commonly used local anesthetic in obstetrics. At dilute concentrations it produces a proportionally greater sensory block than motor block and has limited placental transfer since it is highly protein bound, both of which are desirable characteristics for use in obstetrics. Plain 0.25% bupivacine 10–15 ml produces analgesia in 10–15 minutes that lasts over 60 minutes before the patient requests additional analgesia. Continuous infusions of dilute bupivacaine 0.04–0.125% at rates of 10–15 ml/h with or without opioids and epinephrine provide labor analgesia with minimal side effects.

Ropivacaine and levobupivacaine

Bupivacaine is prepared as a 50/50 racemic mixture of D and L isomers. For unknown reasons, the D-isomer binds cardiac sodium channels more tightly than the L-isomer, and is consequently more cardiotoxic. Commercial preparations of the nearly pure L-isomers, levobupivacaine and ropivacaine, have been developed as replacements for bupivacaine. Bupivacaine, levobupivacaine, and ropivacaine are from the same pipecoloxylidide family and are structural analogs (see *Figure 5.2*). Other than this enantiomeric difference, ropivacaine has a three-carbon side chain while bupivacaine and levobupivacaine have four-carbon side chains.

In addition to being less cardiotoxic than bupivacaine, ropivacaine also reportedly produces less motor block than bupivacaine, although approximately 75% of studies that compare motor block produced by both ropi-

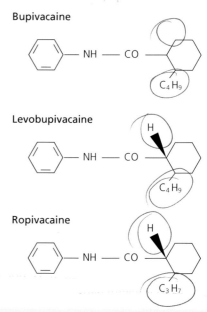

Figure 5.2 The molecular structures of bupivacaine, levobupivacaine and ropivacaine. Bupivacaine is prepared commercially as a 50/50% racemic mixture of the D and L isomers, while levobupivacaine and ropivacaine are prepared in the nearly pure L-isomer forms. Ropivacaine contains a 3-carbon side chain while bupivacaine and levobupivacaine contain 4-carbon side chains.

vacaine and bupivacaine report similar degrees of motor block from each. In addition, recent findings suggest that the ED_{50} of ropivacaine is approximately 40% greater than the ED_{50} of bupivacaine, suggesting that ropivacaine is less potent than bupivacaine. Many clinical studies, however, suggest that the two local anesthetics are clinically indistinguishable. Based on clinical findings, similar concentrations of ropivacaine are recommended if replacing bupivacaine in obstetrics.

Like ropivacaine, levobupivacaine is less cardiotoxic than bupivacaine. However, it is equipotent to bupivacaine, and therefore the two drugs should be clinically indistinguishable. Use similar concentrations of levobupivacaine if replacing bupivacaine in obstetrics.

Although ropivacaine and levobupivacaine are less cardiotoxic than bupivacaine, the dilute concentrations of bupivacaine and safer administration techniques used in contemporary obstetric analgesia have virtually eliminated cardiac arrest in laboring patients.

Lidocaine

Plain 1.0%–2.0% lidocaine 10–15 ml produces labor analgesia in 5–10 minutes that lasts at least 45 minutes before the patient requests additional analgesia. Alkalinization of the lidocaine with 8.4% sodium bicarbonate 1 meq/10 ml of local anesthetic decreases onset time to approximately 3–6 minutes, and the addition of fentanyl enhances analgesia at lower concentrations. Since lidocaine produces more motor block and has greater placental transfer than bupivacaine, and it may have a greater propensity for tachyphylaxis, it is not routinely used as a maintenance agent. Rather, it is more commonly used to test epidural catheters, initiate labor analgesia, treat breakthrough pain, or produce anesthesia for instrumental or operative deliveries.

Chloroprocaine

Plain 2% chloroprocaine 10–15 ml produces labor analgesia in 3–6 minutes that lasts at least 30 minutes before the patient requests additional analgesia. However, chloroprocaine is not routinely used as a maintenance agent because its prohibitively short duration of action makes management difficult. In contrast, chloroprocaine has a rapid onset of action, produces dense sensory and motor block and has a short duration of action, all of which are desirable characteristics when providing anesthesia for relatively short cases like instrumental or operative deliveries. Because chloroprocaine is metabolized by plasma esterases, the plasma half-life is approximately 30 seconds, which makes chloroprocaine one of the least toxic local anesthetics.

Despite these benefits, chloroprocaine has been associated with neurological injury (when administered intrathecally), back pain, and decreased efficacy of epidural opioids. Chloroprocaine-induced neurotoxicity was related to a combination of the preservative sodium metabisulfate and the pH of the commercial preparation. However, since the pH was increased from 3.0 to 7.0 there have been no further reports of neurotoxicity. Nevertheless, avoiding the use of chloroprocaine in cases of an accidental dural puncture with the epidural needle as a precaution is recommended. Chloroprocaine-induced back pain may be related to localized muscle hypocalcemia induced from the preservative EDTA, which theoretically chelates calcium. This back pain has been classically described as severe muscle spasms of the upper back following large doses (>25 ml) of chloroprocaine and occurring when the epidural analgesia is receding. The pain is generally self-limiting but fentanyl 50–100 µg or additional local anesthetic may be required. Because of these problems, preservative free preparations of chloroprocaine are now available. However chloroprocaine also reportedly reduces analgesia from both fentanyl and morphine, even after the block has receded, which is thought to result from chloroprocaine (or one of its metabolites) binding to opioid receptors. Should a patient complain of pain in the recovery room despite epidural opioids after chloroprocaine anesthesia, switching to PCA morphine for postoperative analgesia can circumvent the problem.

Despite these potential problems, the benefits of chloroprocaine clearly outweigh the risks of these rare complications in many situations. Chloroprocaine is probably the best option for routine use for instrumental and operative delivery.

Opioids

Opioids produce analgesia by binding to opioid receptors both in the spinal cord (spinal receptors) and within the brain (supraspinal receptors). Although opioids reliably produce analgesia in early labor, they are less effective during the later phases of labor and for delivery (see Section 4.3.2). Visceral pain fibers (early labor pain) are more amenable to opioid-induced modulation than are somatic pain fibers (late labor and delivery pain), which synapse more deeply within the spinal cord. As a result, opioids are most often co-administered with local anesthetics. The addition of opioids (typically fentanyl 1.5–2 µg/ml) to dilute concentrations of local anesthetic (typically bupivacaine 0.0625–0.125%) reduces local anesthetic use 25–30% through a predominately spinal affect. This is in contradistinction to studies comparing postoperative analgesia from epidural and intravenous fentanyl, which suggest epidural fentanyl offers no advantage over intravenous administration. In these studies, fentanyl use, blood levels, pain scores and side effects are similar between groups. However, patients typically require large doses of fentanyl (>100 µg/h) to treat postoperative pain but receive much lower doses (approximately 20 µg/h) in obstetrics. At the higher doses, epidural fentanyl is absorbed systemically and activates both spinal and supraspinal opioid receptors. In contrast, the lower doses used in obstetrics make it unlikely that enough fentanyl could be absorbed systemically to have a significant supraspinal effect. A recent series suggests that epidural fentanyl, but not intravenous fentanyl, reduces epidural bupivacaine use by 28% in laboring women, indirectly indicating a purely spinal affect.

The lipid soluble opioids, fentanyl (2–4 µg/ml) and sufentanil (0.3–0.5 µg/ml) are the most commonly used opioids in obstetrics. Neuraxial sufentanil is approximately 4–5 times more potent than fentanyl. However, since side effects produced from fentanyl and sufentanil are similar at equipotent doses and since sufentanil costs more than fentanyl, fentanyl is usually a better option for both epidural and CSE solutions. Pruritus is the most frequently encountered side effect (60–100% incidence), but rarely requires treatment. If necessary, pruritus can be treated with an agonist-antagonist such as nalbuphine (5 mg IV). Other rare side effects include nausea, urinary retention, dysphoria and respiratory depression. The lipid soluble opioids have been associated with 'early respiratory depression' occurring 30–45 minutes after administration and may be more likely to occur

following repeat doses; sufentanil appears much more likely to cause respiratory depression when used during labor than fentanyl. All side effects, including respiratory depression, can be reversed with naloxone. Typically, 40 µg boluses are administered and titrated to affect.

The relatively lipid insoluble agents such as morphine and meperidine have been used in obstetrics, but with less success than with the lipid soluble agents. The onset of analgesia from morphine is approximately 1–3 hours. In addition, morphine is associated with 'late respiratory depression' occurring 6–12 hours after administration. This is the time it generally takes morphine to diffuse through the CSF and reach opioid receptors in the brainstem. Theoretically, the incidence of morphine-induced respiratory depression may be increased in parturients that deliver vaginally because they have pregnancy-induced sensitivities to nearly all anesthetics, generally experience less pain than from operative deliveries, and are sent to unmonitored postpartum beds. For these reasons the use of epidural or intrathecal morphine for patients that deliver vaginally is not recommended. Although neuraxial meperidine has local anesthetic-like as well as opioid properties and early reports look promising, additional studies are required before recommendations on its use and safety can be made.

Adjuncts
The α-adrenergic receptor agonist epinephrine, the α_2 adrenergic receptor agonist clonidine, and the anticholinesterase neostigmine have been used as epidural and spinal adjuncts in an attempt to prolong labor analgesia. Advantages of epinephrine include enhanced analgesia, reduced blood levels of local anesthetics, more rapid onset times and longer block duration. Epinephrine is usually administered in concentrations of 1:200 000–600 000 for continuous epidural analgesia. Although infusions of local anesthetic containing epinephrine may increase motor block, using ultra dilute bupivacaine concentrations may reduce this affect. Spinal epinephrine 200 µg

Table 5.9 Summary of spinal analgesia from various CSE solutions

Drugs	Dose	Mean reported duration of spinal (min)	Side effects[a]
Fentanyl	25 µg	90	
Fentanyl Bupivacaine	25 µg 2.5 mg	108	
Sufentanil	10 µg	105	
Sufentanil Bupivacaine	10 µg 2.5 mg	150	
Sufentanil Bupivacaine Epinephrine	10 µg 2.5 mg 200 µg	188	Motor block
Sufentanil Bupivacaine Clonidine	5 µg 2.5 mg 50 µg	205	Sedation Hypotension
Sufentanil Bupivacaine Clonidine Neostigmine	5 µg 2.5 mg 50 µg 10 µg	205	Sedation Hypotension Nausea

[a]Nearly all patients administered spinal opioids experience pruritus although it rarely requires treatment.

significantly increases the duration of spinal analgesia from bupivacaine and sufentanil, but also increases motor block *(Table 5.9)*.

Clonidine should theoretically enhance analgesia from local anesthetics and opioids while minimizing side effects from each. In contrast, 15–50 µg doses administered spinally prolong labor analgesia from bupivacaine and sufentanil, but also increase the incidence of sedation and hypotension *(Table 5.9)*. However, clonidine administered by PCEA at a concentration of 4 µg/ml reduced bupivacaine-fentanyl use in laboring women without significantly increasing side effects. Despite this potential benefit, the routine use of clonidine within the United States cannot be recommended. Clonidine is currently prohibitively expensive and has a Food and Drug Administration (FDA) 'Blackbox Warning' against its use in obstetrics.

Neostigmine is an anticholinesterase that enhances analgesia by indirectly increasing spinal levels of acetylcholine. Although preliminary results from studies on animal and in nonpregnant women looked promising, spinal neostigmine 10 µg failed to enhance labor analgesia while producing severe nausea *(Table 5.9)*.

5.3 Combined spinal epidural (CSE) analgesia

A CSE anesthetic combines both the one-shot spinal and the continuous epidural techniques into one procedure that harnesses the advantages of each while minimizing risks. Although the contemporary 'needle through needle' technique was first described in the early 1980s, concern of inserting the epidural catheter through the newly-made dural puncture at first inhibited widespread use of the CSE technique. However, using small gauge pencil tip spinal needles and blunt tipped large gauge epidural catheters minimizes or eliminates this risk. Series describing thousands of patients administered CSE report a similar incidence of spinal catheters with both the CSE and epidural techniques. Consequently, CSE use in obstetrics is gaining widespread acceptance, both by anesthesia providers and the general public.

5.3.1 Walking epidurals

A 'walking epidural' is simply any epidural or spinal technique that produces analgesia without inhibiting the ability to ambulate. Though it was traditionally thought that minimizing motor block and allowing ambulation during active labor would speed both the progress of labor and reduce the incidence of instrumental or operative deliveries, recent studies fail to support these contentions. Nevertheless, it seems prudent to administer dilute analgesics in an attempt to minimize side effects. In contrast, the use of 'walking epidurals' may actually increase workload since many 'walking epidural' cocktails may require multiple anesthetic interventions. Time is required to not only place and initially dose the anesthetic, but also during subsequent redosing. In addition, allowing patients to ambulate after inducing any regional anesthetic incurs medicolegal risk. Even if the patient performs a deep knee bend prior to ambulating, she could accidentally fall, sustain an injury and later blame the anesthetic. Based on these factors, the use of dilute epidural cocktails to reduce side effects is recommended; however, allowing patients to actually ambulate cannot be actively recommended since studies do not support improved outcome from ambulation. On the other hand, having parturients able to sit in a chair at the bedside or move with only minimal nursing assistance are advantageous and enhance patient satisfaction.

5.3.2 Patient selection

Combined spinal epidural analgesia was originally believed to be particularly beneficial only for patients in either early or late labor. Since spinal opioids produce analgesia without motor block, patients administered spinal opioids in early labor could ambulate and then receive epidural analgesia when requesting

additional analgesia. For patients in later stages of labor, it was hoped that CSE utilization would limit the need for epidural analgesia since these patients would deliver during the spinal analgesia portion of the CSE.

Early CSE research focused on prolonging the duration of the spinal analgesia. Results, however, showed mixed success. Although spinal analgesia was prolonged from little more than one hour to nearly 3.5 hours, the cocktails that produce longer durations of spinal analgesia also produce side effects such as motor block, hypotension, sedation and nausea (*Table 5.9*). Consequently, CSE has evolved from being a technique based primarily on a very long-lasting spinal injection to one truly integrating the spinal and epidural portions of the technique, which increases efficiency, limits side effects and increases patient satisfaction. Contemporary CSE techniques attempt to produce approximately 120 minutes of spinal analgesia with minimal side effects (such as motor block and hypotension); the epidural infusion is started soon after the spinal injection, which allows for the gradual onset of epidural analgesia before the spinal analgesia wears off. CSE increases efficiency by providing more rapid onset analgesia (estimated to be approximately 7 minutes faster onset with CSE compared to epidural analgesia) and avoiding the need for independent dosing of the spinal and epidural portions of the CSE. Less than 20% of patients who eventually develop inadequate analgesia should require additional attention when using this approach.

The primary drawback of the CSE technique is that the epidural catheter remains unproven. As a result, the routine use of CSE anesthetics in parturients at high risk for operative delivery is not recommended. This includes parturients who are morbidly obese or who have preeclampsia, a history of previa or abruption, abnormal presentation, multiple gestation, and fetal macrosomia. Inducing traditional epidural analgesia in high-risk patients is recommended since a well functioning epidural catheter reduces the need for general anesthesia should urgent cesarean section be required.

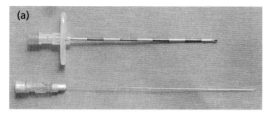

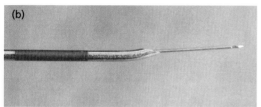

Figure 5.3 (a) Epidural and spinal needles from a standard CSE kit. The epidural needle is a 17G winged needle with a 9 cm barrel. The hub is specially designed to receive this particular spinal needle, which is a 27G 4–11/16 in Whitacre needle. (b) Tips of the epidural and spinal needle using the recommended 'needle through needle' technique. Once the epidural space has been located with the epidural needle, the spinal needle is inserted through the lumen of the epidural needle. The spinal needle tip should extend 11–15 mm past the tip of the epidural needle to facilitate dural puncture. The tip of the spinal needle pictured extends 11 mm past the tip of the epidural needle.

5.3.3 Equipment

Specially designed CSE kits are commercially available and are priced comparably to standard epidural kits. To increase the likelihood of successful dural puncture, the spinal needle tip should extend 11–15 mm past the tip of the epidural needle *(Figures 5.3(a) and (b) and 5.4)*. Distances shorter *(Figure 5.4(c))* or longer than this will increase the chance of failure. Special CSE needles with separate spinal and epidural catheter lumens were designed to theoretically reduce the likelihood of obtaining a spinal catheter. However, evidence suggests that the incidence of a spinal catheter is similar with both CSE and standard epidural techniques, especially when the CSE is technically easy. Because these multilumen needles are expensive and occasionally cumbersome, the 'needle through needle' approach is commonly used *(Figure 5.3(b))*. With this technique a standard

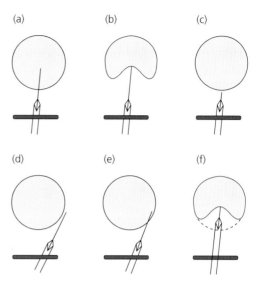

Figure 5.4 Successful CSE anesthetic (a) and possible reasons for failure (b–f). (a) A successful dural puncture. (b) The dura is 'tented' rather than punctured. (c) A short spinal needle fails to reach the dura. (d) Lateral deviation of the epidural needle causing the spinal needle to miss the dural sac. (e) Similar to (d) except that the dura is punctured laterally, which may result in the inability to aspirate CSF. (f) 'Tenting' of the dura with 'too short' spinal needle. Further advancement of the epidural needle may result in the dura rebounding over both the spinal and epidural needle tips causing an accidental 'wet tap' with the epidural needle.

epidural needle is used to identify the epidural space, then a long spinal needle is inserted through the lumen of the epidural needle. Once the spinal solution is administered, the spinal needle is removed and the epidural catheter is inserted as usual.

5.3.4 Technique

Contraindications to regional anesthesia and the guidelines for regional anesthesia previously described *(Tables 5.1 and 5.2)* also apply to CSE techniques. Procedurally, CSE and epidural techniques are similar with only a few exceptions. The sitting position, rather than the lateral decubitus position, usually facilitates CSE placement. The sitting position makes identification of the midline easier, which is essential when attempting a dural puncture.

Furthermore, the sitting position theoretically increases the likelihood of a successful dural puncture by increasing intracranial pressure, which in turn makes the dura more taut. In addition, using air, rather than saline, for loss of resistance is appropriate. When air is used, clear fluid appearing in the spinal needle hub must be CSF. In contrast, this clear fluid may be saline if the spinal needle tip fails to puncture the dura when saline is used for loss of resistance. Once the dura has been successfully punctured *(Figure 5.4(a))*, 1 ml of spinal fluid can be aspirated, if possible, for mixing with the spinal injectate since CSE solutions are actually hypobaric at body temperature. Mixture with CSF makes the injectate more isobaric and limits cephalad spread should epidural catheter insertion be time consuming. During injection, secure the spinal needle by pinching both the spinal and epidural needle hubs between the thumb and index finger. Not doing so increases the failure rate, since the dura does not hold the spinal needle firmly in place like the ligamentum flavum does during a one-shot spinal technique. Once the spinal solution is administered, remove the spinal needle, insert the epidural catheter, remove the epidural needle, secure the catheter, and have the patient immediately move to a lateral decubitus position. Some anesthesiologists advocate immediate testing of the epidural catheter with either plain lidocaine or lidocaine with epinephrine to rule out intrathecal or intravenous placement, though others feel this testing is not routinely necessary. Epinephrine as a test dose may be more useful with the CSE technique since it reliably increases maternal heart rate in patients no longer experiencing painful contractions. In either case, if there are no signs of intrathecal or intravenous cannulation, the epidural infusion should be immediately

---

Table 5.10 Technique for CSE labor analgesia

- Sitting position
- Sterile prep and drape, any interspace between L_2 and S_1
- LOR with air
- CSE kit – ensure spinal needle tip extends 11–15 mm past epidural needle tip
- Small gauge pencil tip spinal needle – 27 G in Whitacre 4–11/16
- Firmly secure spinal and epidural needle hubs with index finger and thumb
- Spinal injectate[a]   Bupivacaine (0.25%) 1.75 mg (0.7ml) +
                  Fentanyl   15 µg (0.3 ml) +
                  Epinephrine   50 µg (0.05 ml)
- If possible, aspirate CSF to total 2 ml prior to injection
- Remove spinal needle, insert multiport epidural catheter 5–6 cm, remove epidural needle
- Secure catheter
- Move patient to lateral position
- Consider testing epidural catheter with 2 ml 2% lidocaine (40 mg) or 3 ml 1.5% lidocaine (45 mg) + epi 15 µg
- Begin epidural infusion via continuous infusion or PCEA technique: Bupivacaine 0.04%–0.125% + fentanyl 1.5–2 µg/ml
- Utilize PCEA at the following settings:

Basal infusion	6–10 ml/h
Bolus dose	5 ml
Lockout	10 min
Hourly limit	30 ml

[a]Alternatively, bupivacaine 2.5 mg (1 ml) + fentanyl 20–25 µg can be substituted as the CSE solution.

initiated. Similar to epidural techniques, the patient must still be observed for 10–15 minutes for side effects such as hypotension or fetal bradycardia. This technique is described in *Table 5.10*.

5.3.5 Reasons for CSE failure

Assuming that an appropriate spinal needle and air (for loss of resistance) were used, the most likely reason for failure is deviation from midline (*Figure 5.4(d)*). When unable to obtain CSF, the spinal needle can be removed, the angle of the epidural needle redirected, and the epidural space reentered at a slightly different angle. If still unable to obtain CSF, abandon the CSE technique and proceed with an epidural technique to increase efficiency. Taking longer to administer spinal analgesia than it would to produce traditional epidural analgesia defeats the purpose of the CSE technique and is counterproductive.

Another potential reason for failure is that the spinal needle only tents rather than penetrates the dura (*Figure 5.4(b)*). One can usually 'feel' the tenting of the dura when this occurs. Rotating the spinal needle rather than bouncing it in and out is recommended since bouncing the spinal needle may result in multiple dural punctures, which in turn increases the likelihood of either a spinal catheter or a post dural puncture headache. Alternatively, the epidural and spinal needles can be further advanced as a unit. This maneuver, however, may increase the likelihood of the dura rebounding over both the spinal and epidural needle tips, resulting in an inadvertent wet tap (*Figure 5.4(f)*). Occasionally, CSF appears in the spinal needle hub, but cannot be aspirated. The most likely cause is a lateral penetration of the dura with the spinal needle and either the dura or nerve root prevents aspiration (*Figure 5.4(e)*). When this occurs, attempt to aspirate while rotating the spinal needle. If still unsuccessful and there is no persistent paresthesia, injecting the spinal solution and proceeding with epidural catheter placement is appro-

priate. If the patient fails to develop spinal analgesia, dose the epidural catheter.

5.3.6 Complications

Risks associated with CSE and epidural analgesia are similar. Whether the CSE technique increases the incidence of post dural puncture headache remains controversial. While it has been estimated that the contemporary CSE techniques produce as many as three extra post dural puncture headaches per 1000 patients, it has also been suggested that the CSE technique actually decreases the risk of post dural puncture headache by reducing the incidence of inadvertent dural punctures with the epidural needle, since the spinal needle can be used to confirm epidural needle placement. Most advocates of the technique do not believe the use of CSE analgesia significantly increases the risk of post dural puncture headache when using small-gauged pencil tipped spinal needles.

Likewise, whether CSE analgesia increases the risk of fetal bradycardia remains controversial. Following initial reports of fetal bradycardia with the technique, it was speculated that fetal bradycardia was related to uterine hypertonicity induced by either a precipitous decrease in circulating maternal catecholamines as a consequence of rapid onset analgesia or through a previously undescribed direct opioid-induced spinal mechanism. Recent prospective studies, however, suggest that the incidence of fetal bradycardia is similar with both CSE and epidural anesthetics and approximates 10%. Fetal bradycardia following either technique is usually self-limiting and generally persists only for a few minutes. Ensuring left uterine displacement and administering maternal oxygen and intravenous ephedrine will help resolve such transient episodes.

Although concerns of meningitis, high spinal block, abscess, permanent neurologic injury, hematoma, and metallic fragments introduced into the spinal space have been suggested as possible complications of the technique, these risks have not been demonstrated in any large study. It is imperative, however, that inter-spaces below the L_2 spinous process be utilized during CSE placement to minimize the risks of permanent neurologic injury, since spinal cord damage can occur if interspaces above L_2–L_3 are utilized.

5.4 Continuous spinal analgesia

Continuous spinal analgesia offers several advantages over either the one-shot spinal or the continuous epidural techniques. Despite these benefits, a continuous spinal anesthetic poses technical challenges, increases the likeli-hood of complications, and may be inherently more dangerous than the other two tech-niques. Although the continuous spinal tech-nique provides rapid-onset, reliable analgesia that can be titrated to varying labor conditions over prolonged durations, the risks for perma-nent neurologic injury or a high spinal block may be increased. Small gauge spinal catheters (< 24 G) were introduced in the late 1980s to reduce the incidence of post dural puncture headache. However, reports of permanent neurologic injuries led to the discontinued use of these catheters within the United States in 1992. These neurological injuries were believed to result from maldistribution of hyperbaric local anesthetic within the CSF. Consequently, relatively large gauge epidural catheters must be used for continuous spinal techniques that can increase the likelihood of a post dural punc-ture headache. In addition, because currently available catheters look like and in fact are 'reg-ular epidural catheters', the potential for acci-dental administration of epidural doses into the CSF increase the likelihood of a high spinal block. A high spinal block in the uncontrolled setting of a labor room potentially increases the risks for catastrophic loss of airway. Because of these risks, at the present time, reserving the use of continuous spinal analgesia for special cases is prudent.

These cases include unintentional dural puncture with the epidural needle in parturi-ents who are about to deliver (multiparous women presenting in late phase labor) or those

in whom locating the epidural space was particularly difficult (multiple attempts in a morbidly obese patient or in a patient with a history of scoliosis surgery, for example). In the former scenario, the catheter will most likely be used for only a limited period of time. In the latter scenario, repeated attempts may incur additional discomfort and a second unintentional dural puncture. In either case, the spinal catheter and the patient's anesthetic record should be boldly marked to clearly stand out from a regular epidural catheter. In addition, all anesthesia care providers in the labor suite should be personally notified. These simple steps should lessen the likelihood of mistakes.

In addition, a planned continuous spinal anesthetic should be considered in patients with an 'unintubatable airway' (a patient with maxillofacial deformities and a history of failed intubation and tracheostomy, for exam-ple) to minimize the chance of losing the air-way. Although an elective tracheostomy may be preferred in these patients, there may not be time to notify a surgeon in urgent situa-tions. A continuous spinal anesthetic reduces the likelihood of a high spinal block from a one-shot spinal technique and reduces the likelihood of inadequate analgesia from a con-tinuous epidural technique by allowing for the careful titration of the anesthetic to a T_6 block.

Continuous spinal anesthesia is typically provided by either intermittent bolus or continuous infusion techniques (*Table 5.11*). When administering opioids, repeat doses may increase the risk of respiratory depression. With the intermittent bolus technique it must be remembered that an epidural catheter and filter may contain up to 1 ml of dead space, therefore flushing each bolus dose with 2 ml of saline is recommended.

The routine use of continuous spinal catheters has also been recommended for morbidly obese patients since obesity may reduce the incidence of post dural puncture headache. However, the increased risks associated with the technique must be balanced against this minor benefit. Therefore, the routine use of continuous

Table 5.11 Solutions for maintenance of spinal catheter analgesia (see also *Table 8.5* for alternative solutions suitable for labor analgesia)

Technique	Solution[a]
Labor analgesia	
Intermittent bolus	0.25% bupivacaine 2.5 mg (1 ml) + fentanyl 15 µg as needed
Continuous Infusion	0.125% bupivacaine + fentanyl 2 µg ml^{-1}, 0.5–2 ml/h and titrated to a T$_{10}$ block
Surgical anesthesia	0.5% bupivacaine 5 mg (1 ml) + fentanyl 15 µg for the initial dose, then administer 0.5 ml of the local anesthetic every 5 min until the desired block height is obtained, then repeat the 0.5 ml dose as needed to maintain the desired block height

[a]The epidural catheter and filter has >1 ml of dead space; therefore, a continuous spinal catheter should be flushed with 2 ml of saline after each bolus dose.

Table 5.12 Recommended epidural local anesthetics for vaginal or assisted vaginal delivery

Agent	Perineal (sitting) dose (%)	Outlet forceps (%)	Mid forceps (%)	Initial dose[a] (ml)
Lidocaine	1.5–2	2	2	10–15
Chloroprocaine	2	2–3	3	10–15
Bupivacaine	0.25	0.25–0.5	0.5	10–15

[a]Dose should be varied to individual patient requirements. A dense T$_{10}$ sensory block is desired for vaginal deliveries or low risk assisted vaginal deliveries while a dense T$_{6}$ sensory and motor block is desired for a mid forceps trial.

epidural analgesia, rather than continuous spinal analgesia, is preferred in these patients. On the other hand, in cases of an accidental dural puncture, a continuous spinal technique should be considered on a case-by-case basis.

5.5 Anesthesia for vaginal delivery

5.5.1 Vaginal delivery

Pain during early labor is primarily visceral in nature and enters the spinal cord at the T$_{10}$–L$_{1}$ levels, while pain during the later stages of labor and during delivery are primarily somatic in nature and enter the spinal cord at the S$_{2}$–S$_{4}$ levels (see Section 4.2.1). These dual pain pathways result in varying analgesic requirements as labor progresses and for delivery. It is not uncommon for patients to experience increasing rectal pressure or perineal pain (sacral sparing) as labor progresses. The S$_{2}$–S$_{4}$ nerve roots (pudendal nerve) are relatively large and may require higher concentrations of local anesthetic to anesthetize than thoracic or lumbar nerve roots. Administering 5–10 ml of 0.25% bupivacaine with fentanyl 25 µg is usually effective; however, occasional patients will require additional local anesthetic. In this circumstance, administering 5–10 ml of 2% lidocaine combined with fentanyl 25 µg may be more effective. If the pain persists, the epidural catheter should be withdrawn so that 3–4 cm remains within the epidural space and additional local anesthetics administered. When vaginal delivery is imminent, perineal anesthesia can usually be produced with 5–15 ml of either 1.5%–2% lidocaine or 2% chloroprocaine (*Table 5.12*).

5.5.2 Forceps or vacuum-assisted delivery

Indications for assisted vaginal delivery include maternal exhaustion, cardiovascular or neurologic disorders that preclude maternal pushing, fetal distress, arrested rotation, and abnormal fetal position. Forceps deliveries are classified as either outlet, low, mid, or high depending on the relation of the fetal head to the introitus and ischial spines, although high forceps deliveries are almost never indicated. Anesthetic requirements vary with the type of forceps delivery attempted. In general, higher fetal stations and rotation of the fetal head require more force by the obstetrician for delivery, which in turn increases the risk of fetal and maternal complications, as well as anesthetic requirements. Although a dense T_{10} sensory block will usually provide sufficient analgesia for a low or outlet forceps delivery, a dense T_6 motor and sensory block may be required for a mid forceps delivery requiring rotation of the fetal head (mid forceps trial). Rarely will the dilute local anesthetic solutions used to provide labor analgesia suffice for forceps delivery, especially those from higher fetal stations. Vacuum deliveries generally require anesthetic levels similar to those of low and outlet forceps. Each patient should be evaluated individually and the dose of local anesthetic titrated to effect (*Table 5.12*).

Although any attempted forceps delivery can result in prolonged fetal bradycardia requiring cesarean section, this is most likely to occur with a mid forceps trial. Therefore, it is recommended that a mid forceps trial be attempted in the operating room prepared for an operative delivery rather than in the labor room. 15–20 ml of 3% chloroprocaine should produce sufficient anesthesia for the forceps trial and for a lower abdominal incision should an urgent cesarean section be required.

5.6 Alternative regional anesthetic techniques

Although alternative regional anesthetic techniques can be used in obstetrics, they do not afford the flexibility of epidural or CSE analgesia. Generally speaking, these alternative techniques are technically more difficult to perform and produce more frequent complications than epidural or CSE techniques. Nevertheless they can be used in patients that are not candidates for epidural or CSE analgesia and who do not have contraindications to regional anesthesia.

5.6.1 Lumbar sympathetic block

This technique produces analgesia for early labor by blocking pain originating in the lower uterine segments and cervix. The technique is ineffective for the later phases of labor and for delivery. With this technique local anesthetic is administered near the lumbar sympathetic chain and provides 2–3 hours of analgesia.

With the patient in the sitting position, the transverse process of the second lumbar vertebrae is identified using a 10 cm, 22 G needle. The needle is then redirected medially below the transverse process and is advanced approximately 5 cm into the anterolateral surface of the vertebral column. At this point the tip of the needle lies just anterior to the medial attachment of the psoas muscle. A loss of resistance technique is then used to identify when the needle has passed beyond the psoas fascia and near the sympathetic trunk. After negative aspiration, 0.5% bupivacaine 10 ml plus 1:200 000 epinephrine is administered and the procedure is repeated on the opposite side. A continuous catheter method has also been described.

Although a lumbar sympathetic block has minimal effects on the fetus and reportedly shortens the duration of labor, it is technically difficult to perform, multiple needle sticks are required and it occasionally produces significant complications. Approximately 20% of patients develop hypotension that requires treatment with ephedrine. In addition, accidental intravascular subarachnoid and epidural injection as well as retroperitoneal hematoma, Horner's syndrome, and post dural puncture headaches have been described with the technique. Because of these risks and the fact that this technique is ineffective for delivery, lumbar sympathetic blocks are rarely utilized in obstetrics.

5.6.2 Paracervical block

This technique produces analgesia by blocking pain originating in the lower uterine segments, cervix and upper vaginal canal by anesthetizing the paracervical (Frankenhauser's) ganglion. Similar to a lumbar sympathetic block, a paracervical block provides analgesia only for early labor. With the patient in the lithotomy position, a special 12–14 cm 22 G needle with a depth guard is introduced 2–3 cm under the mucosa of the vaginal fornix adjacent to the cervix. Approximately 10 ml of dilute anesthetic is injected at both the 3 and 9 o'clock positions. Dilute concentrations are recommended to reduce the risk of intravascular absorption and fetal bradycardia. Analgesia typically occurs within 5 minutes and lasts 45–120 minutes. However, this technique produces a high incidence of maternal and fetal side effects. Maternal toxicity results from systemic absorption or direct intravascular injection, while fetal bradycardia results from direct absorption, vasoconstriction of uterine arteries, or from accidental injection of local anesthetic into the fetal presenting part. In addition, hematoma of the broad ligament and retropsoal or subgluteal abscesses have been reported. Because of these risks, paracervical blocks are rarely utilized in obstetrics.

5.6.3 Pudendal nerve block
This technique blocks the S_2, S_3 and S_4 nerve roots and the pain originating from the perineum, lower vaginal wall and vulva. It is most effective for late phase labor and for delivery. The patient is placed in the lithotomy position and a specialized needle with depth guard is inserted into the vaginal mucosa slightly medial and posterior to the ischial spine. The needle is advanced through the sacrospinous ligament by using a loss of resistance technique. Dilute local anesthetic 10 ml is then administered and the procedure repeated on the other side. Aspiration prior to injection is critical because of the proximity of the pudendal artery. Disadvantages of this technique include risk of systemic toxicity from intravascular injection, potential trauma to the pudendal artery or to the fetal presenting part, formation of vaginal wall hematoma and retropsoal or subgluteal abscesses. In addition, unless the block is timed correctly

many patents do not develop effective analgesia until after delivery since it takes 6–15 minutes to produce analgesia from a pudendal block.

5.6.4 Perineal infiltration
Perineal infiltration is the most commonly used regional anesthetic technique in patients that deliver without preexisting epidural analgesia. It provides anesthesia for repair of lacerations and may also be used to supplement poorly functioning epidural analgesia. The perineum lacks major nerves and therefore the local anesthetic must be injected submucosally to provide local anesthesia. However, anesthetic requirements vary with the amount of injury sustained during delivery. An extensive fourth degree repair will require more local anesthetic than a small first-degree laceration.

5.7 Improving anesthetic efficiency in obstetrics

Maximizing efficiency without compromising patient safety is a worthy goal for any labor epidural service. This discussion focuses on four factors that help accomplish this goal: CSE analgesia, multiport epidural catheters, fentanyl, and the use of PCEA. Recommendations for increasing efficiency are outlined in *Table 5.13*.

5.7.1 CSE
Studies indicate that the CSE technique produces analgesia 7 minutes faster than epidural techniques. Although 7 minutes may not seem significant, on a busy service, the savings add up. A labor service inducing 5000 epidural anesthetics each year can save approximately 600 man-hours of work by using CSE, rather than epidural anesthetics, in all appropriate parturients (the CSE technique is not recommended in patients at high risk for cesarean section). Additionally, the epidural infusion should be initiated immediately following the spinal injection to improve efficiency, otherwise time is required to dose and monitor side effects from both the spinal and epidural

Table 5.13 Recommendations for increased anesthesia efficiency in obstetrics

1. **Use CSE analgesia** in all appropriate patients. If administered efficiently, patients will experience labor analgesia faster than from an epidural technique. However, if CSF is not obtained on the first or second attempt, insert and dose the epidural.

2. **Efficient preparation** of CSE agents is a must.

3. **Minimize side effects** by administering dilute spinal solutions.

4. **Sitting position** to better identify midline and to facilitate dural puncture with the spinal needle during CSE.

5. **Insert multiport epidural catheters 5–6 cm** into the epidural space.

6. **Consider routine use of PCEA** with basal infusion at the following settings: 6–10 ml/h basal rate, 5 ml bolus dose, 10 min lockout, 30 ml/h limit.

7. **Inadequate analgesia**: withdraw the epidural catheter to 3–4 cm within the epidural space and administer additional local anesthetic. If inadequate analgesia persists, remove and replace the epidural catheter.

portions of the CSE in women who do not deliver during spinal analgesia. And finally, the benefits of CSE analgesia are lost if it takes longer to complete the technique than it would to produce epidural analgesia. To increase efficiency, redirect the epidural needle only once when CSF is not observed in the spinal needle hub, and if unsuccessful on the second attempt, insert and dose the epidural catheter.

5.7.2 Multiport epidural catheters

Multiport epidural catheters improve efficiency by reducing the incidence of inadequate analgesia and the number of catheters that require manipulation when compared to uniport epidural catheters. Inserting multiport catheters 5–6 cm into the epidural space reduces the risk of intravenous cannulation and of subsequent catheter dislodgement. If the pain persists for more than 15 minutes after initial local anesthetic administration, withdraw the catheter so that 3–4 cm remains within the epidural space and administer additional local anesthetic. If the patient is not comfortable within 5 minutes, remove and replace the epidural catheter. This maneuver is both time-efficient and more than 90% effective.

Theoretically, multiport epidural catheters risk multi-compartment placement where at least one port lies within the epidural space while the other port(s) lays either intrathecally or in an epidural vein. Should this occur, local anesthetic will theoretically exit different ports depending on the force of the injectate (differential flow) and may in turn increase the risk of toxicity when dosing for instrumental or operative delivery. Despite this theoretical concern and widespread use, no prospective (or retrospective) series have documented this phenomenon.

5.7.3 Fentanyl

Fentanyl, 2 µg/ml, reduces local anesthetic use by approximately 25–30%. Reducing local anesthetic use should reduce side effects, although this benefit has not been demonstrated in a prospective study. Nevertheless, reducing local anesthetic use will at a minimum allow more patients to deliver before the initial container needs to be replaced, thus reducing workload.

5.7.4 PCEA

Although it has been suggested PCEA reduces drug use and increases patient satisfaction, it can also be used to reduce workload. PCEA is used as a continuous infusion device with the capability of administering additional local anesthetic should the patient require additional analgesia. The patient, rather than the anesthesia care provider, then administers the 'top-up' dose, thus saving work and time. One such regimen uses 0.125% bupivacaine + fentanyl 2 µg/ml with the following PCEA settings: 8–10 ml/h basal rate, 5 ml bolus, 10 min lockout, 30 ml hourly limit. More dilute infusions with larger bolus volumes have also been reported effective.

5.8 Epidural analgesia and the progress of labor

Whether epidural analgesia affects the progress of labor or mode of delivery remains controversial. Although epidural analgesia has historically been thought to prolong labor and increase the incidence of instrumental and operative deliveries, these variables are affected by numerous independent maternal, fetal, obstetric and anesthetic factors. Studies addressing this issue are complicated by selection bias, lack of randomization, inability to blind participants, crossover, and ethical issues related to withholding treatment. In addition, women requesting epidural analgesia may be inherently different from those who do not (Table 5.14). Intense pain may actually be a marker for abnormal or dysfunctional labor, which in itself results in longer labor and increases the likelihood for instrumental or operative delivery. Likewise, many epidurals are inserted for fetal and maternal indications that may also prolong labor and increase the likelihood of instrumental or operative delivery (Table 5.14).

Although a large, randomized, prospective study is needed to definitively answer these questions, one will likely never be completed. It would be unethical to withhold safe, effective analgesia from women experiencing pain, but randomized to the placebo group. To that end, one is left sorting through the myriad of retrospective and prospective studies that appear in the literature in an attempt to gain a consensus.

Although retrospective studies generally suffer from selection bias, studies including patients before and after a sentinel event, such as when an epidural analgesia service is initiated in a hospital that previously did not have one, generally offer the best clues to a causal relationship. Nonetheless, variables such as a change in obstetric practice (it is more convenient to perform a forceps delivery in a patient with preexisting epidural analgesia) can confound the results of these studies. Despite this drawback, the majority of these studies indicate little overall affect of epidural analgesia on the progress of labor or the incidence of cesarean section (Table 5.15).

Although it has been traditionally thought that epidural analgesia lengthens the progress of labor and increases the incidence of operative deliveries, many large prospective studies randomizing thousands of patients in total and with minimal crossover fail to support this contention (Table 5.15). In contrast, a recent meta-analysis of 10 trials comparing epidural analgesia to parenteral opioids concluded that epidural analgesia prolongs the first stage of labor by 42 minutes and the second stage of labor by 14 minutes. Despite this prolongation of labor, there were no differences in the rates of instrumental vaginal delivery for dystocia or cesarean section, but there was a significant increase in maternal satisfaction in patients administered epidural analgesia (Table 5.15).

As with epidural analgesia and the progress of labor, it has been traditionally thought that ambulation shortens the duration of labor. Contrary to this belief, a recent study fails to support this contention (Table 5.15). Furthermore, it has been suggested that even when given the opportunity, a majority of parturients choose not to ambulate.

Table 5.14 Characteristics of parturients requesting epidural analgesia

1. Frequently nulliparous
2. Earlier stages of labor and with higher fetal station
3. Slower cervical dilatation prior to requesting analgesia
4. More likely to be receiving oxytocin
5. Deliver larger babies
6. Have smaller pelvic outlets
7. Greater pain of labor (dysfunctional labor)
8. Higher risk of operative delivery (poor fetal status or maternal disease)

Table 5.15 Affect of regional analgesia on labor outcome

Author	Study type	Outcome	No. of patients	Significance
1. Gribble, R.K. (1991)	Retrospective-sentinel	C/S	1084	NSD
2. Lyon, D.S. (1997)	Retrospective-sentinel	Progress of labor, C/S	794	2nd stage: ↑ 10 min C/S: NSD
3. Chestnut, D.H. (1994)	Prospective-early/ late epidural	Progress of labor, C/S	344	NSD
4. Chestnut, D.H. (1994)	Prospective-early/ late epidural/pitocin	Progress of labor, C/S	149	NSD
5. Sharma, S.K. (1997)	Prospective-epidural vs. PCA meperidine	C/S	715	NSD
6. Gambling, D.R. (1998)	Prospective-CSE vs. PCA meperidine	C/S	1223	NSD
7. Bloom, S.L. (1998)	Prospective walking	Progress of labor, C/S	911	NSD
8. Halpern, S.H. (1998)	Meta-analysis (10 trials)	Progress of labor, C/S	2369	1st Stage: ↑ 42 min 2nd Stage: ↑ 14 min C/S: NSD

1. Obstet.Gynecol. **78**: 231; 2. Obstet. Gynecol. **90**: 135; 3. *Anesthesiology* **80**: 1201; 4. *Anesthesiology* **80**: 1193; 5. *Anesthesiology* **87**: 487; 6. *Anesthesiology* **89**: 1336; 7. *N. Engl. J. Med.* **339**: 76; 8. *JAMA* **280**: 2105.

When weighing all the variables that potentially affect the progress of labor and mode of delivery, epidural analgesia probably has a clinically insignificant overall effect. Although the course of labor *may* be slightly prolonged, the substantial benefits of epidural analgesia clearly outweigh these theoretical risks.

Further reading

Beilin, Y., Bernstein, H.H. and Zucker-Pinchoff, B. (1995) The optimal distance that a multiorifice epidural catheter should be threaded into the epidural space. *Anesth. Analg.* 81: 301–304.

Bloom, S.L., McIntire, D.D., Kelly, M.A. *et al.* (1998) Lack of effect of walking on labor and delivery. *N. Engl. J. Med.* 339: 76–79.

Chestnut, D.H., Vincent, R.D. Jr, McGrath, J.M. *et al.* (1994) Does early administration of epidural analgesia affect obstetric outcome in nulliparous women who are receiving intravenous oxytocin? *Anesthesiology* 80: 1193–1200.

Chestnut, D.H., McGrath, J.M., Vincent, R.D. Jr *et al.* (1994) Does early administration of epidural analgesia affect obstetric outcome in nulliparous women who are in spontaneous labor? *Anesthesiology* 80: 1201–1208.

Cook, T.M. (2000) Combined spinal-epidural techniques: review article. *Anaesthesia* 55: 42–64.

D'Angelo, R., Berkebile, B.L. and Gerancher, J.C. (1996) Prospective examination of epidural catheter insertion. *Anesthesiology* 84: 88–93.

D'Angelo, R., Gerancher, J.C., Eisenach, J.C. and Raphael, B.L. (1998) Epidural fentanyl produces labor analgesia by a spinal mechanism. *Anesthesiology* 88: 1519–1523.

Gambling, D.R., Sharma, S.K., Ramin, S.M. *et al.* (1998) A randomized study of combined spinal-epidural analgesia versus intravenous meperidine during labor: impact on cesarean delivery rate. *Anesthesiology* 89: 1336–1344.

Gribble, R.K. and Meier, P.R. (1991) Effect of epidural analgesia on the primary cesarean rate. *Obstet. Gynecol.* 78: 231–234.

Halpern, S.H., Leighton, B.L., Ohlsson, A. *et al.* (1998) Effect of epidural vs parenteral opioid analgesia on the progress of labor: a meta-analysis. *JAMA* 280: 2105–2110.

Hawkins, J.L., Gibbs, C.P., Orleans, M. *et al.* (1992) Obstetric anesthesia workforce survey, 1981 versus 1992. *Anesthesiology* 87: 135–143.

Hawkins, J.L., Koonin, L.M., Palmer, S.K. and Gibbs, C.P. (1997) Anesthesia-related deaths during obstetric delivery in the United States, 1979–1990. *Anesthesiology* 86: 277–284.

Hawkins, J.L., Beaty, B.R. and Gibbs, C.P. (1999) Update on US obstetric anesthesia practices. *Anesthesiology* **91**: A1060.

Hays, R.L. and Palmer, C.M. (1994) Respiratory depression after intrathecal sufentanil during labor. *Anesthesiology* **81**: 511–512.

Holmstrom, R., Rawal, N., Axelsson, K. and Nydahl, P.A. (1995) Risk of catheter migration during combined spinal epidural block: percutaneous epiduroscopy study. *Anesth. Analg.* **80**: 747–753.

Lyon, D.S., Knuckles, G., Whitaker, E. and Salgado, S. (1997) The effect of instituting an elective labor epidural program on the operative delivery rate. *Obstet. Gynecol.* **90**: 135–141.

Meister, G.C., D'Angelo, R., Owen, M. *et al.* (2000) A comparison of epidural analgesia with 0.125% ropivacaine with fentanyl versus 0.125% bupivacaine with fentanyl during labor. *Anesth. Analg.* **90**: 632–637.

Paech, M.J., Pavy, T.J., Orlikowski, C.E. and Evans, S.F. (2000) Patient-controlled epidural analgesia in labor: the addition of clonidine to bupivacaine-fentanyl. *Reg. Anesth. Pain Med.* **25**: 34–40.

Palmer, C.M. (1991) Early respiratory depression following intrathecal fentanyl-morphine combination. *Anesthesiology* **74**: 1153–1154.

Palmer, C.M., Cork, R.C., Hays, R. *et al.* (1998) The dose-response relation of intrathecal fentanyl for labor analgesia. *Anesthesiology* **88**: 355–361.

Palmer, C.M., Maciulla, J.E., Cork, R.C. *et al.* (1999) The incidence of fetal heart rate changes after intrathecal fentanyl labor analgesia. *Anesth. Analg.* **88**: 577–581.

Palmer, C.M., Van Maren, G., Nogami, W.M. and Alves, D. (1999) Bupivacaine augments intrathecal fentanyl for labor analgesia. *Anesthesiology* **91**: 84–89.

Polley, L.S., Columb, M.O., Naughton, N.N. *et al.* (1999) Relative analgesic potencies of ropivacaine and bupivacaine for epidural analgesia in labor: implications for therapeutic indexes. *Anesthesiology* **90**: 944–950.

Power, I. and Thorburn, J. (1988) Differential flow from multihole epidural catheters. *Anaesthesia* **43**: 876–878.

American Society of Anesthesiologists Task Force on Obstetrical Anesthesia (1999) Practice guidelines for obstetrical anesthesia: a report by the American Society of Anesthesiologists Task Force on Obstetrical Anesthesia. *Anesthesiology* **90**: 600–611.

Sharma, S.K., Sidawi, J.E., Ramin, S.M. *et al.* (1997) Cesarean delivery: a randomized trial of epidural versus patient-controlled meperidine analgesia during labor. *Anesthesiology* **87**: 487–494.

Viscomi, C. and Eisenach, J. (1991) Patient-controlled epidural analgesia during labor. *Obstet. Gynecol.* **77**: 348–351.

Chapter 6

Alternative methods of labor analgesia

Michael Paech, FANZCA

Contents

6.1 **Introduction**

There are a remarkable number of views about the relative merit of each of the labor analgesic methods. Indeed, many still question the need for pain relief during labor and delivery. This topic engenders strong emotions among health professionals, organizations and members of the public. Attitudes are divergent and practice varies, at local through international levels, across the full spectrum of possibilities. Despite the justifiable enthusiasm of obstetric anesthesiologists for epidural analgesia, it is sometimes forgotten that pain during labor and delivery is contextually unique and that globally, the vast majority of pregnant women have no access to epidural analgesia or any other form of pharmacological pain relief (see Chapter 17). Not all women want pain eliminated and the extent of relief does not equate with overall satisfaction.

Historically, the traditional religious view that any intervention in the birthing process was contrary to the will of God was abandoned in the 19th century after the introduction of chloroform and ether. Queen Victoria's acceptance of chloroform from Dr John Snow in her eighth confinement in 1853 is considered pivotal to this change of social attitudes. Despite 150 years of advances in labor analgesia and astonishing improvements in maternal and fetal safety, some people remain disillusioned by the level of intervention during childbirth, including the unwanted consequences of pain management. Few would dispute, however, that the quality of regional analgesia is vastly superior to alternatives (see *Figure 6.1*).

Labor pain varies widely in terms of its intensity, duration, and cultural significance within the context of the childbirth experience. This mandates that women are well informed about pain, its consequences and treatment, and that they have flexible plans. Many parturients manage very well with nonepidural analgesia, although in most Western countries up to 90% request some pharmacological or regional technique, if avail-

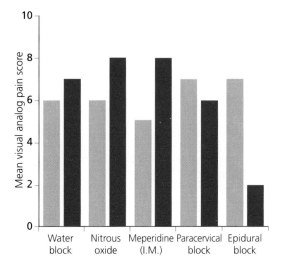

Figure 6.1 Visual pain scores (0–10) before ▨ and after ■ pain management in the first stage of labor in the various pain relief groups. Minimum, lower (25th) quartile, median, upper (75th) quartile, maximum. Reprinted from Ranta, P., Jouppila, P. *et al.* (1994) Parturient's assessment of water blocks, pethidine, nitrous oxide, paracervical and epidural blocks in labour. *Int. J. Obstet. Anesth.* **3**: 196, by permission of the publisher Churchill Livingstone

able. Consequently, epidural rates in many tertiary American obstetric units are 50–90% and alternative methods are reserved as adjuncts or to temporize before regional analgesia is established. In other countries regional analgesia is not as well accepted (in Europe the incidence of epidural analgesia in labor ranges from 5% in The Netherlands to 20% in Germany and 30% in the United Kingdom), and in many hospitals an on-demand service is not available.

Nonepidural analgesic methods (see *Tables 6.1* and *6.2*) retain a very important role, with the popularity of any given technique dependent on cultural, regional and local influences. For example, intramuscular (IM) meperidine (pethidine) is the most commonly used method in much of Europe and Australia, and up to 50% of American parturients receive opioids. Nitrous oxide inhalation is frequently used in Scandinavia, the UK, and Australia. Transcutaneous electrical nerve stimulation (TENS) and 'water blocks' are popular in some

Table 6.1 Alternative methods of labor analgesia

Nonpharmacological
- Childbirth education
- Psychoprophylaxis
- Hypnosis
- TENS/acupuncture/water blocks
- Physical therapies (water baths, massage)

Pharmacological
- Inhaled analgesics – nitrous oxide (N_2O); isoflurane/desflurane in N_2O
- Opioid analgesics – IM, IV or PCIA meperidine, morphine, diamorphine, fentanyl, remifentanil, meptazinol, nalbuphine
- Nonopioid analgesics – ketamine/tramadol

Non-neuraxial regional analgesia
- Paracervical plexus block
- Lumbar sympathetic block
- Pudendal nerve block

Table 6.2 Features of nonpharmacological methods of labor analgesia

In general
Aid relaxation and ability to cope with pain
- no or minimal pain reduction

High levels of maternal satisfaction
- especially if patient-controlled

Popular and widely available
- useful alone or as adjuncts to other methods

Excellent safety record
- avoid hyperventilation during breathing exercises if the fetus is compromised

Specific techniques
Water baths/massage
- readily available; no antenatal preparation required

Learned relaxation techniques/biofeedback/hypnosis
- motivation or investment of time or money essential

Transcutaneous electrical nerve stimulation (TENS)/acupuncture
- mainly a placebo analgesic effect
- safe, but may limit mobility

Water block
- painful injection may need repetition
- modest efficacy and short duration

countries, although in most, pharmacological agents are preferred (opioid, inhalational or nonopioid analgesics). Non-neuraxial regional blocks are also sometimes employed, as is ketamine in India and many developing countries.

6.2 Preparation for childbirth pain

Childbirth educators (lay groups, midwives and nurses, physiotherapists, obstetricians, anesthesiologists) as a rule should encourage parturients to take a holistic approach when preparing for labor pain. The parturient should be presented with all available analgesic options, these discussed factually, and none dismissed. The right of free and informed choice, and the prerogative to change one's mind are tenets of modern society that apply to labor analgesia. Though some decry the poor efficacy of nonepidural methods, provided their safety and cost is acceptable, alternatives increase the range of options. For women opting to deliver at home or in midwifery-model birth units, they may be all that is available.

Women obtain more information about pain relief from friends, relations and the media than from health professionals (and from midwives more often than an obstetrician or anesthesiologist). Although childbirth in a hospital is the norm in many countries, the majority of pregnant women never attend a hospital, health center, or private childbirth preparation class. Nevertheless, anesthesiologists have assumed more prominent roles as educators and have been instrumental in the development of multimedia educational resources about analgesic options.

Intentions regarding labor analgesia are strongly influenced by peers, tradition and local resources. Nulliparous women are more likely to overestimate their ability to tolerate labor pain, and many more request epidural analgesia than plan to do so. Factors important for maternal satisfaction with the experience of childbirth are the perception of personal control, rapport with support staff, and participation in decision making. The feeling of control influences satisfaction, and thus patient-controlled analgesic techniques, whether nonpharmacological, intravenous, inhaled, or epidural, should be encouraged. Modest reductions in pain and a positive experience are more likely for parturients accompanied by a duola (support person) or if patient-controlled techniques (relaxation, breathing exercises, hypnosis) have been practised.

Unfortunately, only a small proportion of women actively prepare for their experience, despite most remaining apprehensive about what is likely to prove one of the most painful experiences of their life.

6.3 Specific alternative methods of labor analgesia

6.3.1 Relaxation, breathing exercises, psychological support and physical therapies

In 1933, Dr Grantly Dick-Read published his theories in the book *Natural Childbirth*, and later in *Childbirth without Fear*. By the 1950s, widespread acceptance of his philosophy had changed the course of labor pain management in the English-speaking world. His premise was that childbirth was not inherently painful, and that pain was due to uterine tension induced by fear. Social expectations induced a fear-tension-pain syndrome, amenable in most instances to muscle relaxation techniques (mainly controlled breathing patterns) for labor. In 1954, Nikoleyev in Russia developed 'psychoprophylaxis', a technique he claimed prevented an 'excitatory-inhibitory cortical and subcortical imbalance', by means of deep breathing patterns, abdominal stroking, and muscular pressure point stimulation. The French obstetrician Lamaze modified this approach, concentrating on breathing exercises and controlled muscle relaxation, believing that 'harmful drugs and anesthetics can be eliminated'. Bradley in the USA (circa 1940) had similar views.

These techniques form the basis of most modern 'natural childbirth' training programs. The essential components are education about pregnancy, labor, and delivery; breathing exercises for relaxation; and the support of a partner or a lay companion (duola). Scientific

evaluation of childbirth training techniques is difficult, but observational studies support reduced opioid use, and possibly pain, during labor. Randomized trials indicate the presence of a duola reduces intervention, shortens labor, and improves mother–infant interaction, possibly by lowering anxiety and maternal catecholamine levels. The French obstetrician Leboyer popularized the concept of 'childbirth without violence', although there are no apparent outcome advantages over a gentle, conventional birth. The use of water at delivery was developed in the 1960s with the introduction of the 'water birth' and warm water baths more recently used for relaxation. Components of all these approaches have now been adopted into conventional modern delivery practice, with emphasis on privacy, familiar home-like surroundings, subdued lighting, and immediate mother–infant contact following delivery.

6.3.2 Biofeedback and physical therapies

Biofeedback training for labor analgesia was first described in the 1980s. Changes in either autonomic (skin) conductance sensed by electrodes on the fingers of the hand, or voluntary muscle relaxation ('electromyographic' method) sensed by electrodes on the abdominal muscles, are represented as clicks. This feedback allows the parturient to concentrate on relaxation, although there is no scientific evidence that labor duration or use of analgesic drugs is reduced. Biofeedback is easily taught by group instruction antenatally, but requires specialized equipment and practice at home, so has never become popular.

In contrast, various physical relaxation therapies are now very popular, especially simple physical interventions that incorporate counter-irritation (skin rubbing, back massage) and relaxation (muscle massage, warmth, water baths). Physical therapies and learned behavior modification techniques can help parturients to cope with labor pain. For motivated women, they have the advantage of being readily available, inexpensive, and safe, and medical staff are not required. Pain is little altered, but maternal satisfaction is high. The only possible adverse effect is prolonged periodic hyperventilation; rarely, severe respiratory alkalosis manifests as maternal dizziness or even tetany, and fetal compromise may result due to uterine artery vasoconstriction and impaired placental oxygen exchange.

6.3.3 Hypnosis

Hypnosis can be effective, and is free of adverse effects. However, only 25% of the population are easily hypnotized and susceptible women require several conditioning sessions with a therapist to learn self-hypnosis. When applied during labor, the pain threshold may be elevated, use of concomitant medication reduced, and rates of post-partum depression are low. Acute anxiety and psychosis are rare complications. Hypnosis is likely more time consuming than other childbirth training techniques. It represents a considerable investment of both time and money and consequently is used infrequently.

6.3.4 Acupuncture, TENS and water blocks

Acupuncture

Acupuncture is a traditional Chinese analgesic method. It is rarely used in China during childbirth, however, despite attempts to resuscitate its use during the Cultural Revolution. Stimulation at meridians according to the

stage of labor may induce a state of lowered pain perception, possibly mediated by endogenous opioids, but success is dependent on careful patient selection and cultural conditioning. Scientific investigation remains inadequate and benefits described in observational studies are confounded by selection bias. Of 12 women in one American study, electroacupuncture had no effect in four, and only two did not eventually request epidural analgesia. A large nonrandomized Scandinavian series found a statistically significant, but clinically unimportant, reduction in use of other analgesics. Pain relief is poor and inconsistent, the technique is time-consuming and restrictive, and electroacupuncture may interfere with electronic fetal monitoring. Not surprisingly, acupuncture is also rarely used in Western society.

Transcutaneous electrical nerve stimulation (TENS)

Transcutaneous electrical nerve stimulation (TENS) was introduced 20 years ago and is readily available in some countries. The TENS stimulator allows patient-controlled variation of both amplitude and rate of current through electrodes placed in a paravertebral position at T_{10}–L_1 and S_2–S_4 levels (see *Figure 6.2*). During contractions, stimulation of the lower electrodes is increased to elicit tingling. Antinociception may result from activation of large afferent myelinated mechanofiber

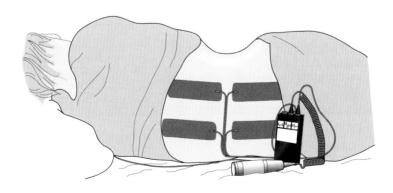

Figure 6.2 Position of TENS electrodes.

stimulation, or the release of endogenous endorphins. Early uncontrolled studies reported a marked analgesic effect in early labor, especially for back pain, but systematic review of subsequent randomized, blinded trials reveals no or minimal analgesic sparing, and may lead to disappointment due to unmet expectations. Interference with continuous fetal heart-rate monitoring is possible and TENS is best considered a more expensive, labor saving alternative to back rubbing.

Water block

A water block involves the injection of sterile water, 0.1 ml, intra- or subcutaneously at four points corresponding to the sacral borders. This method appears limited to Scandinavia, where midwives are licensed practitioners. Pain intensity is reduced for up to 60 minutes compared with TENS, massage and mobilization, 'dry needling', or intradermal saline. However, repeated, transiently painful injections may be necessary, making its appeal very limited.

6.3.5 Inhalational analgesia

History

Professor James Young Simpson, an Edinburgh obstetrician, is credited with the introduction of ether, and subsequently chloroform, for labor analgesia in 1847. Despite opposition from the Church, British society had accepted inhalational analgesia by 1860. In 1880, Klikowitsch in Russia described inhalation of nitrous oxide (N_2O), and during the 1930s the Minnitt apparatus (for patient-controlled N_2O and air inhalation) was developed. Delivery of hypoxic gas mixtures remained possible until a N_2O:oxygen combination was introduced in the 1960s. In the UK, Scandinavia, and Australasia, intermittent inhalation of N_2O in oxygen (or Entonox®, a 50:50 mix) remains popular, whereas this is rare in Continental Europe and North America.

Nitrous oxide

The low blood-gas solubility of N_2O confers a very rapid onset and offset of effect, making it feasible to inhale 30–70% through a demand valve (via a mouthpiece or facemask) in conjunction with contractions (see *Figure 6.3*). Continuous administration in low concentration between contractions via nasal cannula improves analgesia, but increases sedation, and is rarely used. Despite an enviable maternal safety record, the efficacy, side effects, and potential fetal effects have not been well defined (see *Table 6.3*).

Nitrous oxide analgesia shows some concentration-dependent response, but pain-relief is frequently poor. Ten to forty percent of parturients rate their pain relief as superior to, or more satisfactory than IM meperidine, satisfaction possibly being influenced by the patient-controlled delivery of N_2O. A double-blind study found no reduction in pain score after either N_2O or air, although most parturients identified and preferred N_2O. Maternal side effects include reduced awareness, drowsiness, light-headedness, and nausea. Nitrous oxide's sedative effects are potentiated during pregnancy, such that prolonged inhalation of concentrations above 50% may lead to over-sedation or hyperventilation-induced hypocarbia, dizziness, and tetany. Between contractions, compensatory maternal hypoventilation can lead to maternal, and potentially fetal, hypoxemia, especially after systemic opioid analgesia or in the obese parturient. Thus, N_2O is usually reserved for late labor in nulliparous parturients and established labor in multiparous parturients.

The implications of atmospheric pollution within the delivery unit (where N_2O levels may reach 300 p.p.m.) are not fully resolved. Nitrous oxide has fetotoxic effects in rats; in humans, occupational exposure at 100–1000 p.p.m. for over 5 hours per week is associated with decreased fecundity, higher rates of abortion and bone marrow changes. Midwives are often intermittently exposed beyond recommended limits (25–100 p.p.m.) (*Figure 6.4*), because delivery room air changes per hour are not as frequent as in operating room environments. Longitudinal epidemiological review of reproductive problems among female staff exposed to recommended levels are reassuring, but pregnant staff should have the opportunity to work elsewhere.

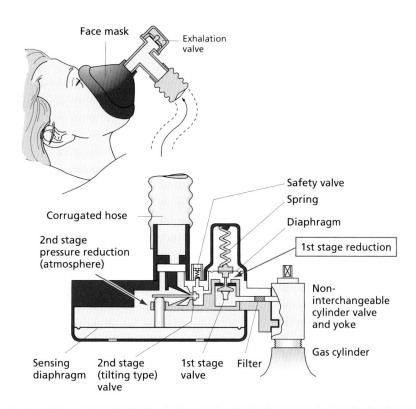

Figure 6.3 The Entonox nitrous oxide/oxygen analgesic apparatus (British oxygen). Reproduced from Crawford, J.S. (1984) *Principles and Practice of Obstetric Anaesthesia* (ed. Crawford, J.S.) 5th edn. With permission from Blackwell Scientific Publications, Oxford, UK, print supplied through the courtesy of the British Oxygen Company Ltd.

Table 6.3 Features of nitrous oxide inhalational analgesia

- Relatively cheap, widely available
- Poor efficacy, possibly placebo only
- Patient-controlled delivery, so maternal satisfaction moderate to good
- Maternal side effects include undesirable drowsiness and reduced awareness
- No significant maternal, fetal or neonatal morbidity, but caution with the compromised fetus
- Atmospheric pollution causes concern about effects on exposed staff

Other inhalational analgesics

In addition to N_2O, sub-hypnotic concentrations of almost all other inhalational anesthetic agents have been investigated for labor analgesia. Trichlorethylene was introduced in 1933 and inhalers developed in the 1950s. The Cardiff inhaler (for methoxyflurane) was popular in the UK in the 1970s–1980s and newer agents continue to be evaluated (e.g. 0.25% isoflurane or 1–4.5% desflurane with 50% nitrous oxide and oxygen). Most provide slightly better analgesia than nitrous oxide alone at the expense of more sedation and amnesia. Practical problems with drug delivery (e.g. specific vaporizers or pre-mixed cylinder gas) and the issues of atmospheric pollution and side effects are significant impediments to the commercial development of this method.

6.3.6 Systemic opioid analgesia

History

The purification of morphine from opium and the invention of the hollow needle led to the

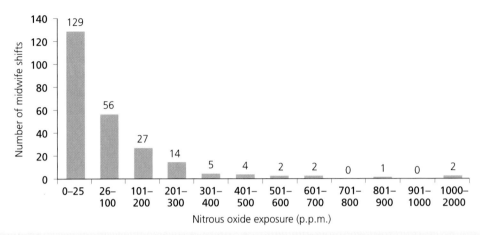

Figure 6.4 Entonox exposure of all midwives working in two hospitals. Reprinted from Mills, G.H. *et al.* (1996) Nitrous oxide exposure on the labour ward. *Int. J. Obstet. Anesth.* **5**: 160–164, by permission of the publisher, Churchill Livingstone.

introduction of morphine and scopolamine injection for labor pain by von Steinbuchel in Austria in 1902. 'Twilight sleep' with morphine was popularized by Gauss in Germany and despite his observation that results were usually unsatisfactory, over subsequent decades larger doses were combined with sedatives (scopolamine, barbiturates) or with general anesthesia. Popular demand shaped medical practice, despite recognition that neonatal depression and hypoxia were common, and systematic evaluation of neonatal effects was difficult before Virginia Apgar developed her simple scoring system in 1953.

Meperidine, morphine and other opioids
Meperidine was synthesized in the late 1930s, used in labor by Bentham in 1940, and ultimately displaced morphine in popularity on the grounds of minimal respiratory depression. It was postulated that equi-analgesic morphine doses had more effect on the newborn respiratory center, based on its poorer blood–brain penetration in adults. However, more recent controlled studies do not support this view. Morphine has more favorable pharmacokinetics, the neonatal half-life is short, and plasma levels remain low or undetectable. During breastfeeding, neonatal effects are undetectable, in comparison to demonstrable effects from

maternal meperidine. In the UK, diamorphine (diacetylmorphine, or heroin) is available by prescription and despite concern about its addictive potential, is occasionally used. It too has more favorable pharmacokinetics, but is no more effective than alternatives. In Europe and the USA, partial μ-receptor agonists or κ-receptor agonists (meptazinol, pentazocine, nalbuphine, butorphanol) and tramadol (a mixed μ-opioid, serotonergic, and α_2-adrenergic agonist) are not controlled drugs, and are used sporadically. A meta-analysis of agonist-antagonists reported equivalent analgesia to meperidine, but less nausea and greater patient satisfaction.

Unfortunately, systemic administration of all these drugs produces poor pain relief. Meperidine is generally the only controlled drug approved for midwifery administration without prescription. It continues to be widely used in the UK, Scandinavia, Australia, and the USA, but in many countries its popularity is in rapid decline (*Table 6.4*).

Intramuscular meperidine in labor
Intramuscular meperidine, 50 mg, has no effect on labor pain; 100–150 mg has a potent sedative effect, such that observers overestimate its analgesic benefit. Additionally, there is great inter-individual variability in drug absorption after IM administration, plasma

Table 6.4 Features of opioid analgesia

Meperidine (pethidine)
- cheap, widely available, midwives legally empowered to administer parenterally
- very poor efficacy
- low levels of maternal satisfaction
- frequent maternal side effects (drowsiness, nausea, dysphoria, reduced awareness)
- minimal maternal morbidity (? delayed maternal gastric emptying and hypoxemia)
- frequent fetal and neonatal effects (reduced FHR variability, respiratory depression, poor neurobehavioral activity)
- initial neonatal effects reversible with naloxone if detected, but delayed effects may persist

Patient-controlled intravenous analgesia
- more reliable opioid pharmacokinetics, but analgesic efficacy poor
- higher maternal satisfaction than IM meperidine
- fentanyl currently recommended, but remifentanil under investigation

the newborn. Accumulation follows repeated dosing and IM administration 2–3 hours before delivery results in greater neonatal depression than dosing nearer delivery (*Figure 6.5*). Many units limit the total dose administered and encourage epidural analgesia if progress of labor is poor.

Prolonged and delayed neonatal effects are due to the markedly increased elimination half-lives in neonates of both meperidine (13–23 hours) and its active metabolite, normeperidine (60 hours). These effects long outlast the activity of the opioid antagonist naloxone, and depression of newborn sucking behavior can persist for up to 4 days. The impact on the establishment of breast-feeding is unknown.

levels rising slowly (30–45 min) and clinical effect being short-lived (90–120 minutes). Surveys consistently report low satisfaction levels and minimal reduction in pain intensity, with a third of patients describing analgesia as poor or inadequate.

Maternal side effects such as confusion, reduced awareness and nausea are common. Delayed gastric emptying (which is not alleviated by co-administration of prokinetic drugs such as metoclopramide) raises concern about the potential for aspiration of gastric content should urgent general anesthesia be necessary. In severe preeclampsia, the proconvulsant activity of normeperidine (the major metabolite of meperidine) is of concern. During labor, maternal respiratory depression is usually modest, but because hypoxemia is possible between contractions, an argument can be made for restricting systemic opioid to multiparous parturients with a good obstetric history.

All opioids cross the placenta rapidly, due to their low molecular weight and lipid solubility. Fetal heart rate variability may diminish. Neonatal exposure is dose-related, but even meperidine 50 mg IM can significantly depress

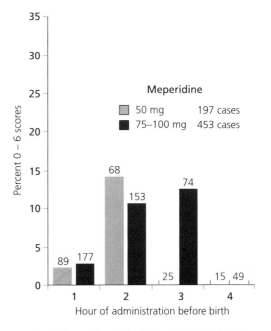

Figure 6.5 Percentage of low neonatal Apgar scores in relation to timing of intramuscular meperidine administration before delivery. Reproduced with permission of Harcourt Health Sciences, Orlando from Shnider, S.M. and Moya, F. (1964) Effects of meperidine on the newborn infant. *Am. J. Obstet. Gynecol.* **89**: 1011.

Intravenous opioid and patient-controlled intravenous analgesia (PCIA)

Intravenous opioids achieve more rapid and predictable plasma levels, and can be titrated by physician, midwife or patient-controlled techniques. Meperidine 25 mg or fentanyl 25–50 µg IV (*Table 6.5*) should not be prohibited in late labor on the grounds of possible neonatal depression, which is dependent on both dose and dose-to-delivery interval. Boluses should nevertheless be given slowly and during contractions, to minimize peak maternal levels and the materno–fetal transfer gradient. Pain scores may be lower after IV than IM opioid administration, but even large IV doses only minimally reduce contraction pain in established labor (*Figure 6.6*). The psychological benefits of patient-controlled intravenous analgesia (PCIA) improve satisfaction.

Nalbuphine has been used, but fentanyl, rather than meperidine or alfentanil is often recommended for PCIA in labor. It has a rapid onset, no active metabolites and causes less nausea and sedation. Typical settings are 20–25 µg demand boluses with a lockout interval of 5 minutes, with or without a continuous infusion. When compared with patient-controlled epidural analgesia using fentanyl-bupivacaine, umbilical cord fentanyl levels are higher and maternal oxygen saturation lower, but neonatal outcome is similar. Total fentanyl doses of more than 600 µg are more likely to

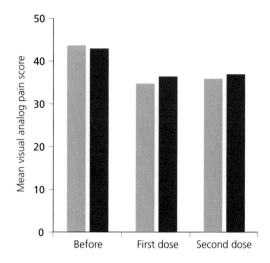

Figure 6.6 Pain intensity before and following intravenous morphine (dose 0.05 mg/kg body weight) or meperidine (dose 0.5 mg/kg body weight). Values are presented in box plot (median with interquartile range). No significant effect was found after each dose. ▪, morphine; ▪, meperidine (pethidine). Reprinted from Olofsson, Ch. *et al.* (1996) Lack of analgesic effect of systemically administered morphine or pethidine on labour pain. *Br. J. Obstet. Gynaecol.* **103**: 969. with permission of Elsevier Science.

depress neonatal respiration and increase the need for naloxone.

The potent, ultra-short acting opioid, remifentanil, has sparked renewed interest in PCIA during labor, which has generally been

Table 6.5 Common opioid doses			
Drug	**Dose IV/IM**	**Onset IV/IM**	**Duration IV/IM**
Meperidine	25/100 mg 10–15 mg PCA bolus	5/20–30 min	20–40/90–120 min
Morphine	5/10–15 mg	5/20–30 min	30–60/120–180 min
Fentanyl	25–50/100 µg 10–25 µg PCA bolus	2/10 min	20–40/30–60 min
Nalbuphine	10–20 mg 1–3 mg PCA bolus	2/15 min	120–240 min
Butorphanol	1–2 mg	5–10/10–30 min	120–240 min
Remifentanil	0.1–0.5 µg/kg PCA bolus	0.5–1 min	2–3 min
Tramadol	100 mg IM	10–30 min	180 min

reserved for specific indications (such as contra-indication to requested epidural analgesia). The effect-site concentration of remifentanil peaks very rapidly and its plasma half-life is independent of the duration of infusion, due to unique tissue and blood esterase metabolism. Remifentanil has rapid placental transfer, but is rapidly metabolized by the fetus with an umbilical artery to vein ratio of 0.3. It may be feasible to allow demand boluses (0.1–0.5 µg/kg with 1–3 minute lockout) coincident with each contraction, without sustaining dangerous drug accumulation. Nevertheless, remifentanil is very expensive, boluses are potentially dangerous (profound respiratory depression and muscle rigidity), and modification of dose according to response, monitoring of oxygen saturation and ready access to naloxone are mandatory. With any opioid, PCIA in labor is likely to cause maternal drowsiness and significant respiratory depression may occur. The safety of remifentanil PCIA in particular needs to be established and the role of PCIA remains uncertain.

An intriguing possibility in future is the development of κ-opioid agonists for labor analgesia. Experimentally, these are particularly effective for polymodal visceral nociception. Neuropharmacological research shows females are more sensitive to their effect, probably because of sexual dimorphism with regard to opioid receptor function.

6.3.7 Non-opioid analgesia

Ketamine in sub-anesthetic doses produces analgesia via antinociceptive mechanisms involving central (notably, serotonergic and N-methyl-D-aspartate receptors) and possibly peripheral activity. Ketamine has the advantage of being cheap and readily available throughout the world, making it appealing in poorer countries, but convincing evidence for its efficacy is lacking. Small IV doses have a 3–5 minute effect and have been used in late labor or at delivery, but can cause amnesia and aspiration has been reported. Observational experience with IV ketamine infusion (0.25 mg/kg/h), after a bolus of 0.25 mg/kg, in Asia and Africa, suggests reduc-

tion of mid-labor pain scores from a median of 8 to 2.5 (scale 0–10). Psychomimetic effects have been a major disadvantage of ketamine in anesthetic doses, although pregnancy confers significant protection and preliminary descriptive studies suggest delirium and unpleasant dreaming is infrequent.

Other sedative drugs (e.g. the benzodiazepines and barbiturates) and those antiemetics causing significant sedation (e.g. promethazine) have no place in modern labor analgesia, yet continue to be used.

Further reading

Aly, E.E. and Shilling, R.S. (2000) Are we willing to change? (editorial). *Anaesthesia* **55**: 419–420.

Bramwell, S. (1993) Systemic medications for labor analgesia. In: *Obstetric Anesthesia* (ed. Norris, M.C.), pp. 281–296. Lipincott Co., Philadelphia.

Carroll, D., Tramer, M., McQuay, H., Nye, B. and Moore, A. (1997) Transcutaneous electrical nerve stimulation in labour pain: a systematic review. *Br. J. Obstet. Gynaecol.* **104**: 169–175.

Carstoniu, J., Levytam, S., Norman, P., Daley, D., Katz, J. and Sandler, A.N. (1994) Nitrous oxide in early labor. Safety and efficacy assessed by a double-blind, placebo-controlled study. *Anesthesiology* **80**: 30–35.

Clyburn, P.A. and Rosen, M. (1993) The effects of opioid and inhalational analgesia on the newborn. In: *Effects on the Baby of Maternal Analgesia and Anaesthesia* (ed. Reynolds, F.), pp. 169–190. W.B. Saunders Company, London.

Elbourne, D. and Wiseman, R.A. (2000) Types of intra-muscular opioids for maternal pain relief. In: *The Cochrane Database of Systematic Reviews*. The Cochrane Library, Volume (Issue 2).

Freeman, R.B.M., Macaulay, A.J., Eve, L., Chamberlain, G.V. and Bhat, A.V. (1986) Randomized trial of self-hypnosis for analgesia in labour. *Br. Med. J.* **292**: 657–658.

Huffnagle, H.J. and Huffnagle, S.L. (1999) Alternatives to conduction analgesia. In: *Obstetric Anesthesia* (ed. Norris, M.C.), 2nd edn, pp. 251–282. J.B. Lippincott Co., Philadelphia.

Kennell, J., Klaus, M., McGrath, S., Robertson, S. and Hinkley, C. (1991) Continuous support during labor in a US hospital. *JAMA* **265**: 2197–2201.

Melzack, R., Taenzer, P., Feldman, P. and Kinch, R. (1981) Labour is still painful after prepared childbirth training. *Can. Med. Assoc. J.* **125**: 357–363.

Mills, G.H., Singh, D., Longan, M., O'Sullivan, J. and Caunt, J.A. (1996) Nitrous oxide exposure on the labour ward. *Int. J. Obstet. Anesth.* **5**: 160–164.

Minnich, M.E. (1999) Childbirth preparation and nonpharmacological analgesia In: *Obstetric Anesthesia – Principles and Practice* (ed. Chestnut, D.H.) 2nd edn, pp. 336–345. Mosby, St. Louis.

Nikkola, E.M., Ekblad, U.U., Kero, P.O., Alihanka, J.M. and Salonen, M.A.O. (1997) Intravenous fentanyl PCA during labour. *Can. J. Anaesth.* **44**: 1248–1255.

Olofsson, Ch., Ekblom, A., Ekman-Ordeberg, G., Hjelm, A. and Irestedt, L. (1996) Lack of analgesic effect of systemically administered morphine or pethidine on labour pain. *Br. J. Obstet. Gynaecol.* **103**: 968–972.

Oster, M.I. (1994) Psychological preparation for labor and delivery using hypnosis. *Am. J. Clin. Hypn.* **37**: 12–21.

Paech, M.J. (1991) The King Edward Memorial Hospital 1000 mother survey of methods of pain relief in labour. *Anaesth. Intensive Care* **19**: 393–399.

Ranta, P., Jouppila, P., Spalding, M., Kangas-Saarela, T., Hollmen A. and Jouppila, R. (1994) Parturients' assessment of water blocks, pethidine, nitrous oxide, paracervical and epidural blocks in labour. *Int. J. Obstet. Anesth.* **3**: 193–198.

Report to the Medical Research Council of the Committee on nitrous oxide and oxygen analgesia in midwifery (1970) Clinical trials of different concentrations of oxygen and nitrous oxide for obstetric analgesia. *Br. Med. J.* **1**: 709–713.

Robinson, P.N., Salmon, P. and Yentis, S.M. (1998) Maternal satisfaction. *Int. J. Obstet. Anesth.* **7**: 32–37.

Ross, J.A.S., Tunstall, M.E., Campbell, D.M. and Lemon, J.S. (1999) The use of 0.25% isoflurane premixed in 50% nitrous oxide and oxygen for pain relief in labour. *Anaesthesia* **54**: 1166–1172.

Chapter 7

Anesthesia for cesarean section

Michael Paech, FANZCA

Contents

7.1 History and indications for cesarean section

Although the Roman law, *lex caesarea*, of 715 BC decreed that women dying in late pregnancy should have the infant delivered through an abdominal incision, the term 'cesarean section' (CS) derives neither from this nor the birth of Julius Caesar in 100 BC. It arose in the Middle Ages from the Latin verb *caedare* 'to cut' and its derivative *caesura*, 'a cut or pause in a line or verse'. The word 'section' also comes from Latin *secare* 'to cut', making the term 'cesarean section' somewhat redundant. The first successful cesarean delivery probably occurred late in the Middle Ages, although it was almost always fatal until the nineteenth century. With improved surgical techniques, CS is in many situations now the delivery mode of choice.

Indications for CS in the first half of the 20th century were mainly 'fetopelvic disproportion', 'dysfunctional labor' (dystocia), abnormal presentation, cord prolapse, placenta previa, and placental abruption. Ensuing decades saw an increase in CS for 'fetal distress' (especially after the introduction of electronic fetal heart rate monitoring in the early 1970s) and dystocia. It has become widely used for multiple pregnancy, breech presentation, delivery of the preterm infant, and a number of obstetric and medical disorders. In the 1970s and 1980s, a dramatic rise in the incidence of CS occurred in many countries, with rates below 10% increasing to over 20% in Australia, Canada and the United States, and over 30% in Brazil. In the absence of any obvious improvement in perinatal mortality, this high rate of intervention has raised concern in both medical and lay communities. It has been estimated that in the USA, changing obstetric indications, increasing maternal age, and birth weight accounted for only 20% of the total increase. The most common indication for CS in multipara is now previous CS.

Contributing to the rise in CS rates are factors such as greater safety, medical training, social expectations, and medicolegal pressure.

Attempts to control the rise in CS rate have been implemented and rates appear to have stabilized, although significant overall reduction has been difficult except in isolated examples. Strategies such as increased use of vaginal birth after cesarean delivery, active management of labor, strict policies for the diagnosis and management of dystocia in nulliparous labor, and publicizing of individual obstetrician's CS rates, have all proven useful.

7.2 Trends in anesthetic technique for cesarean section

7.2.1 Regional anesthesia – increasing utilization

Regional anesthesia, either *de novo* or using an epidural catheter inserted during labor, is increasingly used and predominates in most countries. This trend is underpinned by evidence (epidemiological and expert opinion) of greater maternal safety, fetal benefits, higher parental satisfaction, and consumer demand (see *Table 7.1*). Regional anesthesia permits active participation in childbirth and early

---

Table 7.1 Advantages of regional anesthesia for cesarean section

Maternal safety
- airway reflexes intact, so aspiration unlikely
- spontaneous respiration avoids airway manipulation, loss of airway and hypoxia

Fetal and neonatal safety
- reduced fetal drug exposure and depression
- neonatal resuscitation less likely

Parental satisfaction
- less maternal pain (intraoperative)
- earlier mother–infant bonding and breast-feeding
- paternal involvement
- best postoperative analgesia (intraspinal opioids)

Reduced morbidity
- reduced intraoperative blood loss
- reduced thromboembolic risk
- better respiratory function
- no sore throat
- less postoperative nausea and vomiting
- earlier return of gastrointestinal function

infant bonding, and the presence of a spouse or other support person, has become accepted as the norm in many communities.

General anesthesia (GA) was once the mainstay of anesthesia for CS. In some developed countries, Germany, Austria and Malaysia for example, and in developing countries, GA remains the usual approach. However, a large survey in the UK noted a decline in the use of GA from 77% in 1982 to 22% in 1997, with similar trends in Latin and North America and Australasia (*Table 7.2*). Tertiary centers in several countries now report GA rates as low as 3–5%.

Currently, GA is infrequently used for elective CS, being reserved for specific indications (see Section 7.9.1). It is most often used in the emergency setting, where it remains the fastest method of allowing immediate operative delivery. In Germany, 85% of urgent CS is conducted with GA, yet in many countries practice changes have reduced this proportion to less than 10%. These changes include redefinition of the appropriate use of regional anesthesia, greater use of regional analgesia in labor, earlier maternal anesthetic assessment, and greater willingness to employ spinal anesthesia (SA) in emergency situations. The American College of Obstetricians and Gynecologists has stated that when risk factors are identified '. . . the obstetrician (should) obtain antepartum consultation from an anesthesiologist . . . and that strategies (such as early intravenous access and placement of an epidural or spinal catheter) be developed . . .

to minimize the need for emergency induction of GA in women in whom this would be especially hazardous'.

Historically, although GA with ether and chloroform was first used for CS, SA with cocaine was described in Europe and North America in the early 1900s. Continuous spinal anesthesia (CSA) with a malleable needle was introduced in 1940 and, subsequently, catheter techniques were introduced. Epidural anesthesia (EA) appeared in the 1930s, but was only widely introduced for CS in the 1950s, a decade in which it almost replaced SA in many large centers.

Currently, preference for a specific regional anesthetic technique varies widely internationally, locally and between individuals, although the past decade has witnessed a global trend favoring spinal anesthetic techniques (see *Table 7.2*). This surge in the popularity of subarachnoid block followed rediscovery of the pencil-point style spinal needle, highlighted by Sprotte in 1987. Subsequent technological advances in spinal needle design and production have reduced the complication of post-dural puncture headache PDPH, and changes in perioperative management have improved control of hemodynamic changes. In the UK, USA and Australasia, single-shot SA is the most popular technique, followed by EA and combined spinal-epidural anesthesia (CSEA).

Little is known of technique demographics in developing countries, although in the Far East the use of regional anesthesia appears to parallel the economic status of the country and SA predominates (see Chapter 17). In poorer countries, conventional GA, ketamine-based GA or even open ether inhalation GA is used. Regional anesthesia, where available, is invariably SA or local infiltration regional block. The latter involves progressive infiltration of the layers of the abdominal wall and intraperitoneal instillation of large volumes of dilute local anesthetic (LA) combined with sedation and/or a field block of the lower abdomen (bilateral iliohypogastric and ilioinguinal nerve blocks) (*Figure 7.1*).

Table 7.2 Utilization of anesthetic techniques for elective cesarean section

	UK (1997)	USA (1992–1993)
General anesthesia	24%	26%
Spinal anesthesia	68%	53%
Epidural anesthesia	3%	47%
Combined spinal-epidural anesthesia	15%	–

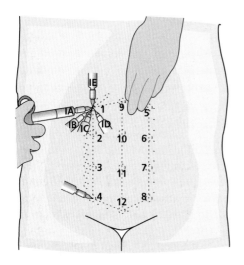

Figure 7.1 Method of local field block of the lower abdominal wall. Reproduced with permission of the American College of Obstetricians and Gynaecologists from Ranney, B. and Stanage, W.F. (1975) Advantages of local anesthesia for cesarean section. *Obstet. Gynecol.* **45**: 165.

7.2.2 Maternal mortality and choice of anesthesia

Reduction in anesthetic-related maternal mortality in the past two decades has been linked to the declining use of GA. Between 1970 and 1996, the Confidential Enquiries into Maternal Deaths (CEMD) in the UK (the most comprehensive national audit of anesthetic-related mortality) reported 214 maternal deaths directly related to anesthesia, of which only 14 were associated with regional anesthesia. Between 1991 and 1993, seven of eight maternal deaths directly attributed to anesthesia (and all deaths associated with CS) followed complications of GA, usually difficult airway management with subsequent hypoxic cardiac arrest and/or aspiration of gastric contents. The CEMD has no denominator data, but this strongly suggests a disproportionate number of deaths associated with GA. A review of data in the USA between 1979 and 1990 noted that, although anesthetic-related mortality had declined, the estimated risk of death associated with GA (especially for urgent CS) between

1985 and 1990 was over 16 times that of regional anesthesia. Reviews of closed claims databases show GA associated with more severe injuries and higher payment, and obstetric admissions to intensive care units are also dominated by complications of GA.

With the increased incidence of CS, the number of emergency cesareans has also risen, so the absolute number of general anesthetics performed in the UK has probably remained constant. Despite this, there were 19 deaths related to GA in the 1970–72 CEMD and none in 1994–1996. It is thus likely that other factors (improved obstetric and perioperative care; better use of resources, manpower and greater supervision; heightened awareness of risks; better anesthetic assessment and patient preparation) have also contributed to declining anesthetic-related maternal morbidity and mortality there. In the USA the estimated death rate from complications of GA increased between the early and late 1980s, and a major reduction in mortality appeared to be in the regional anesthesia cohort. This difference probably reflects selection bias, with GA reserved for the most urgent situations and for parturients with serious comorbidity (hemorrhage, coagulation abnormalities, etc.).

7.2.3 Neonatal outcome and choice of anesthesia

Much of the data relating fetal outcome to method of anesthesia is unreliable, being based on nonrandomized retrospective or prospective series. The fetus is more exposed to pharmacological effects with GA, and consensus opinion is that regional anesthesia has some minor short-term advantages for the neonate. At emergency CS for fetal acidosis or hypoxemia, neonatal acid-base balance improves after either regional or general anesthesia (*Figure 7.2*). Following GA for CS, a larger proportion of neonates require resuscitation, and have low Apgar scores and poorer neurobehavioral assessments, although these are transient and long-term outcome is similar. Inhalational agents can cause sedative effects,

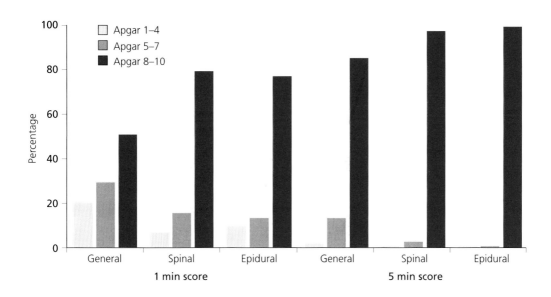

Figure 7.2 Influence of anesthetic technique on neonatal condition after urgent cesarean section for fetal distress. Data derived from Marx, G.F. *et al.* (1984) Fetal-neonatal status following cesarean section for fetal distress. *Br. J. Anaesth.* **56**: 1011. Reproduced from Reisner, L.S. and Lin, D. (1999) Anesthesia for cesarean section. In: *Obstetric Anesthesia* (Chestnut DH ed.) 2nd edn. With permission from Mosby, Inc., St. Louis.

Table 7.3 Neonatal acid-base status after general, epidural or spinal anesthesia for elective cesarean section

	General (*n* = 30)	Epidural (*n* = 30)	Spinal (*n* = 30)
Maternal			
pH	7.36 (0.04)[a]	7.44 (0.06)	7.42 (0.03)
pO$_2$ (kPa)	30.80 (1.37)	31.73 (1.56)	32.10 (1.50)
Base deficit (mmol/l)	5.10 (1.82)	2.43 (2.13)	3.21 (1.79)
Umbilical vein			
pH	7.33 (0.05)	7.34 (0.04)	7.34 (0.05)
pO$_2$	5.80 (0.33)	5.67 (0.36)	5.92 (0.51)
Base deficit	4.00 (2.10)	4.80 (1.81)	4.78 (2.23)
Umbilical artery			
pH	7.28 (0.04)	7.29 (0.07)	7.28 (0.02)
pO$_2$	2.90 (0.19)	2.91 (0.23)	2.87 (0.23)
Base deficit	4.31 (1.79)	4.58 (1.99)	4.53 (2.01)

Values are mean (SD). [a]*P* < 0.01 compared with other groups. Reproduced with permission of Churchill Livingstone from Mahajan, J. *et al.* (1993) Anaesthetic technique for elective caesarean section and neurobehavioural status of newborns. *Int. J. Obstet. Anesth.* 2: 91.

especially with a prolonged interval between induction of GA and delivery. Assuming sustained or profound hypotension is avoided during regional anesthesia, the biochemical and metabolic condition of the healthy fetus will be unaffected (*Table 7.3*). The effects of absorbed epidural LA and opioid are minimal, although uncorrected hypotension may produce subtle changes in infant sucking and behavior.

7.3 Preparation of the patient for cesarean section

7.3.1 The preoperative visit and consent

Preoperative assessment

The obstetric anesthesiologist may be faced with unique challenges when preparing parturients for CS. Ideally, multidisciplinary antenatal assessment clinics would be used to evaluate all parturients, and those scheduled for, or likely to require CS would meet with an anesthesiologist and a detailed perioperative plan organized. In reality, the anesthesiologist may be faced with an emergency where fetal demise is impending, the patient is unknown to them, and preparation is limited to a few critical actions.

In any setting, optimal care is impossible without good communication between the obstetrician and the anesthesiologist. While only about 50% of CS are planned in advance, in less than 20% is there *no* prior indication that operative delivery may prove necessary. Very few parturients require true emergency delivery within minutes, so those scheduled for elective CS, or in labor and at risk of CS, should be identified and assessed by the anesthesiologist well in advance. Even in emergencies, the anesthesiologist must determine the current maternal and fetal condition and effects of therapy, ascertain the time frame before delivery, and most importantly, assess the maternal airway. Some national obstetric organizations have suggested that the time from decision to perform a CS to surgical incision should not exceed 30 minutes; in this setting preparation will be short.

Preparation of the parturient for CS begins with the anesthetic assessment (*Tables 7.4* and *7.5*). In the direst emergency, when an unknown patient with fetus in extremis is met, this assessment must be focused and conducted simultaneously with rapid patient preparation. In elective settings, the establishment of good rapport is important, as this may be a stressful time for prospective parents, who may have had little time to adjust to changing circumstances.

Table 7.4 Preparation of the healthy parturient prior to elective cesarean section

Perform anesthetic assessment
- history, examination and investigations such as blood type and screen

Obtain informed consent

Provide aspiration prophylaxis
- typically 30 ml 0.3 M sodium citrate orally within 30 minutes of surgery
- prokinetic, anti-reflux and antiemetic drugs, histamine$_2$-receptor antagonists, antacid (e.g., ranitidine 150–300 mg orally 2 h preoperatively and/or metoclopramide 10 mg intravenously)

Avoid aortocaval compression
- during transfer to the operating room (left lateral position, or semierect with 15° pelvic tilt)

Prepare drugs and equipment
- vasopressors, emergency drugs and general anesthetic drugs
- Intravenous and airway equipment

Secure intravenous access
- one or more 14–16 gauge cannula

Institute monitoring
- maternal vital signs, pulse oximetry, fetal heart rate

Cesarean section is one of the few operations where a patient is expected to undergo major surgery without anxiolytic premedication or sedation. These drugs are usually avoided to prevent fetal exposure, although little evidence supports the practice. In contrast, animal studies suggest that relief of anxiety (and lowering of endogenous catecholamine levels) may improve placental perfusion. If so informed, many women are willing to accept anxiolytics, but further study is needed.

Preparation for CS should be tailored to the patient's past and current medical condition. There is no evidence to support routine preoperative laboratory testing, including hemoglobin or platelet count, or blood typing and screen. The American Society of Anesthesiologists (ASA) Task Force Practice Guidelines recommend decisions be based on individual assessment. The incidence of blood transfusion for CS is less than 1%, so availability of blood can be reserved for specific situations

Table 7.5 Principles of maternal assessment for cesarean section

Previous anesthetic history
- emphasis on airway management, especially ease of intubation, and patient recovery

Previous and current medical history
- special interest in cardiorespiratory disease and function, but also other co-morbidity

History of allergy, medication, smoking, dentition

Past and current obstetric history
- especially delivery outcomes, problems in this index pregnancy and current fetal condition

Fasting status
- note: gastric emptying effectively ceases at the onset of painful contractions

Current analgesia
- function of an epidural catheter

Airway examination
- Difficult intubation is not always predictable and airway anatomy may change during labor

Examination of other relevant organ systems
- emphasis on cardiac, respiratory systems and surface anatomy relevant to regional anesthesia

where the risk of hemorrhage is increased. The severe preeclamptic patient may warrant multiple laboratory investigations, including hematological and coagulation status, renal function and electrolytes, liver function and blood sugar, pulse oximetry or arterial blood gas levels, electrocardiography, or echocardiography.

Premedicant drugs are usually confined to those for aspiration prophylaxis (see below). Drug therapy that has been required for other conditions during pregnancy (asthma, diabetes, etc.) should be continued.

Fasting guidelines are based on expert opinion rather than specific evidence. The ASA practice guidelines recommend fasting intervals of at least 6 hours (for solids) prior to elective CS, avoidance of solids during labor, and restriction of clear fluids during labor only in those parturients with additional risk factors for aspiration or operative delivery.

Consent

In an elective setting, most obstetric patients want full disclosure of the anesthetic process, events, complications, consequences and alternatives. This should be respected, as good communication usually benefits both parturient and anesthesiologist, and litigation is less likely in the event of a complication. The other elements of informed consent are comprehension (the process of weighing risks, benefits and outcomes) and voluntary choice (free of coercion).

Rarely, problems arise when the anesthesiologist meets a patient who, for example, insists on GA despite knowledge and comprehension of its disadvantages and risks. Patient autonomy must be respected, but the anesthesiologist is placed in a difficult position, especially if the level of risk is high (for example, if difficult intubation is anticipated) or if, in their opinion, the choice is unacceptable (for example severe uncontrolled asthma). The anesthesiologist can withdraw from care, but has an obligation to organize an alternative anesthesiologist. Parturients in labor presenting for CS should be considered capable of providing informed consent, although in an emergency, anesthetic care must be provided and some compromise may need to be reached. Important ethical principles are autonomy (the right of self-choice by the patient), nonmaleficience (avoid doing harm), justice (give the patient what they deserve) and beneficence (duty to work for the good of the patient). The latter may need to be invoked in true emergencies to do what is felt to be in the patient's (and their infant's) best interest.

Minimization of aortocaval compression

In 1972, Crawford in the UK demonstrated an increased incidence and degree of fetal acidosis and lower Apgar scores in the newborn of parturients kept supine rather than tilted during CS. In the supine position, the gravid uterus may obstruct the inferior vena cava (IVC), reducing venous return and cardiac output. The aorta may also be obstructed near its bifurcation, reducing uterine arterial blood flow and placental circulation. This effect is possible in the second trimester, but increases in likelihood as pregnancy progresses, with IVC obstruction evident in 90% of pregnant women lying supine at term. This may lead to maternal symptoms (nausea and syncope), or fetal compromise, from reduced placental perfusion. Normally, compensatory responses occur, such as diversion of blood through the azygous venous system, vasoconstriction and increased cardiac work. These may be overwhelmed by GA-induced myocardial depression and vasodilatation or regional anesthesia-induced splanchnic and lower limb sympathectomy (with venous pooling) and loss of cardio-accelerator tone from the upper thoracic segments. It is thus routine to avoid aortocaval compression prior to and during CS (*Table 7.6*). An important point is that aortocaval compression may occur despite normal brachial BP measurement. Unfortunately, it is often not possible to entirely eliminate aortocaval compression until after delivery, particularly when the uterus is overdistended (multiple pregnancy, polyhydamnios).

Prophylaxis against pulmonary aspiration of gastric contents

The gastrointestinal changes of pregnancy, especially increased reflux and regurgitation, and delayed gastric emptying during labor, predispose to an increased risk of pulmonary aspiration of gastric contents. Both esophageal reflux and regurgitation are common and symptomatic heartburn peaks in the third trimester, due to hormone-induced relaxation of the lower esophageal sphincter and alteration of the gastro-esophageal angle from compression by the gravid uterus.

Hall, in 1940, and subsequently Mendelson in 1946, drew attention to the risk of pulmonary aspiration of solids or gastric acid in pregnant women. All pregnant women should be considered at risk of pulmonary aspiration from (at latest) mid-pregnancy, although no data are available to quantify the level of risk. At the time of GA for CS, the incidence of aspiration detected clinically is 1 in 660, which is several times higher than in the general surgical population. The overall incidence at CS is thought to be about 1 in 1600, with emergency CS at 2–4-fold higher risk. However, serious morbidity does not usually occur. Perioperative aspiration is no longer a major cause of morbidity or mortality (recent deaths in the CEMD have involved over-sedation, post-ictal vomiting and regurgitation in intensive care). This is likely due to the widespread adoption of prophylactic measures against aspiration (see Chapter 15, Section 15.8.1 and Figure 15.6). Fatal aspiration is far less common at present than during previous eras when GA via facemask for CS was the norm. Other factors contributing to the lower morbidity and mortality are the greater use of regional anesthesia (preservation of airway reflexes); increased awareness of the risk; policy changes (restriction of food consumption in labor, pharmacological prophylaxis); and rapid sequence induction for GA.

Fasting guidelines remain important, but frequently CS is indicated for patients with a possible 'full stomach' (solid or semi-solid gastric content). Pain from uterine contractions is a potent inhibitor of gastric emptying, and this is compounded by concurrent opioid analgesia. Policies with respect to oral intake during labor remain hotly debated, but from an anesthetic standpoint, caution is warranted because once labor commences, solid intragastric material may remain despite fasting

---

Table 7.6 Precautions against aortocaval compression

Maintain normovolemia

Appropriate positioning
- transport parturients to the operating room in the lateral position without truncal flexion, or in the semi-erect position with pelvic tilt
- after regional block, place the parturient in the lateral or left tilted supine position
- maintain pelvic tilt, at least 15 degrees, during surgery
- left tilt or left uterine displacement usually results in the best neonatal outcome, but occasionally right tilt proves more satisfactory

periods beyond 24 hours. Aspiration of solids may cause upper or lower airway obstruction with immediate severe hypoxemia.

Since all parturients should be considered at risk for aspiration, nonparticulate antacid (0.3 M sodium citrate, 30 ml orally) is the most important prophylactic drug. Although the pH–volume relationship for serious pneumonitis is unknown, gastric fluid of pH <3.5 and volumes of >30 ml generate concern, and sodium citrate reliably neutralizes over 200 ml of liquid of pH 1 for at least 30–45 minutes. This should be given just prior to surgery.

Several other drugs may also be useful in terms of reducing stomach fluid volume and acidity or increasing esophageal sphincter tone. Prokinetic drugs promote gastric emptying, although metoclopramide is of poor efficacy, especially in the presence of opioids. At the time of decision to proceed to urgent CS, some anesthesiologists also administer IV metoclopramide (10 mg) and ranitidine (50 mg raises gastric pH above 3 within 30–45 minutes and the duration of effect is several hours). Parenteral metoclopramide is used by some for its activity as an antiemetic and for increasing lower esophageal sphincter tone. Side effects (dystonic reactions, akasthisia and arrhythmias) are very uncommon. The histamine$_2$-receptor antagonists, especially ranitidine (150–300 mg orally either the night before surgery and/or 1–2 hours preoperatively), reliably suppress acid secretion, but are of less value in the acute setting. Side effects are rare, although rapid intravenous bolusing has caused arrhythmia. The gastric parietal cell proton pump inhibitor, omeprazole, has no significant advantage over ranitidine and is more expensive. Anticholinergic drugs such as glycopyrrolate have similar effects, but increase the potential for reflux and are now rarely used.

Insertion of an orogastric tube to empty the stomach is recommended intraoperatively during CS under GA.

Airway assessment

Difficult intubation (see Chapter 15, Section 15.8.2) is arguably the greatest concern of the obstetric anesthesiologist. Although not always predictable, several factors are associated with an increased risk and multiple factors magnify the degree of risk (*Table 7.7*). Routine airway assessment is mandatory, systematically evaluating anatomical structures and function (*Table 7.8*). Adequate neck movement, particularly extension at the atlanto-occipital joint, is an integral function when aiming to align the axis from the mouth to larynx. Reduced mouth opening, external tissues or poor positioning can limit oral access. The nasal route is generally avoided because of nasal mucosal edema during pregnancy and

---

Table 7.7 Risk factors for difficult intubation at cesarean section[a]

- Poor view of oropharyngeal structures
- Short neck
- Obesity
- Single or missing maxillary incisors
- Receding mandible
- Protruding maxillary teeth

[a]Multiple factors increase risk significantly.

Table 7.8 Airway assessment in the parturient

History
- previous anesthesia and intubation
- stridor in severe preeclampsia or airway infection

Mouth opening and access
- unrestricted neck extension, especially atlanto-occipital
- normal temporomandibular joint function
- access limited by size of neck and breasts; large hair knots or buns; other pathology

Dentition (prostheses, caps, crowns and implants, loose and missing teeth)
- missing incisors and prominent maxillary teeth make manipulation of laryngoscope and equipment difficult
- caries increase the risk of dental injury

Oropharyngeal view (Mallampati score)
- tongue and airway edema with preeclampsia, prolonged straining, infection

Other parameters
- nasal passages, adequate distance between thyroid cartilage or sternal notch and chin

the increased risk of serious epistaxis. The state and configuration of dentition impacts on the introduction of a laryngoscope and direct laryngoscopic view. A large tongue or recessive mandible cause concern and a 'Mallampati score' (based on visualization of oropharnygeal structures while the patient is in a seated position with the mouth open without phonation) is commonly assigned to estimate ease of intubation (*Figure 7.3*). A short thyro- or sternomental distance is an indicator of a potentially difficult view.

If difficulty is anticipated, advance preparation and planning is mandatory. Early placement of an epidural catheter during labor is likely to circumvent the need for emergency GA; appropriate equipment (the 'difficult intubation cart') should always be available, assistance organized, and a management plan formulated (see Chapter 15, Section 15.8 and *Figure 15.7*).

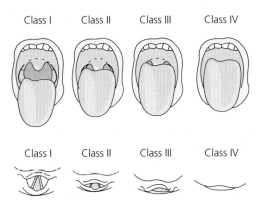

Figure 7.3 Airway assessment. Upper panel: classification of view of the pharyngeal structures during airway assessment (modified from Mallampati, S.R. *et al.* (1985) A clinical sign to predict difficult intubation: a prospective study. *Can. Anaesth. Soc. J.* **32**: 429–434). Lower panel: Classification of direct laryngoscopic view (modified from Cormack, R.S. and Lehane, J. (1994) Difficult intubation in obstetrics. *Anaesthesia* **39**: 1105–1111). Reproduced with permission of BMJ Publishing Group, London, UK from Samsoon, G.L.T. and Young, J.R.B. (1987) Difficult tracheal intubation: a retrospective study. *Anaesthesia* **42**: 488.

7.3.2 Monitoring during cesarean section

Respiratory monitoring (ventilation and oxygenation)

During GA for CS, in addition to measurement of inspired and expired oxygen and inhalational anesthetic concentration, patient ventilation and oxygenation are monitored using expired airway gas analysis, ventilator parameters and pulse oximetry. Arterial gas analysis and other pulmonary function tests (flow-volume and pressure-volume loops, compliance) may be used for specific indications. End-tidal nitrogen measurement prior to induction may be used to indicate the degree of denitrogenation produced by pre-oxygenation with 100% oxygen. In addition to many other diagnostic capabilities, a normal capnograph trace is an early and invaluable confirmation of tracheal (as opposed to esophageal) intubation.

A number of changes in respiratory physiology during pregnancy (see Section 2.3) influence monitoring and the anesthesiologist's response to measured variables. Monitoring of end-tidal carbon dioxide (CO_2) tension during GA is used to adjust ventilation to maintain normocarbia for pregnancy (30–32 mmHg), recognizing that the alveolar-arterial difference is small in the healthy parturient due to their higher minute ventilation and lower alveolar dead space. End-tidal volatile anesthetic concentration provides a guide to adequacy of anesthetic depth and to the timing of arousal for return of protective airway reflexes prior to extubation. Pulse oximetry is mandatory and should preferably be 99–100% prior to delivery and above 95% during anesthesia.

During regional anesthesia, clinical observation of respiratory rate and depth and arterial hemoglobin oxygen saturation measured with pulse oximetry can be supplemented if desired by capnography using a sampling line connected into a face mask. This is not of benefit quantitatively, but gives additional information about respiratory frequency and pattern. Regional block to T_3–T_4 reduces vital capacity and coughing is weakened. Higher levels of block may lead to dyspnea, especially if significant intercostal muscle weakness results. Nevertheless, provided oxygenation is maintained and the patient is reassured, regression of sensory and motor deficit is usually prompt and intervention to assist with ventilation rarely necessary (approximately 1 in 2000–5000).

Cardiovascular monitoring

In most healthy parturients, a noninvasive blood pressure (BP) device, pulse oximeter plethysmograph, electrocardiogram (ECG) and clinical assessment are adequate means of monitoring the circulation. The accuracy of non-invasive BP devices is reduced during pregnancy, with diastolic BP readings from automated devices being about 10 mmHg lower than phase 4 Korotkoff sounds, and these show further variability in the presence of hypertension.

Patient shivering may interfere with automated measurement, so assessment of BP by auscultation of Korotkoff sounds should also be available. After insertion of regional block, regular BP monitoring at frequent intervals (each minute) is essential to detect rapidly developing hypotension.

Benign and transient arrhythmias are very common during CS, but serious arrhythmias are rare. ECG changes in ST segments are also very common, although they appear inconsequential in the vast majority of cases. There is no direct evidence that they are caused by myocardial ischemia in this population, and may instead reflect autonomic nervous system imbalance. Another phenomena that is common (incidence up to 50%), but also apparently benign except in rare circumstances is venous air embolism. Small emboli, particularly when the uterine venous sinuses are open, can be detected with great sensitivity using a precordial Doppler probe. Most anesthesiologists do not routinely use this monitor, however, because of its intrusive nature and

the fact that serious air embolism has only rarely been reported. Such an event is likely to be detected rapidly by fall in end-tidal CO_2 tension, hypotension, oxygen desaturation and clinical signs.

In some obstetric conditions (severe pre-eclampsia, hemorrhage) and medical disorders (morbid obesity, cardiac disease) invasive hemodynamic monitoring with arterial BP and central venous pressure or pulmonary artery cannulation may be indicated. In parturients with severe bleeding disorders, marked thrombocytopenia or coagulopathy (secondary to massive hemorrhage, placental abruption, amniotic fluid embolism, sepsis or prolonged fetal death *in utero*) a peripherally inserted central venous catheter is safest. Pulmonary artery catheters may provide useful information in those with poor cardiac function, severe pulmonary edema, pulmonary hypertension and renal failure. The indications for pulmonary artery catheterization are widely debated, based on a lack of evidence of benefit in the obstetric population and a low but potentially serious complication rate. Rates of utilization vary with local circumstances, particularly intensive care resources.

Fetal monitoring

Monitoring of fetal condition should continue after the decision is made to deliver by CS, and FHR should be at least briefly assessed immediately prior to elective CS. It should be appreciated that cardiotocographic (CTG) heart rate monitoring is less useful and more difficult to interpret in severe prematurity (<28 weeks). Nevertheless, continuous electronic fetal heart rate monitoring or intermittent monitoring (by Doppler ultrasound or direct auscultation) is prudent while preparing the parturient for anesthesia or surgery. The presence of a normal heart rate, pattern and variability after anesthesia has been instituted is reassuring (see also Section 3.6).

7.4 Spinal anesthesia for cesarean section

7.4.1 Introduction

With any central neuraxial block for CS, adequate surgical conditions will require block of the pudendal nerves $(S_2–S_4)$ and the somatic and visceral sensation from the surgical field $(T_4–L_1)$. Exteriorization of the uterus tends to be more uncomfortable, and a cephalad block to T_2 is preferred (*Figure 7.4*). This can be achieved with small doses of LA (bupivacaine 8–12.5 mg) for subarachnoid block or spinal anesthesia (SA), larger volumes and doses for epidural anesthesia (EA) (15–30 ml) or combinations of both approaches (combined spinal-epidural anesthesia or CSEA). Spinal anesthesia usually regresses more rapidly than EA and depending on the technique chosen, a variety of options are available for postoperative analgesia (see Chapter 8).

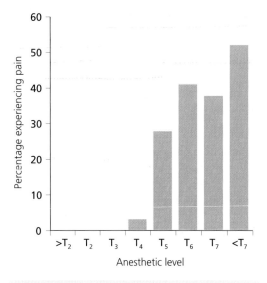

Figure 7.4 The number of parturients attaining a particular level of analgesia or anesthesia after spinal or epidural anesthesia and the number of women subsequently experiencing pain within that subgroup. Reprinted from Russell, I.F. (1995) Levels of anaesthesia and intraoperative pain at caesarean section under regional block. *Int. J. Obstet. Anesth.* **4**: 74. With permission from the publisher Churchill Livingstone.

Patient positioning for central neuraxial block is determined by the anesthesiologist's preference, although it is occasionally dictated by obstetric factors (the sitting position is inadvisable, for example, when the umbilical cord is presenting). The sitting position is preferable for the obese parturient (see Chapter 11). It allows better spinal flexion, is associated with higher arterial oxygen tension and favors identification of midline structures. More reliable dural puncture during CSEA and rapid return of cerebrospinal fluid (CSF) into the needle hub are also advantages of the sitting position; however, some parturients are more comfortable in the lateral position, and the incidence of hypotension may be reduced.

7.4.2 Spinal anesthesia compared with epidural anesthesia

In terms of resources and patient well-being, SA has several advantages and few disadvantages in the healthy parturient compared with EA (*Tables 7.9* and *7.10*). These relate to the speed of patient preparation for CS, the quality of anesthesia and the elimination of LA toxicity. Preparation time is determined by the time taken to prepare for and perform the anesthetic, and the time from drug injection to

Table 7.9 Advantages of spinal anesthesia (SA) compared with epidural anesthesia (EA)

Time to anesthesia
- Insertion usually faster
- LA spread to mid-thoracic level more rapid with SA
- Risk of failure lower

Patient comfort
- Less preoperative shivering
- Reduced pre-incision anxiety
- Less intraoperative pain
- Lower rate of conversion to GA

Costs
- Cheaper equipment

Complications
- No LA toxicity
- No epidural catheter-related complications (venous trauma, subdural block, skin site infection)

Table 7.10 Disadvantages of spinal anesthesia

Single injection of local anesthetic in predetermined dose
- Failure to reach adequate cephalad level (1%)
- Excessive sensory block involving upper thoracic (20–50%) and cervical dermatomes (5%)
- Excessive sensory and motor block requiring intubation (1 in 1–5000)
- Finite duration occasionally exceeded by duration of surgery

Maternal hypotension
- Common (60–70% despite avoiding aortocaval compression and fluid loading; 10–50% with prophylactic or early vasopressors; higher vasopressor requirements)
- Fetal acidosis and neurobehavioral impairment if hypotension severe or prolonged (>5 min)

Postdural puncture headache
- 1 in 150–200 with 27 gauge Whitacre-style needles, but up to 1 in 5 with large gauge cutting bevel needles

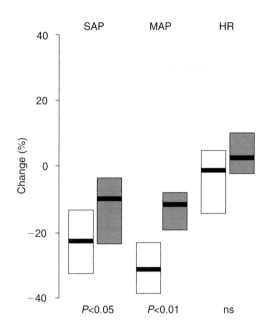

Figure 7.5 Maximum percentage change in hemodynamic measurements during spinal anesthesia for elective cesarean section. SAP, systolic arterial pressure; MAP, mean arterial pressure; HR, heart rate; (□, $n = 16$) and epidural (■, $n = 16$) Median 95% confidence intervals. Modified with permission of Oxford University Press, from Robson, S.C. *et al.* (1992) Maternal and fetal haemodynamic effects of spinal and extradural anaesthesia for elective caesarean section. *Br. J. Anaesth.* **68**: 58.

onset of adequate anesthesia. Spinal techniques may be marginally quicker to perform than epidural, although preparation of subarachnoid adjuncts to LA can be time-consuming and the difference in insertion time is minimal in experienced hands. Unless epidural chloroprocaine is used, subarachnoid block almost invariably develops faster, normally in 5–15 minutes, particularly as sacral block is an early rather than late component. This is of little consequence for elective CS except for cost-efficiency, allowing more efficient use of personnel and operating room time, but the 10 to 20 minutes gained in the face of severe fetal compromise may be vital.

Maternal satisfaction with SA is high, low doses of LA remove the hazard posed by accidental intravenous injection during EA, and the neonatal outcome is comparable to EA. Although PDPH remains a problem, the incidence has been reduced to acceptable levels (1 in 150–200) with 26 or 27-gauge pencil point needles (see Section 15.1). The management of hypotension has also improved considerably.

The hemodynamic changes after SA differ from those with EA. After fluid loading, cardiac output, measured by Doppler and cross-sectional echocardiography at the aortic valve, increases. It then decreases with SA, but remains elevated with EA, and maximal changes in arterial pressure are greater with SA. Large falls in cardiac output may be reflected by changes in the uteroplacental bed, with increased umbilical placental vascular resistance, and greater fetal acidemia (*Fig 7.5*).

7.4.3 Techniques for spinal anesthesia
Spinal anesthetic techniques are performed in a low lumbar interspace, below the termination of the spinal cord (usually about the body of L_2 vertebra), so that direct neurological

trauma to the cord is unlikely. However, anatomical variability and difficulty in determining the exact intervertebral space using surface landmarks makes it crucial that the anesthesiologist aims for L_3–L_4 or below. To avoid complications (see Section 15.5), this means choosing an interspace at or below 'Tuffier's line', joining the top of the posterior iliac crests. During pregnancy, subarachnoid drug requirements for SA fall by about 30%, probably because of hormonal effects on neuronal sensitivity. Determining an ideal drug dose for each individual is not possible, because factors such as height, weight and vertebral column length are poor predictors of subarachnoid spread and the main determinant, the volume of CSF within the lumbar intrathecal compartment, is not accessible for measurement. On average, parturients with high body mass index and those with multiple pregnancy have greater segmental spread, but individual variability is great.

The behavior of hyperbaric drugs depends on patient positioning and the anatomical shape of the spinal column, with pooling in dependent regions. When the pregnant woman lies supine and lateral, the slope of the thoracolumbar spine is about 10 degrees cephalad and pooling occurs in the T_5–T_6 area. Initial spread to midthoracic level is more rapid when the sitting position is used, but time to T_4 block is similar. Injection of hyperbaric solutions in the right lateral position, followed by turning to supine with left lateral tilt, ensures better block than left lateral followed by tilt. If the left lateral position is used, turning to full right lateral is recommended to guarantee bilateral spread. The injection of plain (isobaric) bupivacaine with the patient seated is associated with higher cephalad spread than with lateral positioning, and worrisome high thoracic and cervical block may be more likely.

When SA is instituted after failed EA or epidural analgesia during labor, caution is required because of the possibility of unexpectedly high spread. The mechanism is thought to be compression of the lumbar intrathecal sac and reduced CSF volume secondary to fluid distention of the epidural space. Although total spinal block has been reported, worrisome high block is infrequent. Most anesthesiologists consider it safe to proceed using a dose of LA at the lower end of the effective range (for example 8–10 mg hyperbaric bupivacaine) and with left tilt positioning with shoulders elevated to accentuate the thoracic curve.

7.4.4 Drugs for spinal anesthesia

Bupivacaine is a readily available LA in developed countries and is widely considered the drug of choice. Other amide LAs such as tetracaine, 8 mg (less reliable sensory block), ropivacaine, 10–15 mg (less reliable sensory and motor block) and lidocaine, 60–80 mg (short duration) are less satisfactory. Despite similar outcomes (although possibly more high and low blocks) with equivalent doses of plain 0.5% (termed isobaric, although slightly hypobaric in CSF at body temperature) or hyperbaric 0.5–0.75% bupivacaine (in 8–8.25% dextrose), the hyperbaric preparation appears most popular. A dose of 10–12.5 mg has a rapid onset (5–15 min) and surgical anesthesia lasts 90–120 minutes (*Figure 7.6*). The incidence of intraoperative visceral pain during SA with bupivacaine is dose-related and lower after bupivacaine doses at the upper end of the therapeutic range. When injected with the patient sitting, hyperbaric bupivacaine 10 mg is usually less satisfactory than 12.5 mg; compared with 15 mg, 12 mg in the lateral position (followed by turning) is reliable and associated with fewer cervical blocks. Satisfactory anesthesia can also be achieved by using a high volume method (plain bupivacaine 0.125%, 10 ml or 0.25%, 5 ml).

Although low rates of intraoperative pain occur with bupivacaine alone, the addition of subarachnoid fentanyl, 10–20 µg, or sufentanil, 2–3 µg, reduces both pain (incidence 2–4%) and nausea, and improves early postoperative analgesia. Intrathecal morphine (100–150 µg) may also improve intraoperative analgesia if CSF morphine concentration has

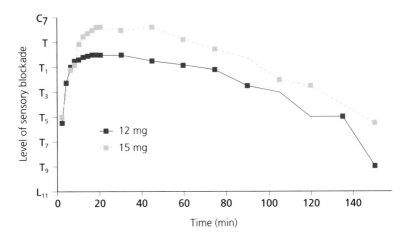

Figure 7.6 Onset and duration of sensory block after subarachnoid hyperbaric bupivacaine, 12 mg or 15 mg, showing more spinal segments blocked for a significantly longer time with the higher dose. Reproduced with permission of WB Saunders, Orlando from De Simone, C.A. *et al.* (1995) Spinal anesthesia for cesarean delivery. A comparison of two doses of hyperbaric bupivacaine. *Reg. Anesth.* **20**: 91.

peaked (45–90 minutes). In the UK, subarachnoid diamorphine, 300–500 µg, is used to improve intraoperative conditions and decrease postoperative opioid requirements. The addition of opioid or epinephrine (adrenaline) alters the baricity of spinal LA, but has no important impact on distribution. Clonidine, 75 µg, combined with fentanyl, 12.5 µg, improves intraoperative analgesia and prolongs postoperative analgesia more than either drug alone (see also Chapter 8).

7.4.5 Management of hypotension during spinal anesthesia

Introduction
The principles of BP management during SA apply to other regional anesthetic techniques. Hypotension associated with regional anesthesia is more likely at elective CS than when parturients have been in labor, probably because of differences in hydration, levels of atrial natriuretic peptide and endogenous catecholamines. Clinically, maintenance of BP within 20% of baseline, or a systolic blood pressure of 90–100 mmHg, appears reasonable. The primary concern with decreased BP is decreased uteroplacental perfusion; placental blood flow is perfusion pressure-dependent

and not autoregulated, so lower blood pressures warrant intervention empirically to ensure adequate perfusion.

After obstetric regional block, modest BP reduction should be anticipated due to sympathectomy, although the magnitude varies widely. Large falls in BP may reflect reduced cardiac output and vital organ perfusion, manifesting as fetal heart rate and acid-base changes (uteroplacental circulation) and nausea, dizziness or syncope (maternal cerebral circulation). During the onset of SA, blood pressure often falls rapidly, within 3–10 minutes. Bradycardia is uncommon (2%), but nausea very common (25–60%). Nausea and vomiting should always be assumed to be due to hypotension and poor perfusion of the relevant brainstem centers until proven otherwise. Nausea may also arise from surgical stimulation, and preoperative antiemetics (ondansetron, droperidol and metoclopramide) will reduce the perioperative incidence.

Complete hemodynamic stability and a low incidence of hypotension are difficult to achieve with single-shot SA, and several preventative strategies have been suggested (*Table 7.11*). Providing hypotension is avoided, the supine position with 20 degree left lateral tilt

Table 7.11 Strategies against maternal hypotension after spinal anesthesia

Ambulation
- immediately prior to insertion (to stimulate secretion of atrial natriuretic hormone)

Thromboembolic stockings or leg wrapping in elastic bandages
- to prevent venous pooling

Injection in the lateral position
- followed by supine with left tilt

Intravenous fluid loading

Elevation of the lower limbs

Prophylactic or early vasopressor

Slow injection of subarachnoid local anesthetic
- over several minutes

is sufficient to prevent aortocaval-induced changes in neonatal Apgar scores and blood gases after SA.

Intravenous fluid

Intravenous (IV) fluid preloading with crystalloid has long been considered mandatory, but it is only of minor benefit and its prophylactic use is being questioned. The volume of crystalloid that should be used for preloading is controversial. Though no clinical benefit has been proven from volumes greater than 10 ml/kg, some advocate routine use of volumes as high as 2000 ml. With rapid extracellular redistribution, blood volume rises by only 10–30% of the volume administered. A rapid increase in central venous pressure and reduction of colloid osmotic pressure and hematocrit are theoretical disadvantages of greater volumes. High volume preloading does augment renal blood flow and urine output, and its hemodilutional effects may help decrease the need for transfusion in certain situations. Atrial natriuretic peptide levels rise in response to fluid loading and subsequent vasodilatation may be counterproductive. In an urgent setting, SA should never delayed to permit preloading. Dextrose-containing fluids should be avoided, because maternal hyperglycemia and hyperinsulinemia predispose to subsequent neonatal hypoglycemia.

Colloids have a longer intravascular half-life, more effectively expand the blood volume (80–100%) and increase cardiac output, and modestly reduce hypotension (incidence 20–50%). They are less popular because of additional cost and occasional anaphylactoid reactions (0.06% with hydroxyethyl starches and higher with gelatins and dextrans).

Vasopressors

The early administration of ephedrine in response to an initial drop in BP, or prophylactic intramuscular injection or intravenous infusion has become a popular strategy (also see Section 14.1). However, if used alone, ephedrine may result in fetal acidemia. With frequent monitoring, prophylactic IV ephedrine (5–10 mg and a titrated infusion) to maintain baseline systolic BP reduces nausea and the incidence of hypotension. Ephedrine has been considered the vasopressor of choice, because its indirect mechanism of action does not increase uterine artery resistance. Despite direct α-sympathomimetics being more likely to increase vascular resistance and reduce uteroplacental flow, clinical studies show that titration of small doses of phenylephrine (50–100 µg) or metaraminol (0.25 mg) are safe for the healthy fetus. These alternatives are warranted for hypotension unresponsive to ephedrine or in parturients for whom the inotropic or chronotropic effects of ephedrine may be detrimental (for example, severe valvular stenosis or hypertrophic obstructive cardiomyopathy).

7.5 Epidural anesthesia for cesarean section

7.5.1 Introduction and advantages

Despite the advantages of SA (see *Table 7.9*), EA is an effective method of regional anesthesia for CS. If established using LA alone, mild or moderate intraoperative pain occurs in up to 25% of parturients, falling to about 10% with adjunctive epidural fentanyl. Conversion to GA is more common than with spinal anesthetic techniques, but maternal safety and expediency recommend EA in most cases where the decision to perform CS is made after an epidural catheter has been placed for labor analgesia (see Sections 7.2.1 and 7.2.2). Thus, although EA is not available in many poorer countries, and despite the popularity of SA in the UK, Australasia, North America and Europe, EA retains an important place in the obstetric anesthesiologist's armamentarium (*Tables 7.12* and *7.13*).

The greatest advantage of EA is its flexibility, although it can be argued that sequential CSEA (see Section 7.6 later) offers similar potential. Unlike single-shot SA, epidural catheterization allows ready prolongation of anesthesia when necessary. In the unusual circumstance of prolonged operative time (for example, an unplanned cesarean hysterectomy or the incidental discovery of major intra-abdominal pathology), GA may be avoided. If surgical anesthesia is deliberately established very slowly over 45–90 minutes, compensatory mechanisms markedly diminish the risk of hypotension. This approach is an effective means of avoiding IV fluid loading, the potentially serious consequences of sudden fall in pre- or afterload and the chronotropic and inotropic effects of ephedrine in parturients with severe preeclampsia, cardiac failure, cardiomyopathy, or certain cardiac diseases (see Chapters 9 and 13). Epidural anesthesia or CSEA also offer the option of high quality postoperative analgesia, in either the short-term as a routine or for several days in complicated cases.

The principal application of EA for CS in current practice is the urgent CS when epidural analgesia has already been instituted during labor. Conversion to epidural block appropriate for surgery is a safer alternative than conversion to GA or to SA (both unnecessary and

---

Table 7.12 Comparison of epidural anesthesia and single-shot spinal anesthesia

Mechanism of block
- Spread of spinal solution within CSF determined mainly by drug dose, baricity and patient posture, compared with lumbar epidural solution spread determined mainly by drug dose (volume and concentration) and minimally affected by patient position
- Anatomically less reliable spread of epidural solution increases failure rate
- Spinal nerve root, with some subarachnoid effect, from epidural local anesthetic

Onset
- Usually slower with epidural anesthesia by 10–20 minutes, creating advantages (better hemodynamic stability) and disadvantages (less efficient use of operating time)

Efficiency
- Less dense sensory and motor block with epidural anesthesia, resulting in increased risk of mild operative pain (1 in 5–10 vs 1 in 25–40)

Complications
- Incidence of hypotension similar, though cardiac output fall is more likely and maximum change greater with spinal anesthesia. Slow titration of epidural local anesthetic can reduce hypotension very significantly
- No LA toxicity with spinal anesthesia
- Post-dural puncture headache possible with both
- Shivering less common or severe with spinal anesthesia
- Incidence of serious infection possibly lower with spinal anesthesia
- Incidence of neurological injury uncertain with both

Table 7.13 Situations in which epidural anesthesia may be preferable to spinal anesthesia

Severe preeclampsia

Cardiac failure
- cardiomyopathy
- severe preeclampsia

Cardiac disease
- pulmonary hypertension
- severe aortic or mitral stenosis
- hypertrophic obstructive cardiomyopathy
- myocardial ischemia

Central nervous system pathology
- raised intracranial pressure

Anticipated prolonged surgery
- difficult repeat CS
- co-existing abdominal pathology or procedure
- planned or possible cesarean hysterectomy

requiring caution because of the potential for unexpectedly high block). Conversion to dense regional anesthesia can be readily and rapidly achieved. Several options exist (see below), but it is usually possible to establish surgical anesthesia to T_4–T_7 and to start surgery within 10 minutes of drug injection, irrespective of the last time of epidural drug injection or its nature.

7.5.2 Epidural drugs

There are several local anesthetics suitable for EA, with 3% 2-chloroprocaine (available in the USA) or 1.5–2% lidocaine (lignocaine) with epinephrine (adrenaline) 1:200–400 000, popular for urgent CS because of their rapid onset. Plain lidocaine should probably be avoided because of a higher incidence of unsatisfactory block and greater risk of accumulative LA toxicity. Both bupivacaine and ropivacaine are suitable, but are slow in onset, with 20–30 ml of the plain 0.5% concentration of either providing good conditions. Some studies have combined bupivacaine and lidocaine, although there is no significant clinical advantage. Ropivacaine, 0.5–0.75%, or levobupivacaine, 0.5%, are clinically similar and arguably safer than racemic bupivacaine when a plain LA is chosen.

Epinephrine, as an adjunct to lidocaine, reduces lidocaine's systemic absorption and increases the quality (probably by a direct α_2-adrenergic spinal and nociceptive effect) and duration of anesthesia. This is useful because high doses (300–600 mg) are often required and plain lidocaine is more likely to lead to toxic plasma levels. In contrast, the absorption and clinical characteristics of bupivacaine and ropivacaine are not significantly affected by epinephrine.

Absorbed epinephrine has β-agonist vasodilator, chronotropic and inotropic effects that are best avoided in maternal cardiac disease (see Chapter 13.3) and preeclampsia (maternal hypertension and uteroplacental effects, see Chapter 9), or where there is evidence of fetal compromise from increased placental vessel resistance (elevated systolic/ diastolic ratios or pulsatility indices reflecting increased resistance tend to deteriorate). Clonidine is an α_2-agonist that prolongs the duration of anesthesia and is associated with hypotension, sedation and postoperative analgesia of 4–10 hours duration after large doses. Its role in this setting remains investigational.

Three percent 2-chloroprocaine works the most rapidly (less than 5 minutes), has low toxicity risk because of an elimination half-life of less than a minute secondary to plasma pseudocholinesterase metabolism, and is the only ester LA available for EA. It has limited availability outside the USA and although concerns about neurotoxicity have been dispelled following reformulation of the preparation, postpartum backache (possibly from calcium chelation in paraspinal muscles) and antagonism of epidural opioid analgesia remain problems.

If chloroprocaine is unavailable, strategies are available to hasten the onset of EA in urgent situations. In 1967, Bromage showed that carbonation decreased the latency of lidocaine and prilocaine by a quarter to a third, but had little effect on bupivacaine. Over the past decade the fresh addition of 8.4% sodium bicarbonate (approximately 1 ml per 10 ml to avoid precipitation) has become a popular means of alkalinization of 2% lidocaine with epinephrine. Elevation of the pH, from about 4.5 to 7 or more, increases the unionized proportion of LA; more unionized lipid soluble free base is available to penetrate the nerve sheath and the onset of action is hastened and depth of anesthesia increased (see Section 4.3.1). Surgical anesthesia can usually be achieved within 5 minutes with alkalinized 1.5–2% lidocaine with epinephrine (adrenaline) (20–25 ml over 2–4 minutes). Finally, warming the epidural solution speeds onset by about 20%, but is of little practical application.

In the late 1980s the benefit of combining epidural fentanyl with LA for elective CS was recognized, although initially some reserved this until after delivery. Fentanyl improves the efficacy of EA, reduces intraoperative pain, nausea and shivering, and enhances patient satisfaction. A dose of 100 µg has no neonatal effect, although an analgesic ceiling effect may be reached at about 50 µg. Fentanyl is also an appropriate adjunct when converting from labor epidural analgesia to surgical anesthesia, although frequently it may already have been administered. Sufentanil is an alternative, but neither provides a useful duration of postoperative analgesia.

7.5.3 Epidural techniques

Epidural catheters may be inserted with the patient either seated or in the flexed lateral position depending on parturient and anesthesiologist preference and obstetric considerations. Consensus opinion now favors loss- of-resistance to saline versus air as the identification technique, with respect to a reduction of both accidental dural puncture and other potential minor complications of air injection (see Chapter 15.1). These include subcutaneous emphysema and intrathecal air injection, subscapular and occipital pain, paradoxical embolism, and unsatisfactory spread of solution. Injection of at least 10 ml of saline through the epidural needle before threading the catheter reduces venous cannulation and paresthesia, but may dilute subsequent LA. Injection of LA through the needle arguably improves the spread of solution and reliability of the block, but is not recommended. Anesthesia does not develop any more rapidly than after incremental injection through the catheter, hemodynamic disturbance requiring intervention is more common, and safety is reduced because intravascular or subarachnoid injection may occur. Minor complications appear similar whether 16 or 18 gauge epidural needles are used.

The question of whether a test dose should be administered routinely, and what is the optimal method of safely detecting both intravascular and intrathecal placement, has been investigated for many years without consensus being achieved. In many countries, no single LA preparation is ideal and many drugs and techniques (for example, 3 ml 1.5% lidocaine with epinephrine 1:200 000 with ECG monitoring or epidural air with thoracic Doppler monitoring) have been advocated. The routine use of test-doses remains controversial, though most support the concept of 'every dose is a test dose', catheter aspiration, slow drug injection and selective test dosing based on a thorough understanding of the limitations and risks in a given situation.

Following placement of an epidural catheter for CS, the patient can be positioned in the full left lateral position to avoid aortocaval compression, without compromising the spread of epidural solution. A slight head-up position may assist sacral spread. There is wide interindividual variability in spread of LA, but usually 20–25 ml of LA administered slowly, in divided doses of 3–5 ml per increment, results in anesthesia to T_3–T_5 within 10 minutes (chloroprocaine), 10–20 minutes (lidocaine) or 15–45 minutes (bupivacaine and ropivacaine). For emergency CS, a slow bolus of 10–20 ml, 3% 2-chloroprocaine or alkalinized 1.5–2% lidocaine with epinephrine, with frequent aspiration to detect intravascular injection, will augment epidural analgesia and usually provides satisfactory anesthesia within 5–10 minutes.

During the CS, the administration of an increased inspired oxygen fraction using a face mask will increase fetal oxygen stores and acid-base values. Although logically this may help the fetus withstand unexpected oxygen deprivation, there is no evidence that outcome is improved. Mild hypothermia is common during regional anesthesia due to exposure of body surfaces and fluid administration, and can be significantly reduced by measures such as warming of intravenous fluids and forced air–skin surface warming.

7.6 Combined spinal-epidural anesthesia (CSEA)

7.6.1 History

Combined spinal-epidural anesthesia (CSEA) was first described in 1937. A double intervertebral space approach was applied to anesthesia for CS in 1979 in Eastern Europe and independently by Brownridge in Australia in 1981.

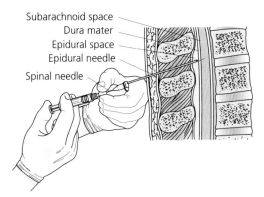

Subarachnoid space
Dura mater
Epidural space
Epidural needle
Spinal needle

Figure 7.7 Combined spinal-epidural insertion using the single intervertebral space needle-through-needle approach. Reprinted from Rawal, N. *et al*. (2000) The combined spinal-epidural technique. In: *Textbook of Obstetric Anesthesia* (Birnbach, D.J., Gatt, S.P., Datta, S. eds.), p.166, with permission from the publisher Churchill Livingstone.

Further developments were the single inter-space needle-through-needle technique (*Figure 7.7*) suggested for CS in 1984, and sequential methods in 1988 and 1992. The popularity of CSEA for CS grew in the UK particularly, and was further boosted by the introduction of pencil-point spinal needles. As the popularity of EA has waned, many units in the UK, parts of Continental Europe and Australasia, but very few in North America, Germany and Asia, have adopted CSEA, rather than single-shot SA. Other modifications to CSEA equipment in the past decade have included passage of the spinal needle through a 'back-eye' rather than the bevel of the epidural needle, standardization of the protrusion distance of the spinal needle (12–15 mm), and the introduction of locking devices to prevent displacement of the spinal needle tip from the subarachnoid space after dural penetration.

7.6.2 Advantages and disadvantages of CSEA for cesarean section

It can be argued that the combination of both SA (for rapid onset and quality of block) and EA (for hemodynamic stability and flexibility, plus postoperative opioid analgesia), is the ideal regional anesthetic for CS (*Table 7.14*). CSEA combines the advantages of SA with the flexibility afforded by epidural catheterization. This increases its reliability compared with EA or SA, with a very low incidence of perioperative conversion to GA because of inadequate anesthetic quality.

A variety of initial concerns about the CSEA approach have proven unfounded. Metallic particle fragmentation due to friction and shearing of the needles, with implantation into the vertebral canal, does not occur. Unrecognized epidural catheter penetration or later migration through the dural hole made by the spinal needle might result in high spinal block or severe respiratory depression after injection of epidural drugs, but these are rare events clinically. Based on cadaver and epiduroscopic studies, catheter movement from the epidural to the subarachnoid space only appears possible after dural damage by the epidural needle or multiple passes of large spinal needles. Rotation of the epidural needle within the space after penetration of the ligamentum flavum is inadvisable, because it increases the accidental dural puncture rate.

The transdural drug transport of epidural drugs into the subarachnoid compartment during CSEA depends principally on the size of

Table 7.14 Advantages of combined spinal-epidural anesthesia (CSEA) for cesarean section

- Lower failure rate (<1%) compared with spinal (1–4%) or epidural (4–10%) anesthesia
- Speed of onset and quality of spinal anesthesia
- Lower risk of local anesthetic toxicity than epidural anesthesia
- If desired, initial low spinal block, augmented or extended to mid-thoracic level with epidural local anesthetic (sequential CSEA)
- Better hemodynamic stability than spinal anesthesia (sequential CSEA)
- Ability to prolong anesthesia using epidural local anesthetic increments
- High quality postoperative epidural analgesia
- Lower post-dural puncture headache risk

the dural hole, the drug lipophilicity, and pressure dynamics in the vertebral canal. When small gauge pencil-point spinal needles are used, epidural LA spread in a caudal direction may increase, but this does not appear clinically significant and, experimentally, epidural contrast medium does not enter the subarachnoid space. Although drugs do pass into the CSF, only a very small percentage of even poorly lipid-soluble (hydrophilic) drugs like morphine cross into CSF.

The risk of meningitis must always be considered when the dura is breached; however, the literature suggests epidural abscess (secondary to epidural catheterization) is actually more common, more difficult to treat, and more likely to cause permanent injury. Combined spinal-epidural techniques are very safe, and meningitis has not been documented despite experience with tens of thousands of CSEA cases in many institutions. The incidence of meningitis, which may also follow skin and subcutaneous infection at the epidural site, has been difficult to quantify, but appears to be in the range of 1 in 6–10 000 after obstetric neuraxial block and is associated with a good prognosis.

7.6.3 Technique for combined spinal epidural anesthesia

The double interspace insertion method for CSEA has two principal advantages, one being that the epidural catheter can be placed first, avoiding the potential problem if it proves difficult to thread after injection of spinal solution in a needle-through-needle method. Rarely, when a high vertical abdominal incision, rather than Pfannensteil, is needed for CS, the epidural catheter can be positioned in a higher interspace (or even a low thoracic level) before conventional low-lumbar subarachnoid block. This optimizes delivery of local anesthetic and opioid for postoperative analgesia.

Patient preference, convenience, and the commercial availability of a number of purpose-designed kits, have seen the single intervertebral space needle-through-needle method come to dominate, however. It is faster and more comfortable for the patient, the disadvantages being that testing of epidural catheter position is problematic, and should the catheter prove difficult to insert through the epidural needle, the distribution of subarachnoid drug may be restricted. There are other single interspace insertion methods, including a needle-beside-needle technique, and dual needles that allow the epidural catheter to be sited prior to performing SA.

For CS, CSEA is usually performed by inserting the epidural needle at $L_3/_4$ or below, passing a long spinal needle through the epidural needle until free flow of CSF is confirmed, stabilizing the spinal needle and then injecting the spinal solution. The required protrusion distance varies with the level of insertion, flexion of the spinal column, midline entry and the direction of the spinal needle, but in most CSEA kits is up to 13–15 mm. When performed with the patient seated, efflux of CSF is more rapid. In up to 10% of parturients a small amount of cerebrospinal fluid becomes visible in the epidural needle hub, but should not be interpreted as evidence of accidental dural puncture. Failure to enter the subarachnoid space occurs in about 4–5% of insertions (see Section 7.8 and *Figure 7.9* below). Following withdrawal of the spinal needle, the epidural catheter is inserted and secured.

7.6.4 Management of CSEA for cesarean section

There are two principal methods of CSEA for CS, the first using conventional spinal drug doses (e.g. bupivacaine 10–12.5 mg) to establish SA, with the epidural catheter employed only if required to extend sensory block in the case of inadequate block. To prolong anesthesia in the situation of prolonged surgery (more than 90–120 minutes) and for postoperative analgesia, the epidural catheter is employed. The second method is a sequential CSEA technique, with lower dose of LA used for SA, and epidural LA administered incrementally to extend the block to the desired level (*Figure 7.8*). At the expense of slower onset, sequential CSEA

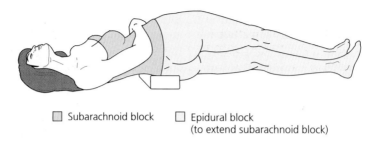

☐ Subarachnoid block   ☐ Epidural block
(to extend subarachnoid block)

Figure 7.8 Sequential combined spinal-epidural approach, with limited spinal block extended by increments of epidural local anesthetic. Reproduced from Rawal, N. *et al.* (2000) The combined spinal-epidural technique. In: *Textbook of Obstetric Anesthesia* (Birnbach, D.J., Gatt, S.P., Datta, S. eds.), p.167, with permission from the publisher Churchill Livingstone.

provides good operative conditions, a low incidence of hypotension and nausea (both 10–30% versus up to 50–70% with conventional SA or CSEA), using very small doses of subarachnoid bupivacaine and fentanyl (e.g. 5 mg bupivacaine plus 25 µg fentanyl).

There is circumstantial evidence that CSEA reduces the risk of accidental dural puncture with the epidural needle. Post-dural puncture headache rates as low as 0.13% have been reported

7.7 Continuous spinal anesthesia

Continuous spinal anesthesia (CSA) is infrequently used in most countries except parts of Continental Europe. The technique of CSA was first introduced using a malleable needle in 1940 and has been refined extensively since. The advantage of CSA is greater control, reducing the likelihood of hemodynamic instability often seen with SA. This feature makes CSA particularly attractive where rapid reduction in afterload is dangerous (for example, parturients with severe pulmonary hypertension, aortic or subaortic stenosis); when access to the epidural space is difficult or impossible; or when spread of the spinal solution is unpredictable (for example, severe spinal deformity or previous spinal surgery). Cardiac filling and output can be preserved without the use of inotropes or vasopressors.

Plain bupivacaine 0.5% in 0.5–1 ml increments is most often used and subarachnoid opioid may be added. A renewal of interest in CSA in the USA was dampened by the withdrawal of microspinal catheters less than 24 gauge by the Federal Drug Authority in 1992, after reports of cauda equina syndrome; this complication appeared to arise because of maldistribution of hyperbaric lidocaine and local neurotoxicity. New styles of small gauge intrathecal catheter are commercially available in some countries. These appear to be associated with better mixing of LA and CSF and some are designed to minimize post-dural puncture headache (PDPH) (see Section 15.1) by introducing the catheter over the spinal needle (rather than through it).

The occasional use of CSA in obstetrics has mainly followed the deliberate insertion of an epidural catheter intrathecally, either electively or after accidental dural puncture. This approach has become more popular for analgesia when dural puncture occurs during labor, and should the parturient require later CS, a CSA technique is used. Despite some attractions, CSA has a number of significant disadvantages that preclude its routine use, the most obvious being a high incidence of PDPH when performed with epidural needles and catheters. Neuraxial infection is a concern, although it is not a significant risk with short-term catheterization. CSA is unlikely to become popular if technical problems and PDPH remain consistently higher than alternative regional techniques. It can be very useful in selected patient populations, however (see Section 11.7.3).

7.8 Failure of regional anesthesia

7.8.1 Introduction

In a recent survey conducted in the UK, conversion of regional anesthesia to GA occurred in about 10% of CSs, although the conversion rate of SA to GA was less than 2%. Conversion rates varied widely, possibly reflecting the organization of services and level of anesthetic expertise and supervision. Failure is usually due to technical problems. After insertion, epidural catheter tips are mainly located in the lateral epidural space or near the proximal intervertebral foramen, rather than in the posterior (or anterior) epidural space. Occasionally patients have anatomical variants such as dural folds and tissue barriers. It is thus not surprising that, although epidural solution usually spreads bilaterally to cover all segmental nerve roots, sometimes unilateral, asymmetric, or restricted spread occurs or block of larger roots such as L_5 and S_1 is inadequate. Spinal needles may not reach or may be misdirected or deflect past the dural sac (*Figure 7.9*), and during injection into the subarachnoid space minimal movement of the needle tip may result in failure to deposit the desired drug dose intrathecally.

Most studies, depending on the size and nature of the hospital, report overall conversion rates of 0.5–4% for SA and 4–13% for EA. The reliability and quality of spinal techniques, and their lower failure rate, are principal reasons for their popularity.

7.8.2 Failure of regional anesthesia due to intraoperative pain

Introduction and assessment

During EA performed with LA alone, visceral pain can be frequent (20–50%). Dramatic improvement in the quality of block (incidence of intraoperative pain 5–10%) follows

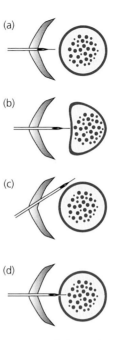

Figure 7.9 Position and direction of the spinal needle during combined spinal-epidural anesthesia. (a)–(c) result in technical failure. Similar mechanisms may apply for failure of spinal anesthesia. Reproduced from Rawal, N. *et al.* (2000) The combined spinal-epidural technique. In: *Textbook of Obstetric Anesthesia* (Birnbach, D.J., Gatt, S.P., Datta, S. eds.), p.176, with permission from the publisher Churchill Livingstone.

the routine addition of opioid adjuncts such as fentanyl, and better understanding of block requirements and assessment. The resurgence of SA, especially with added intrathecal fentanyl, sufentanil or morphine, has led to greater confidence that the parturient will be pain free. The likelihood of discomfort with SA is less than 1 in 30–40. In a blinded comparison of EA and CSEA, both techniques were highly effective, although pain was more likely and of greater severity with EA.

Intraoperative pain is not uncommon during regional anesthesia for CS, so all patients should be forewarned and complaints of pain responded to. Unrelieved pain is a source of anxiety for all concerned and poor communication, especially failure to act, is a potential reason for litigation.

Before starting surgery, it is mandatory to test the upper level sensory block; confirmation of adequate sensory block (bilateral spread to mid thoracic level) prior to surgery is reassuring before surgical incision. If loss of light touch extends above T_5, intraoperative pain is very unlikely, even when intraspinal opioid is omitted. When unilateral or asymmetric block remains unresolved, an alternative method must be instituted. In an occasional urgent situation when epidural catheter function in labor has been good, it is acceptable to proceed with emergency CS when anesthesia has reached above T_{10}, but sensory block to T_4 is still developing.

Initial evaluation of intraoperative pain during CS requires checking of pain intensity and the current level of anesthesia, and exclusion of surgical or epidural complications. Pain may arise from inadequate anesthesia (block below T_2, regression of block and incomplete block of L_5, S_1 and S_2) or due to subcostal or referred shoulder tip pain (from subdiaphragmatic fluid after delivery). An attempt to diagnose the etiology not only assists with treatment, but also can provide a prognosis to guide further management. Pain at skin incision is clearly undesirable and unless sufficient time is available to defer, conversion to GA is extremely likely. Breakthrough pain, especially at delivery and thereafter, may be due to an inadequate upper sensory level for the degree of visceral stimulation (peritoneal pain mediated by the greater splanchnic nerve may occasionally require T_1 block) or inadequate low block of bladder and uterosacral ligaments. Referred pain to the chest or shoulder mediated by the phrenic nerve C_3–C_5 occurs in up to 5% due to diaphragmatic irritation by blood or amniotic fluid and may respond to head-up positioning (5–10 degrees) or counter-irritation by vigorous shoulder tip massage. Precordial pain is usually referred visceral pain, but ischemic and other pathological pain should be considered.

Management

Mild breakthrough pain can be managed by a sympathetic expectant approach, reassuring

Table 7.15 Drug treatment of intraoperative pain during cesarean section under regional anesthesia

- Intravenous fentanyl 1–2 µg/kg or alfentanil 5–10 µg/kg
- Nitrous oxide 50% in oxygen
- Midazolam (or similar) 1–3 mg
- Epidural fentanyl 50–100 µg or sufentanil 20–30 µg
- Epidural local anesthetic (2% lidocaine with epinephrine or 3% 2-chloroprocaine) 3–5 ml increments
- Ketamine 5–10 mg increments (maximum 0.5 mg/kg)
- Surgical injection of local anesthetic into wounds or the peritoneal cavity

the parturient the discomfort is transient while awaiting spontaneous resolution. Analgesia with low dose intravenous opioid or nitrous oxide inhalation, and occasionally anxiolysis may be helpful (*Table 7.15*). The level of sensory block should be augmented if necessary, with further epidural LA or opioid. More severe pain may require larger doses of intravenous opioid, or intravenous ketamine. The latter is given with great caution, in 5–10 mg increments, titrated against response. Over-sedation with loss of consciousness and airway reflexes are worrisome possibilities, and a warning about psychotomimetic side effects and amnesia should be given. The obstetrician should be asked to be gentle, and LA can be instilled intraperitoneally, applied topically, or infiltrated into the wound. Depending on the stage of surgery, discussion of conversion to GA may be necessary.

7.8.3 Failure of regional anesthesia due to complications

Unexpected complications of regional anesthesia may require resuscitative intervention (*Table 7.16*). At CS, this may require urgent induction of anesthesia or conversion to GA. Adequate regional anesthesia is associated with effects on respiratory function, mainly reduced peak expiratory pressures and flows. The parturient may notice mild dyspnea or

Table 7.16 Complications that may require conversion of regional anesthesia to general anesthesia

High spinal, subdural or epidural block
- Cervical or cranial nerve block with impaired swallowing and phonation
- Thoracic motor block with significant impairment of ventilation
- Unconsciousness, respiratory depression

Severe syncope or cardiovascular collapse

Incorrect drug administration

Surgical complications
- Massive hemorrhage
- Amniotic, massive air or pulmonary embolism

Table 7.17 Disadvantages of general anesthesia for cesarean section

Reduced maternal safety
- Difficult or failed tracheal intubation
- Esophageal intubation
- Pulmonary aspiration of gastric content
- Hemodynamic instability
- Adverse physiological effects in some medical conditions
- Increased thromboembolic risk
- Increased intraoperative blood loss

Lower parental satisfaction
- Missed experience of childbirth
- Lower quality of postoperative analgesia
- Maternal awareness

Neonatal effects
- Increased neonatal sedation
- Greater exposure of breast fed infant to opioid analgesics

reduced power to cough, especially with sensory block to pinprick above T_2. In most cases, arterial oxygen tension remains normal, so reassurance and monitoring of ventilation and oxygenation will suffice.

High regional block can arise through several mechanisms, including exaggerated spread or inadvertent injection of drugs into the incorrect space (for example, subarachnoid injection of epidural solution). Additionally, patient variability is such that segmental spread of sensory and motor block is never entirely predictable, especially with techniques such as single-shot SA. Titrated injection techniques (EA, CSEA, CSA) also offer no guaranteed predictability.

7.9 General anesthesia for cesarean section

7.9.1 Indications
General anesthesia has a diminishing role (see Section 7.2 above and *Table 7.17*), but it remains essential for true emergency CS, and it has distinct benefits in a number of situations (*Tables 7.18* and *7.19*). One of the most common indications for GA is deteriorating fetal condition (nonreassuring fetal heart rate trace) or potential sudden death (cord prolapse). In practice, 'fetal distress' is rarely unheralded and GA can usually be avoided by early anesthetic involvement, including the use of

Table 7.18 Advantages of general anesthesia for cesarean section

- Speed for emergency surgery
- Reliability, reproducibility, and control
- Avoidance of dural puncture
- Greater hemodynamic stability in some cardiac conditions when urgent CS is required
- Safety when regional anesthesia is contraindicated

epidural analgesia in labor for high-risk parturients. Indeed, the American College of Obstetricians and Gynecologists has acknowledged the dangers inherent with GA for emergency CS: '. . . cesarean deliveries that are performed for a non-reassuring fetal heart rate pattern do not necessarily preclude the use of regional anesthesia'. Many tertiary units have reduced the use of GA for CS to less than 10% by embracing this philosophy, by means of education and improved service provision.

In both elective and urgent settings, indications for GA include patient refusal, unfavorable risk-benefit assessment for complications of regional anesthesia, failed regional anesthesia and certain maternal disease (*Table 7.18*). Patient refusal is most often based on fear of

Table 7.19 Situations in which general anesthesia may be preferable to regional anesthesia

Emergency CS – immediate delivery desirable for fetal survival

Anatomic abnormality
- Failed regional anesthesia or severe back pathology

High level of concern about risk of serious infective complications (e.g. epidural abscess, meningitis or encephalitis)
- Insertion site skin lesions/infection, severe sepsis, active systemic viral disease

High level of concern about risk of intraspinal hematoma
- Uncorrected or uncontrolled bleeding and dilutional coagulopathy
- Severe thrombocytopenia, coagulation disorder or disturbance; therapeutic anticoagulant or antithrombotic therapy, inherited or acquired bleeding disorders

High level of concern about hemodynamic consequences of regional block
- Obstetric hemorrhage with cardiovascular instability
- High-risk of anticipated massive hemorrhage (placenta accreta, increta and percreta; anterior placenta previa and previous myometrial scar)
- Pulmonary hypertension; severe valvular stenosis; cardiac failure

High level of concern about potential effects of regional block on the central nervous system
- Raised intracranial pressure

The uncooperative patient
- Recent or imminent eclampsia
- Severe anxiety, psychiatric or other mental disturbance
- Refusal of regional anesthetic

backache or needle insertion and may be amenable to reassurance. 'Contraindication to regional block' can rarely be used to justify GA, because of the safety of central neuraxial block. Allergy to LA is very rare, but alternative drugs can be used for regional anesthesia (for example, meperidine for spinal anesthesia). An individual risk-benefit assessment is warranted in some maternal conditions, including the hereditary and acquired bleeding and coagulation disorders, primary viral

infection, severe back pathology, and certain neurological, neuromuscular and cardiac disorders (see *Chapter 13*).

7.9.2 General anesthetic technique and drugs

History

The problems of aspiration pneumonitis, fetal depression, and obstetric hemorrhage led to the abandonment of face-mask techniques and the adoption of rapid sequence induction by the 1960s (*Figure 7.10*). The introduction of volatile inhalational anesthetics (such as halothane) in the 1970s, led to a consistent approach to GA technique in most developed countries (*Table 7.20*). Interestingly, rapid sequence induction with application of cricoid pressure is considered mandatory in the USA, UK, and Australasia, yet in France high standards of maternal safety are maintained without the use of cricoid pressure at GA for elective CS.

The pre-induction phase

The pre-induction phase (see also Section 7.2 above) is used to address the aim of rapidly securing control of the airway (*Figures 7.10 and 7.11*) and prevention of hypoxemia. Several activities may need to be performed over a

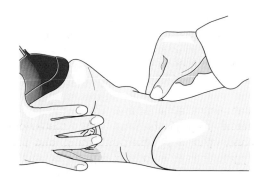

Figure 7.10 Application of cricoid pressure to prevent regurgitation of gastric content into the pharynx. Reproduced with permission of The Lancet, London, UK from Sellick, B.A. (1961) Cricoid pressure to control regurgitation of stomach contents during induction of anaesthesia. *Lancet* **2**: 405.

Table 7.20 Typical anesthetic drugs for general anesthesia for cesarean section

- Sodium pentothal 4–5 mg/kg intravenous bolus
- Succinylcholine 1–1.5 mg/kg intravenous bolus
- Isoflurane (or sevoflurane) and nitrous oxide 50% in oxygen until near completion of surgery
- Rocuronium (0.2–0.3 mg/kg) or atracurium (0.2–0.3 mg/kg) intravenous bolus prn or succinylcholine infusion (1–4 mg/min)
- Morphine (0.1–0.2 mg/kg) or fentanyl (3–5 μg/kg) intravenous bolus post-delivery
- Oxytocin 5 iu intravenous bolus post-delivery
- Neostigmine 0.25 mg /kg and glycopyrrolate 0.4 mg intravenous bolus (near completion of surgery)

Table 7.21 Preparing the parturient for general anesthesia for emergency cesarean section

- Prepare induction and neuromuscular blocking drugs, airway and ancillary equipment
- Secure good intravenous access
- Obtain brief patient and obstetric history and perform brief examination, especially airway
- Ensure nonparticulate antacid (e.g. 0.3 M sodium citrate 30 ml) has been administered
- Commence monitoring and pre-oxygenation
- Optimize patient position
- Pelvic tilt to minimize aortocaval compression
- Thorax, head and neck support to optimize access to airway and laryngoscopic view
- Anesthetic assistant ready to apply cricoid pressure

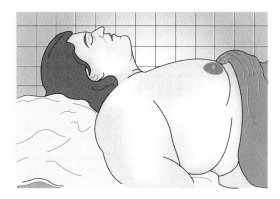

Figure 7.11 Positioning of the obese parturient to improve access to the neck and mouth and the view at direct laryngoscopy at induction of anesthesia. Note elevation of the upper torso and head and neck.

Table 7.22 Strategies and planning for possible difficult intubation

Aim for regional anesthesia
- Early epidural catheter in labor

Promote early obstetrician referral of parturients when difficulty is anticipated

Plan airway management for general anesthesia
- Consider awake fiberoptic intubation; other awake intubation techniques if airway assessed as difficult
- Consider post-induction intubation method, avoiding aspiration and paralysis until adequate ventilation with mask confirmed

Obtain appropriate equipment, drugs and assistance for induction phase

Optimize patient position with pillows under upper thorax and head

Learn and practice a 'failed intubation drill'

Positioning

The uterus must be displaced from the IVC and aorta with a wedge placed under the right hip or table tilt to prevent aortocaval compression and fetal compromise prior to delivery. Left tilt (5–15%) is more effective than right, and it may be difficult to avoid aortocaval compression in some parturients, especially those with a large abdominal mass (for example, multiple pregnancy or polyhydramnios).

short time frame (*Tables 7.21* and *7.22*): antacid prophylaxis, large bore intravenous access, optimal patient positioning, and pre-oxygenation are essential. Drugs to obtund the response to laryngoscopy and intubation may be considered (*Table 7.23*). This strategy is advisable for patients with severe hypertension (e.g. severe preeclampsia, Section 9.6.2), cardiac disease (e.g. valvular stenoses, ischemic heart disease, Section 13.3.2) and some neurological disease (e.g. raised intracranial pressure, Section 13.5.4).

Table 7.23 Drugs for obtunding the response to intubation at cesarean section

Opioid
- alfentanil 15–30 μg/kg
- fentanyl 5–10 μg/kg
- remifentanil 0.5–1 mg/kg

Magnesium sulfate
- 40–60 mg/kg (depending on previous magnesium loading)

Beta-blocker
- esmolol 0.5–1 mg/kg

Vasodilator
- hydalazine 5–20 mg
- labetolol 5–25 mg
- nitroglycerin infusion 0.25–3 μg/kg min
- sodium nitroprusside 0.1–2 μg/kg min

Local anesthetic
- lidocaine 1 mg/kg

Positioning of the upper body should facilitate the application of cricoid pressure, and insertion of the laryngoscope should optimize the view at direct laryngoscopy. As well as flexion of the cervical spine with extension of the atlanto-occipital joint ('sniffing position'), the obese parturient in particular should have the upper thorax elevated and the head supported with pillows (*Figure 7.11*). The cricoid cartilage should be identified by the assistant, to minimize the risk of distortion of laryngeal and hypopharyngeal anatomy during intubation.

Preoxygenation
At the onset of apnea, arterial oxygen tension falls at approximately twice the normal non-pregnant rate, because of increased oxygen consumption and reduced oxygen storage in the functional residual capacity of the lung. Hypoxemia is compounded by small airway closure at normal tidal volume in the supine position, particularly in the obese and/or smoking parturient. Maternal oxygen tension below 100 mmHg during GA is associated with adverse fetal outcomes (lower Apgar score and time to sustained respiration). Preoxygenation to maximize maternal and fetal arterial oxygen tension and increase oxygen storage buys valuable time while securing the airway after induction and paralysis. Oxygen tension above 300 mmHg is ideal and achieved by deep inhalation of 100% inspired oxygen through a close fitting face mask and nonrebreathing circuit for about 3 minutes. In an emergency, four to six vital capacity breaths raise oxygen tension to similar levels of about 350 mmHg and denitrogenates the lungs satisfactorily (expired oxygen more than 95%).

The induction phase
In addition to airway protection to prevent gastric aspiration, adequate ventilation and oxygenation, adequate anesthesia, and maintenance of normal placental perfusion are important considerations. In order to minimize fetal drug exposure, hypnotic adjuncts such as intravenous benzodiazepines (e.g. midazolam) and opioids (e.g. fentanyl) are not administered routinely prior to intravenous induction. These and some other drugs (see *Table 7.23*) are reserved for specific circumstances. If used, the doctor responsible for neonatal resuscitation must be advised so that potential fetal effects can be assessed and appropriate antagonists (naloxone for opioids, flumazenil for benzodiazepines) administered.

Intravenous anesthetics
Based on a good safety record (in preventing maternal awareness and neonatal depression), sodium pentothal 4–5 mg/kg has remained the intravenous anesthetic of choice for CS for several decades. Despite rapid placental transfer that continues for up to 10 minutes, IV sodium pentothal does not reach fetal brain levels sufficient to sedate the newborn, due to the rapid fall in the materno-fetal concentration gradient after bolus injection, fetal liver uptake and dilution within the fetal circulation.

Despite propofol's popularity and advantages in many other settings, it has not generally replaced sodium pentothal. A flatter dose–response relationship makes prediction of a reliable induction dose at rapid sequence induction more difficult. After bolus administration of propofol, 2 mg/kg, bolus, autonomic signs of 'light' anesthesia are more common than after sodium pentothal. Both a 2.5 mg/kg bolus and total intravenous anesthesia with propofol at 6–9 mg/kg/h have been associated with some neonatal depression. Pain on injection and excitation (e.g. hiccups) may occur, but the intubation response is obtunded more effectively, and recovery similar or slightly more rapid to sodium pentothal. Propofol induction should be reserved for specific patients, such as for severe asthmatics, in whom airway reflexes are depressed more effectively, or parturients at risk of malignant hyperthermia, for whom total intravenous anesthesia is indicated.

Compared with sodium pentothal ketamine (1.5 mg/kg IV) is an effective agent characterized by a good maternal and fetal safety profile, hemodynamic stability (although sympathetic stimulation renders ketamine less suitable if hypertension is undesirable) and low rates of intraoperative awareness without recall (see Chapter 15). Nevertheless, it is rarely used in developed countries, because, although less frequent in the pregnant woman, psychotomimetic side effects are undesirable. Elsewhere, ketamine (1.5–2 mg/kg IV or 5–10 mg/kg IM) is valuable and sometimes used as a sole agent, taking advantage of its profound analgesic properties and reduced depression of upper airway reflexes. Other potential induction drugs are etomidate 0.3 mg/kg and midazolam (0.2–0.3 mg/kg). Disadvantages include pain on injection, myoclonus, postoperative nausea and suppression of neonatal adaptive adrenal responses with etomidate, and neonatal depression and slower recovery from midazolam.

Rapid sequence induction, cricoid pressure and muscle relaxants

As patient consciousness wanes, the lower and upper esophageal pressures decline and cricoid pressure should be applied, occluding the esophagus against the cervical vertebrae (see *Figure 7.9*). This is uncomfortable and can cause retching, so light pressure is increased with loss of consciousness; about 30 Newtons

(3 kg) force is probably sufficient to prevent passive regurgitation. Improper application may lead to potential regurgitation (inadequate force) or laryngeal displacement, airway obstruction and neck flexion that makes intubation more difficult (excessive force or inaccurate finger position). Once the airway is secured, cricoid pressure is released, although in the event of difficult intubation, and provided depth of anesthesia is adequate, the temporary release or reapplication of cricoid pressure is reasonable if it assists with airway management. A two-handed technique supporting at the back of the cervical spine may be better than a single-hand technique, but is less popular.

Rapid paralysis of the muscles of the upper airway, including the larynx, is achieved by the use of a rapid-acting muscle relaxant. The depolarizing muscle relaxant succinylcholine (suxamethonium), 1–1.5 mg/kg remains the drug of choice. Excellent intubating conditions result within 60 seconds and spontaneous reversal (due to plasma pseudocholinesterase enzymatic metabolism) follows in 4–10 minutes. During pregnancy, an increase in the volume of distribution is balanced by a fall in plasma pseudocholinesterase metabolism, such that duration is similar to the nonpregnant state. Like other highly ionized neuromuscular blockers, placental transfer is minimal. Myalgia is less common during pregnancy (incidence 3%), possibly due to hormonal influences, contrasting with an incidence of over 20% in ambulatory patients. Undesirable features are prolonged duration with atypical or low levels of pseudocholinesterase, bradycardia with readministration, and several contraindications (especially certain muscle and neuromuscular disorders and hyperkalemic states).

The search for a nondepolarizing blocker with similar characteristics has been a 'Holy Grail' of modern anesthesia. Rocuronium is an aminosteroid nondepolarizing neuromuscular blocker of rapid onset (satisfactory intubating conditions in 60–90 seconds after 0.6 mg/kg) that is free of cardiovascular effects, and has become an option when succinylcholine is contraindicated, despite more prolonged duration. The new nondepolarizer rapacuronium (2.5 mg/kg) appeared promising, combining rapid speed of onset to succinylcholine with short duration of action (return of adequate neuromuscular function in 15–30 minutes). Due to the effects of histamine release the future of this drug is currently in doubt. A longer duration remains a potential disadvantage of neuro-precursor blockers in the difficult intubation scenario.

Following intubation, the endotracheal tube cuff is inflated, and esophageal intubation and endobronchial intubation are excluded by auscultation, direct observation, and capnography.

The maintenance phase

Prior to delivery, the maintenance of normal physiological parameters, fetal gas exchange and prevention of maternal awareness are necessary. Muscle relaxation can be maintained with small doses of a nondepolarizing relaxant of short to medium duration (for example vecuronium 0.01–0.02 mg/kg, atracurium 0.2–0.3 mg/kg, or rocuronium 0.1–0.2 mg/kg) or succinylcholine infusion. Rapid and complete reversal of neuromuscular block at the end of the operation is the aim, so that awake extubation occurs in the presence of full airway protection and normal respiratory function.

Fetal and neonatal condition

The uterine vascular bed is maximally dilated at term, but GA can reduce placental blood flow by up to a third due to vasoconstriction (secondary to catecholamine release in response to laryngoscopy and intubation), or reduced cardiac output (due to anesthetic-induced myocardial depression). Ventilation should be regulated to maintain a normal arterial carbon dioxide (CO_2) tension (28–32 mmHg or 4–4.5 kPa at term). Both hypoventilation with hypercarbia and hyperventilation with severe hypocarbia adversely affect fetal gas exchange. Fetal acidosis may occur if maternal pCO_2 falls below 25 mmHg, due to uterine artery vasoconstriction and impaired oxygen release with maternal alkalosis.

Good maternal and fetal oxygenation (equilibration of oxygen tension occurs in 3–6 minutes) is maintained by administration of a high maternal inspired oxygen fraction, although the optimum percentage is controversial. Convention recommends 50% (with nitrous oxide), based on a ceiling effect with maternal O_2 above 300 mmHg (*Figure 7.12*). However, in severe fetal hypoxemia, although the dose–response relationship may not be linear, 100% oxygen is recommended despite a lack of evidence that it improves outcome. With this approach, increased inhalational anesthetic is required to avoid both an inadequate depth of anesthesia leading to maternal recall, and the vasoconstrictive effects of rising catecholamines on uterine blood flow.

Adequate depth of anesthesia and inhalational anesthetics

The period of volatile anesthetic uptake while intravenous anesthetic (sodium pentothal) effect wanes has the highest risk of inadequate depth of anesthesia. Most volatile anesthetics (halothane, isoflurane, sevoflurane and desflurane) are suitable and widely used, usually in

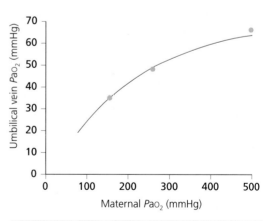

Figure 7.12 Scatter graph showing relationship between maternal arterial oxygen tension (PaO_2) and umbilical venous PaO_2 during general anesthesia for cesarean section. Reproduced with permission of Oxford University Press from Baraka, A. (1970) Correlation between maternal and foetal PO_2 and PCO_2 during caesarean section. *Br. J. Anaesth.* **42**: 435.

conjunction with nitrous oxide. Pregnancy reduces minimum alveolar concentration (MAC) by about 25%. Prior to delivery, volatile anesthetic end-tidal concentration is kept to about 0.5 MAC. Increased levels may be associated with reduced uterine tone (and increased blood loss), hypotension and poorer neonatal outcome. However, it should be noted that conscious recall rates at 0.5 MAC are above 1%, and blood loss is not increased at 1 MAC volatile anesthetic. With transient initial 'overpressure' (high inspired concentration of isoflurane (~2%) or sevoflurane (~3%) to rapidly achieve at least 0.5 MAC, which is then maintained), the incidence of recall ('awareness') can be reduced to less than 1%. Isoflurane and sevoflurane have lower blood-gas partition coefficients than halothane, ensuring more rapid uptake, and agent concentration monitoring allows adequate alveolar concentration to be rapidly obtained and adjusted for adequate depth of anesthesia. Equilibration with the fetal circulation approaches 90% for nitrous oxide in 15–20 minutes (but only 60% for the volatile anesthetics) and may cause neonatal sedation. 'Induction-to-delivery' times of less than 10 minutes are optimal, although more prolonged exposure to inhalational anesthetics does not adversely effect neonatal parameters in the absence of hypotension, aortocaval compression, or low inspired oxygen fraction. A more important determinant of neonatal condition is the 'uterine incision-to-delivery' interval, due to the impact of uterine manipulation on placental and fetal blood flow. Delays of over 90 seconds (or 180 seconds under regional anesthesia) lead to acidosis and lower Apgar scores.

Following delivery, intravenous opioids are administered for intra- and postoperative analgesia. Choices include fentanyl 3–5 μg/kg or morphine 0.1–0.15 mg/kg. Maintenance of muscle relaxation facilitates surgical closure and control of ventilation. Nitrous oxide concentration can be increased to 70% if tolerated, which may permit the concentration of volatile agent to be decreased. The object is to attain early arousal (to permit awake extubation) in the presence of an analgesic plasma opioid concentrations that provides comfort and a smooth transition to postoperative analgesia. Oxytocic drugs are also administered (see Chapter 14) to facilitate uterine contraction. Aspirating the stomach contents is recommended during emergency CS, recognizing that solid or semi-solid matter from recent ingestion will not be removed.

The extubation phase

Near completion of surgery, volatile anesthetics should be discontinued to facilitate awake extubation that minimizes the risk of regurgitation and aspiration on emergence. Unless monitoring confirms satisfactory spontaneous recovery (e.g. the ratio of the fourth to first twitch in a train-of-four stimulus is greater than 0.7, or there is no post-tetanic fade), neuromuscular block should be reversed. Once adequate spontaneous ventilation has resumed and after airway suctioning, the parturient is extubated awake, an oxygen mask is applied, and suction apparatus kept available during initial recovery.

Further reading

American Society of Anesthesiologists Task Force on Obstetrical Anesthesia (1999) Practice guidelines for obstetrical anesthesia. *Anesthesiology* **90**: 600–611.

Aveling, A. and Howell, P. (1999) Heavy bupivacaine has no advantage over plain bupivacaine in spinal anaesthesia for caesarean section. *Int. J. Obstet. Anesth.* **8**: 260–265.

Barnardo, P.D. and Jenkins, J.G. (2000) Failed tracheal intubation in obstetrics: a 6-year review in a UK region. *Anaesthesia* **55**: 685–694.

Ben-David, B., Miller, G., Gavriel, R. and Gurevitch, A. (2000) Low-dose bupivacaine-fentanyl spinal anesthesia for cesarean delivery. *Reg. Anesth. Pain Med.* **25**: 235–239.

Blumgart, C.H., Ryall, D., Dennison, B. and Thompson Hill, L.M. (1992) Mechanism of extension of spinal anaesthesia by epidural injection of local anaesthetic. *Br. J. Anaesth.* **69**: 457–460.

Boldt, J. (2000) Volume replacement in the surgical patient – does the type of solution make a difference? *Br. J. Anaesth.* **84**: 783–793.

Capogna, G. and Celleno, D. (1994) Improving epidural anesthesia during cesarean section:

causes of maternal discomfort or pain during surgery. *Int. J. Obstet. Anesth.* **3**: 149–152.

Dahlgren, G., Hultstrand, C., Jakobsson, J. *et al.* (1997) Intrathecal sufentanil, fentanil, or placebo added to bupivacaine for cesarean section. *Anesth. Analg.* **85**: 1288–1293.

Davies, S.J., Paech, M.J., Welch, H., Evans, S. F. and Pavy, T.J.G. (1997) Maternal experience during epidural or combined spinal-epidural anesthesia for cesarean section: a prospective, randomized trial. *Anesth. Analg.* **85**: 607–613.

Engelhardt, T. and Webster, N.R. (1999) Pulmonary aspiration of gastric contents in anaesthesia. *Br. J. Anaesth.* **83**: 453–460.

Fan, S-Z., Susetio, L., Wang, Y-P., Cheng, Y-J. and Liu, C.-C. (1994) Low dose of intrathecal hyperbaric bupivacaine combined with epidural lidocaine for cesarean section – a balanced block technique. *Anesth. Analg.* **78**: 474–477.

Finucane, B.T. (1994) Spinal anesthesia for cesarean delivery. The dosage dilemma. *Reg. Anesth.* **20**: 87–89.

Gaiser, R.R., Cheek, T.G. and Gutsche, B.B. (1994) Epidural lidocaine versus 2-chloroprocaine for fetal distress requiring urgent cesarean section. *Int. J. Obstet. Anesth.* **3**: 208–210.

Greiff, J.M.C., Tordoff, S.G., Griffiths, R. and May, A.E. (1994) Acid aspiration prophylaxis in 202 obstetric anaesthetic units in the UK. *Int. J. Obstet. Anesth.* **3**: 137–142.

Hawkins, J.L., Gibbs, C.P., Orleans, M., Martin-Salvaj, G. and Beaty, B. (1997) Obstetric anesthesia work force survey, 1981 versus 1992. *Anesthesiology* **87**: 135–143.

Hawkins, J.L, Koonin, L.M, Palmer, S.K. and Gibbs, C.P. (1997) Anesthesia-related deaths during obstetric delivery in the United States, 1979–1990. *Anesthesiology* **86**: 277–284.

Lussos, S.A. and Datta, S. (1992) Anesthesia for cesarean delivery. Part II: Epidural anesthesia. Intrathecal and epidural opioids. Venous air embolism. *Int. J. Obstet. Anesth.* **1**: 208–221.

Lussos, S.A. and Datta, S. (1992) Anesthesia for cesarean delivery. Part I: General considerations and spinal anesthesia. *Int. J. Obstet. Anesth.* **1**: 79–91.

Lyons, G. and May A. (1995) Epidural is an outmoded form of regional anaesthesia for elective caesarean section. *Int. J. Obstet. Anesth.* **4**: 34–39.

McIntyre, J.W.R. (1998) Evolution of 20th century attitudes to prophylaxis of pulmonary aspiration during anaesthesia. *Can. J. Anaesth.* **45**: 1024–1030.

Morgan, B.M., Magni, V., Goroszenuik, T. (1990) Anaesthesia for emergency caesarean section. *Br. J. Obstet. Gynaecol.* **97**: 420–424.

Morgan, P. (1995) Spinal anaesthesia in obstetrics. *Can. J. Anaesth.* **42**: 1145–1163.

Muir, H.A. (1994) General anaesthesia for obstetrics, is it obsolete? *Can. J. Anaesth.* **41**: R20–R25.

Mulroy, M.F., Norris, M.C. and Liu, S.S. (1997) Safety steps for epidural injection of local anesthetics: review of the literature and recommendations. *Anesth. Analg.* **85**: 1346–1356.

Norris, M.C. (1990) Patient variables and the subarachnoid spread of hyperbaric bupivacaine in the term parturient. *Anesthesiology* **72**: 478–482.

Paech, M.J. (1996) Obstetric airway management. In: *Airway Management* (Hanowell, L.H., Waldron, R.J. eds.), pp. 343–355. Lippincott-Raven Publishers, Philadelphia.

Paech, M. (2000) Opposer. The use of combined spinal epidural anaesthesia for elective caesarean section is a waste of time and money. *Int. J. Obstet. Anesth.* **10**: 30–35.

Palmer, C.M., Norris, M.C., Guidici, M.C. *et al.* (1990) Incidence of electrocardiographic changes during cesarean delivery under regional anesthesia. *Anesth. Analg.* **70**: 36–43.

Palmer, C.M., Voulgaropoulos, D. and Alves, D. (1995) Subarachnoid fentanyl augments lidocaine spinal anesthesia for cesarean delivery. *Reg. Anesth.* **20**: 389–394.

Peyton, P.J. (1992) Complications of continuous spinal anaesthesia. *Anaesth. Intensive. Care* **20**: 417–438.

Plumer, M.H. and Rottman, R. (1996) How anesthesiologists practice obstetric anesthesia. Responses of practicing obstetric anesthesiologists at the 1993 meeting of the Society for Obstetric Anesthesia and perinatology. *Reg. Anesth.* **21**: 49–60.

Price, M.L., Reynolds, F. and Morgan, B. (1991) Extending epidural blockade for emergency cesarean section. Evaluation of 2% lignocaine with adrenaline. *Int. J. Obstet. Anesth.* **1**: 13–18.

Rawal, N., Van Zundert, A., Holmstrom, B. and Crowhurst, J.A. (1997) Combined spinal-epidural technique. *Reg. Anesth.* **22**: 406–423.

Robson, S.C., Boys, R.J., Rodech, C. and Morgan, B. (1992) Maternal and fetal haemodynamic effects of spinal and extradural anaesthesia for elective caesarean section. *Br. J. Anaesth.* **68**: 54–59.

Rocke, D.A. and Rout, C.C. (1995) Volume preloading, spinal hypotension and Caesarean section. *Br. J. Anaesth.* **75**: 257–259.

Rocke, D.A., Murray, W.B., Rout,C.C. and Gouws, E. (1992) Relative risk analysis of factors associated with difficult intubation in obstetric anesthesia. *Anesthesiology* **77**: 67–73.

Russell, I.F. (1995) Levels of anaesthesia and intra-operative pain at caesarean section under regional block. *Int. J. Obstet. Anesth.* **4**: 71–77.

Schneck, H. and Scheller, M. (2000) Acid aspiration prophylaxis and caesarean section. *Curr. Opin. Anesthesiol.* **13**: 261–265.

Soreide, E., Bjornstad, E. and Steen, P.A. (1996) An audit of perioperative aspiration pneumonitis in gynaecological and obstetric patients. *Acta Anaesthesiol. Scand.* **40**: 14–19.

Tsen, L.C., Pitner, R. and Camann, W.R. (1998) General anesthesia for cesarean section at a tertiary care hospital 1990–1995: indications and implications. *Int. J. Obstet. Anesth.* **7**: 147–152.

Ueyama, H., He, Y.-L., Tanigami, H., Mashimo, T. and Yoshiya, I. (1999) Effects of crystalloid and colloid preload on blood volume in the parturient undergoing spinal anesthesia for elective cesarean section. *Anesthesiology* **91**: 1571–1576.

Weeks, S. (2000) Reflections on hypotension during Cesarean section under spinal anesthesia: do we need to use colloid? *Can. J. Anaesth.* **47**: 607–610.

Chapter 8

Postoperative analgesia

Craig M. Palmer, MD

Contents

8.1 Introduction

Cesarean delivery is the most frequently performed in-patient operation in the United States and probably throughout the world. Given our vast knowledge of postoperative pain management in this population, planning an anesthetic for cesarean delivery should also include planning for adequate postoperative analgesia.

For many years, intramuscular narcotics were the mainstay of analgesia after cesarean delivery, and in some settings they still are. The last two decades, however, have seen a major shift in methods of postoperative analgesia in obstetric patients, due to our improved understanding of CNS pharmacology, and improvements in technology.

8.2 Epidural morphine

In 1979, epidural morphine was reported effective for analgesia in cancer patients. Shortly thereafter, a number of series reported epidural morphine effective for post-cesarean analgesia in doses ranging from 2 to 10 mg.

Analgesia following epidural morphine for post-cesarean analgesia follows a consistent dose–response relationship. As the dose of epidural morphine increases, analgesia improves until the dose reaches about 4 mg (Figures 8.1 and 8.2). Increasing the dose beyond this level does not further improve analgesia, but does increase side effects. Volume of diluent is not a significant factor in epidural morphine analgesia; a volume of 5 – 10 ml is generally adequate.

Morphine is currently the most widely used epidural opioid for analgesia after cesarean section. The optimal dose is approximately 4 mg, which provides 18 – 24 hours of good to excellent analgesia. Even at this dose, due to inter-individual differences, some patients will require supplementation with other systemic analgesics (see Section 8.5). A higher failure rate (i.e. diminished analgesia) becomes apparent if the dose is reduced below 3 mg.

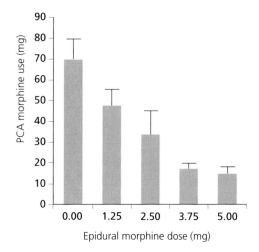

Figure 8.1 Total 24-hour PCA morphine use after varying doses of epidural morphine. Data are mean (± S.E.M.) Adapted from:Palmer, C.M., Nogami, W.M., Van Maren, G. and, Alves, D. (2000) Post-cesarean epidural morphine: a dose response study. *Anesth. Analg.* 90: 887–891.

8.2.1 Side effects of epidural morphine

Pruritus

While an effective analgesic, epidural morphine does have a few significant side effects. Pruritus is the most consistently reported. It is characteristically mild, and occurs most often on the face or trunk, although it may be generalized. In the clinically utilized range, it is not significantly dose-related (*Figure 8.3*).

The exact mechanism by which epidural morphine causes pruritus is unknown. The available evidence indicates it to be more complex than a simple μ-receptor-related issue. The role of opioid receptors in pruritus may be primarily by facilitation of other excitatory neuronal pathways and protective reflexes. A full understanding of the phenomenon awaits further investigation.

Nausea and vomiting

Nausea and vomiting are less frequent after epidural morphine than pruritus. The reported incidence ranges from 11% to about 30%, but

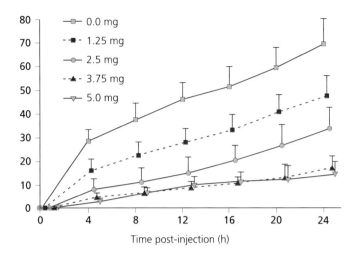

Figure 8.2 Cumulative PCA morphine use over time after varying doses of epidural morphine. Data are mean (± S.E.M.), and are slightly offset for clarity. Adapted from: Palmer, C.M., Nogami, W.M., Van Maren, G., and, Alves D. (2000) Post-cesarean epidural morphine: a dose response study. *Anesth. Analg.* **90**: 887–991.

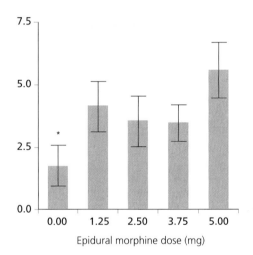

Figure 8.3 Cumulative 24-hour pruritus scores after varying doses of epidural morphine. Data are mean (standard error). *The control group, group 0, was significantly lower than the four epidural morphine groups, which were not different from each other. Unpublished data from Palmer, C.M.

has also been reported to be no different from placebo.

Epidural morphine can cause nausea and vomiting by stimulating the chemoreceptor trigger zone located in the base of the fourth ventricle of the brain. Morphine, which is highly hydrophilic, remains free (unbound) in the cerebrospinal (CSF) fluid for a significantly longer time than more lipophilic opioids (i.e. fentanyl or sufentanil). Morphine concentration in cervical CSF peaks 3–4 hours after injection (*Figure 8.4*). Radiographic studies of other water-soluble compounds confirm that cephalad migration in the CSF does occur.

Respiratory depression

Respiratory depression was recognized as a complication of epidural morphine shortly after its introduction to clinical use. The risk at clinically used doses is quite low, however. A retrospective review of 4880 parturients receiving epidural morphine after cesarean delivery found a respiratory rate below 10 in only 12 patients, or 0.25%. A prospective study of 1000 parturients who received morphine, 5 mg epidurally, reported four patients with a respiratory rate of below 10 (0.4%). The incidence of clinically significant respiratory depression after epidural morphine at doses of 5 mg or less in the obstetric population is at most 0.2–0.3%.

Respiratory depression following epidural morphine is usually described as 'late', with an

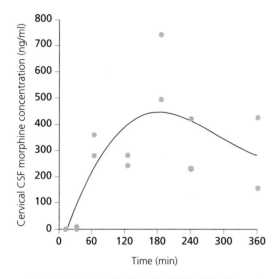

Figure 8.4 Cervical cerebrospinal fluid (CSF) morphine concentrations vs. time in patients after lumbar epidural administration of 10 mg epidural morphine. Adapted from Gourlay, G.K. et al. (1985) Cephalad migration of morphine in CSF following lumbar epidural administration in patients with cancer pain. *Pain* **23**: 317–326.

onset between 6 and 12 hours after administration. This 'delayed' depression is due to the slow cephalad migration of epidurally administered morphine, which can cause direct central depression of respiration. Untreated, a gradual decline in respiratory rate leads to progressive respiratory acidosis. Based on case reports, the risk of respiratory depression probably rises as dose increases, at least beyond 5 mg.

Early respiratory depression after epidural morphine is also possible. This event probably arises from rapid systematic uptake or intravascular injection of the drug.

8.2.2 Treatment of side effects

Most cases of pruritus are mild and do not require treatment (*Table 8.1*). Diphenhydramine, 12.5–25 mg intravenously, usually provides adequate symptomatic relief. The sedation associated with diphenhydramine may be as instrumental in providing relief as its antihistaminergic effect. Nalbuphine (5 mg intravenously) is also an effective treatment for pruritus without significant side effects. In rare cases, naloxone may be necessary to relieve severe pruritus (0.04–0.2 mg intravenously, followed by a continuous infusion starting at 0.4–0.6 mg/h and titrated as needed). Other treatments, including propofol, droperidol, and ondansetron have been reported effective in treating pruritus, but are generally either too costly or have significant side effects themselves.

Treatment options for nausea and vomiting include antiemetics and opioid antagonists (*Table 8.1*). As noted above, nausea and vomiting in this setting are often not due to the epidural morphine and conventional

Table 8.1 Side effects of epidural morphine

Side effect	Incidence	Treatment	Comments
Pruritus	Up to 100%	Nalbuphine 5 mg IV or diphenyhdramine 12.5–25 mg IV or naloxone 0.04–0.2 mg IV	Usually mild Naloxone rarely necessary
Nausea and vomiting	10–30%	Droperidol 0.625 mg IV or ondansetron 4 mg IV or nalbuphine 5–10 mg IV	Usually not related to epidural morphine
Respiratory depression	<0.25%	Naloxone 0.2–0.4 mg IV Assisted ventilation if necessary	Very rare in healthy parturients

antiemetics should be the first option. Intravenous ondansetron, 4 mg, or droperidol, 0.625 mg, are generally effective treatments. Intravenous nalbuphine, 5–10 mg, or very low-dose naloxone can relieve narcotic-induced nausea and vomiting.

Early or late, the treatment of choice for respiratory depression is intravenous naloxone. Institute artificial or mechanical support of ventilation immediately if the patient is obtunded while waiting for naloxone to have effect.

Preemptive therapy to prevent the side effects of epidural morphine has been largely disappointing. While a number of treatments can prevent side effects, they generally also either decrease analgesia or cause side effects of their own. Intravenous naloxone and oral naltrexone can prevent side effects, but both decrease analgesia in a dose-dependent fashion. Epidural butorphanol modestly decreases side effects, but causes somnolence. Prophylactic transdermal scopolamine decreases the incidence of nausea and vomiting during the first 24 hours after cesarean delivery, but must be applied several hours in advance, and causes dry mouth.

8.3 **Other epidural opioids**

8.3.1 Fentanyl
Epidural fentanyl, 50–100 µg, rapidly provides profound analgesia for up to 4 hours (*Figure 8.5*). Increasing the dose further neither improves nor prolongs pain relief. Epidural fentanyl can cause all the same side effects as morphine, though in a shorter time frame. While useful as an intraoperative adjunct during epidural anesthesia for cesarean delivery (*Figure 8.6*), the short duration limits fentanyl's utility as a post-operative analgesic.

8.3.2 Sufentanil
Like fentanyl, the major advantage of epidural sufentanil over epidural morphine is its rapid onset. The incidence of side effects is comparable to, or higher than, equianalgesic doses of epidural morphine. Larger doses (up to 50 µg)

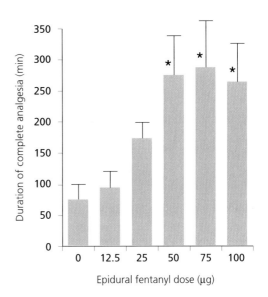

Figure 8.5 Duration of complete analgesia (visual analog pain score of 0) after doses of epidural fentanyl ranging from 0 to 100 µg. Data are mean (standard error). Adapted from : Naulty, J.S., Datta, S., Ostheimer, G.W., *et al.* (1985) Epidural fentanyl for post-cesarean delivery pain management. *Anesthesiology* **63**: 694–698.

provide analgesia for up to 4 hours. Little data is available to evaluate the risk of respiratory depression. When given intravenously at these doses, sufentanil can produce profound respiratory depression.

8.3.3 Others
The speed of onset and duration of analgesia from epidural meperidine (pethidine) increase as the dose increases up to about 25 mg, but further increasing the dose provides no additional benefit (*Table 8.2*). Pain relief lasts about 2.5 hours, and while side effects are infrequent, clinical utility is limited by its short duration.

Hydromorphone is a semisynthetic derivative of morphine. A dose of 1 mg provides analgesia comparable to 5 mg epidural morphine, but the duration of action is considerably shorter – about 12 h. The side effect profile is similar to morphine.

Epidural methadone has a more rapid onset than epidural morphine, but the duration of analgesia after 4 – 5 mg is only 5 – 6 h.

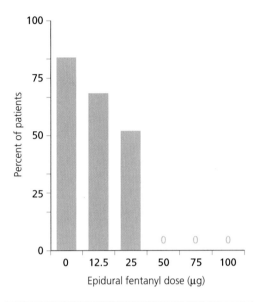

Figure 8.6 Percentage of patients feeling pain during cesarean delivery under epidural anesthesia vs. dose of epidural fentanyl. At doses above 50 μg, no patient complained of pain.

Diamorphine (heroin) has been used as an epidural analgesic, but reports of the duration of analgesia are inconsistent, ranging from 5 – 15 h after 2.5 – 5 mg.

Among mixed agonist/antagonist opioids, epidural butorphanol has a faster onset but a shorter duration than epidural morphine. The low incidence of pruritus after epidural butorphanol is its major advantage, but the short duration and high incidence of somnolence are significant shortcomings. Nalbuphine is another mixed opioid agonist/antagonist. The duration of analgesia increases as the dose is increased from 10 mg to 30 mg from about 1 hour to 3 hours. Its only significant side effect is somnolence, seen in up to 50% of patients after 30 mg. The safety of neuraxial nalbuphine has not been carefully evaluated, however, so its use cannot be recommended.

8.4 Nonopioid analgesics

8.4.1 Clonidine

Clonidine is an α-adrenergic type-2 receptor agonist. After oral administration, it has significant antihypertensive actions. After epidural or spinal injection, it produces significant analgesia from activation of α-adrenergic receptors within descending inhibitory pathways of the spinal cord (see Chapter 4). In volunteers, the bolus administration of 700 μg epidural clonidine results in significant sedation (*Figure 8.7*) and decreased blood pressure. At a dose of 150 μg, epidural clonidine has been shown to modestly augment intrathecal morphine analgesia after cesarean section. In nonobstetric populations, the addition of clonidine to local anesthetic infusions improves postoperative analgesia, but at the cost of greater sedation and lower blood pressure. Due to a relatively short duration of action, for postoperative analgesia, it is best administered via continuous infusion. For this reason, it is probably most appropriate for use in the setting of patient-controlled epidural analgesia (see Section 8.9.1).

Table 8.2 Summary of epidural opioid options

Opioid	Dose	Reported duration (hours)	Comments
Morphine	3.5–4 mg	18–24	'Gold standard'
Fentanyl	50 μg	Up to 4	Useful as an intraoperative analgesic
Sufentanil	10–20 μg	Approx. 3	Also useful intraoperatively
Meperidine	25 mg	2–3	Local anesthetic effects
Hydromorphone	1.0 mg	Approx. 12	
Methadone	4–5 mg	5–6	
Diamorphine	2.5–5 mg	? 5–15	Heroin – not available in the USA

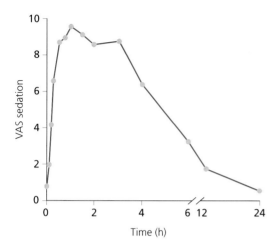

Figure 8.7 Visual analog sedation scores (0–10) after epidural injection of 700 µg clonidine in nonpregnant volunteers. Adapted from Eisenach, J. *et al.* (1993) Hemodynamic and analgesic actions of epidurally administered clonidine. *Anesthesiology* **78**: 277–287.

8.4.2 Epinephrine

Epinephrine, a naturally occurring catecholamine with both α- and β-adrenergic agonist actions, has been used with a variety of epidural analgesics. The primary aim of this combination is to prolong analgesia, and secondary goals are to decrease the incidence of side effects and decrease systemic uptake. Alpha-2 agonism is likely responsible for most of epinephrine's intrinsic analgesic properties. Administered with lidocaine, epinephrine results in not only prolonged anesthesia, but also enhanced analgesia (*Figure 8.8*). In parturients, epinephrine may prolong the analgesic effects of shorter-acting opioids. This prolongation often comes at the expense of an increased incidence or severity of side effects. If used as a component of a continuous epidural infusion, epinephrine may reduce the infusion rate and total amount of opioid.

8.5 Summary of epidural analgesics

There are a variety of ways to provide epidural analgesia after cesarean delivery. Fentanyl,

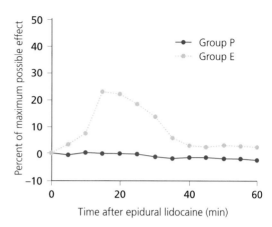

Figure 8.8 Epinephrine augmentation of epidural lidocaine anesthesia. When added to epidural lidocaine 1%, sensory block of an electrical stimulus was not merely prolonged, it was enhanced, illustrating epinephrine's intrinsic analgesic/anesthetic properties. (Group P, plain lidocaine 1%; Group E, lidocaine 1% with epinephrine 1:200 000). From Sakura, S. *et al.* (1999) The addition of epinephrine increases intensity of sensory block during epidural anesthesia with lidocaine. *Reg. Anesth. Pain Med.* **24**: 541–546.

50–100 µg, mixed with the local anesthetic, enhances intraoperative comfort and provides early postoperative analgesia. Despite the occurrence of side effects, morphine is still the longest-lasting epidural opioid available, and is the mainstay of single-shot epidural postoperative analgesia. Immediately after delivery, administer 4 mg, in a volume of 8 ml. For the infrequent patient who requires significant amounts of additional analgesics in the early postoperative period, PCA is a useful option for additional analgesia (see Section 8.9).

Because of the theoretical risk of respiratory depression and the occurrence of side effects, standard postoperative orders are very useful (*Table 8.3*). Nurses should check and record respiratory rates hourly for 18 – 24 h after epidural morphine. If respiratory rate falls below eight breaths per minute, the nurse should immediately inject naloxone and notify the anesthesiologist. In the absence of other sedatives or narcotics, respiratory depression of this degree is extremely uncommon.

Table 8.3 Postoperative neuraxial opioid orders

1. Epidural/intrathecal _____, _____ mg, administered at _____ hours on _____ (date).

2. No sedatives or narcotics administered except by order of anesthesiologist.

3. One ampule naloxone at bedside at all times.

4. Main IV access or heparin-lock at all times.

5. Measure and record respiratory rate q 1 h; for respiratory rate <8/min, give naloxone, 0.2 mg IV slowly over 2 min; notify anesthesiologist.

6. Supplemental analgesia: Morphine 2 mg IV q 1–2 h PRN
                              or
                              Ketorolac 15 mg IV q 6 h PRN
                              or
                              Ibuprofen 400 mg PO q 6 h PRN

7. For pruritus: nalbuphine, 5 mg IV q 4 h PRN itching.

8. For nausea/vomiting: ondansetron 4 mg IV q 6 h PRN nausea and vomiting.

9. For pain, pruritus, or nausea/vomiting unresponsive to above, page anesthesiologist on call.

10. This protocol covers 24 h after each dose of neuraxial narcotic.

8.6 Intrathecal morphine

The past decade has seen the resurgence of spinal anesthesia for cesarean delivery. As the use of spinal anesthesia has increased, so has the use of intrathecal opioids for postoperative analgesia.

As with epidural analgesia, morphine is the mainstay of intrathecal post-cesarean analgesia. In parturients, intrathecal morphine produces excellent pain relief after cesarean section after surprisingly small doses. When self-administered PCA morphine is used to quantify analgesia, no improvement in analgesia is seen despite increasing the dose of morphine from 0.1 to 0.5 mg (*Figure 8.9*). Interestingly, patients will continue to self-medicate with PCA morphine at a constant rate despite a five- to ten-fold increase in the dose of intrathecal morphine. This suggests that optimal analgesia requires occupation of opioid receptors at two distinct sites within the CNS; intrathecal morphine occupies spinal receptors, and parenteral (PCA) morphine acts at supraspinal receptors. Support for this spinal-supraspinal receptor synergy can be found in animal models (see also Chapter 4).

Side effects after intrathecal morphine are comparable to those seen after administration of epidural morphine. Pruritus occurs in 40%–80% of patients and appears dose-dependent (*Figure 8.10*). Vomiting occurs

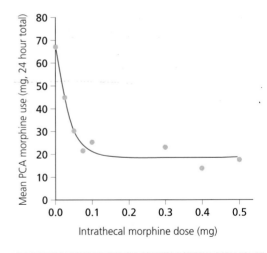

Figure 8.9 Mean 24-hour PCA morphine use after doses of intrathecal morphine from 0 to 0.5 mg in parturients after cesarean delivery. Data are mean (standard error). After Palmer, C.M. *et al.* (1999) Dose-response relationship of intrathecal morphine for post-cesarean analgesia. *Anesthesiology* **90**: 437–444.

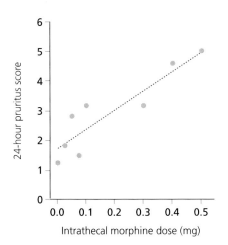

Figure 8.10 Mean 24-hour pruritus scores in parturients after doses of intrathecal morphine from 0 to 0.5 mg. After Palmer, C.M. *et al.* (1999) Dose-response relationship of intrathecal morphine for post-cesarean analgesia. *Anesthesiology* **90**: 437–444.

rarely after low doses (0.1 mg) of morphine. Clinically significant respiratory depression is rare, but can occur. At clinically relevant doses, the respiratory response to carbon dioxide challenge is not depressed.

Based on the very steep dose–response curve of intrathecal morphine, the optimal dose of intrathecal morphine for post-cesarean analgesia lies between 0.1 mg and 0.2 mg, which should provide over 18–20 hours of good analgesia while avoiding excessive side effects. As with epidural morphine, standardized postoperative orders are very useful. Intrathecal morphine cannot completely eliminate the need for supplemental analgesics, however, and the best way to insure excellent analgesia may be through a combination of intrathecal morphine and PCA supplementation.

8.7 Other intrathecal opioids

8.7.1 Fentanyl

Fentanyl can be used for analgesia at cesarean delivery and the maximal clinical benefit can be obtained with very low doses. The duration of effective analgesia from intrathecal bupi-

vacaine increases from 71.8 minutes without fentanyl to 192 minutes with 6.25 µg of fentanyl (*Figure 8.11*), but 24-hour supplemental narcotic usage is not affected. In conjunction with lidocaine anesthesia, fentanyl has similar effects, but the duration of analgesia is shorter. The short duration of effective analgesia even at high doses limits the value of intrathecal fentanyl as a postoperative analgesic. Pruritus occurs frequently, but rarely requires treatment, and fentanyl can actually *decrease* the incidence of nausea and vomiting intraoperatively.

8.7.2 Others

Subarachnoid sufentanil, up to 10 µg, has very similar analgesic properties to fentanyl. Like fentanyl, a short duration limits the usefulness of sufentanil as a postoperative analgesic. Subarachnoid buprenorphine, 0.045 mg, also prolongs the pain-free interval after bupivacaine spinal anesthesia, perhaps as long as 6 – 7 hours; its only advantage would seem to be a lower incidence of pruritus. Other subarachnoid opioids that have been

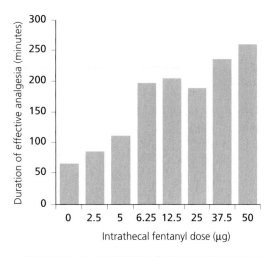

Figure 8.11 Duration of effective analgesia after fentanyl doses ranging from 0 to 50 µg in parturients after cesarean delivery. Adapted from Hunt, C.O. *et al.* (1989) Perioperative analgesia with subarachnoid fentanyl-bupivacaine for cesarean delivery. *Anesthesiology* **71**: 535–540.

used in nonpregnant populations include methadone and oxymorphone. Methadone produces analgesia of shorter duration and less consistent quality than morphine, even at doses as high as 20 mg. Oxymorphone provides approximately 16 hours of analgesia when administered intrathecally, with predictable side effects of pruritus, nausea, and vomiting (*Table 8.4*).

Nalbuphine has been combined with intrathecal morphine to attempt to decrease morphine's side effects. It has no effect on the incidence or severity of pruritus, or postoperative analgesic use, but tends to increase nausea.

8.7.3 Nonopioid intrathecal analgesics
While epinephrine can be added to intrathecal local anesthetics to prolong the duration of anesthesia, it does not augment intrathecal morphine post-operative analgesia. The addition of epinephrine to intrathecal morphine, 0.2 mg, does not increase the duration of postoperative analgesia or decrease supplemental analgesic requirements after cesarean delivery.

8.7.4 Summary
For spinal anesthesia for cesarean delivery, 0.1–0.2 mg of morphine with 15 µg of fentanyl (combined with either lidocaine or bupivacaine) remains the best choice of postoperative analgesic. Morphine provides 18 – 24 hours of good to excellent postoperative analgesia for most parturients, but if a patient is having significant discomfort, supplemental analgesia is appropriate. This may be PCA morphine, but as many parturients are able to handle oral

Table 8.4 Summary of intrathecal opioid options

Opioid	Dose	Reported duration
Morphine	0.1–0.2 mg	18–24 hours
Fentanyl	10–20 µg	3–4 hours
Sufentanil	Up to 10 µg	3–4 hours
Buprenorphine Methadone → Oxymorphone	Limited experience. Doses and durations not well characterized	

analgesics within hours after their surgery, oral pain medications can be equally effective. Fentanyl enhances intraoperative comfort and provides some early postoperative analgesia. Because of the very small volumes of opioids used with this technique, it is prudent to measure these drugs in tuberculin syringes to minimize the risk of accidental overdose. As with epidural morphine analgesia, close postoperative monitoring of patients is essential.

8.8 Continuous intrathecal analgesia

Continuous intrathecal analgesia can be used in those patients who have an intrathecal catheter in place. Such a technique has the advantage of allowing medications to be readily titrated to patient comfort, and additional boluses given for breakthrough pain. Generally speaking, the highly lipid-soluble opioids, with their fast onset and relatively short duration of action, are the best-suited agents. Sufentanil, 5 µg/h, will provide adequate analgesia for most parturients after cesarean delivery. A combination of bupivacaine and fentanyl can also be used (fentanyl 15 µg/h with bupivacaine 1.5 mg/h). This latter combination may be associated with greater motor block than the sufentanil infusion (*Table 8.5*).

8.9 Patient-controlled analgesia (PCA)

Patient-controlled analgesia (PCA) is effective for post-cesarean analgesia. While epidural or intrathecal morphine analgesia is rated superior (by patients) to that provided by PCA morphine, overall patient satisfaction with PCA is as high, probably due to the feeling of control that PCA provides parturients. Both PCA and neuraxial morphine are markedly more effective than intramuscular injections.

The choice of opioid for use with PCA does not make any difference in patient satisfaction or side effects, when equipotent doses are used. Likewise, use of a basal infusion does not change 24-hour opioid usage, but may

Table 8.5 Continuous intrathecal analgesia

Medication	Initial bolus	Infusion	Comments
Sufentanil	5 µg	5–7.5 µg/h	Mix as 1 µg/ml infusion
Fentanyl/ bupivacaine	Fentanyl 25 µg with bupivacaine 2.5 mg	Fentanyl 15 µg/h Bupivacaine 1.5 mg/h	Mix infusion with fentanyl 5 µg and bupivacaine 0.5 mg/ml. Run at 3 ml/h

[a]To mix infusion: Begin with 50 ml normal saline; withdraw 15 ml; add 5 ml 0.5% bupivacaine and 5 ml fentanyl. **Note:** Most commercial infusion bags are slightly overfilled, therefore these numbers are very close approximations.

decrease pain scores with movement; this minor advantage is offset by the fact that the incidence of nausea is higher when a basal infusion is used. Finally, PCA is an excellent choice to use in combination with neuraxial techniques for post-cesarean analgesia, and an effective way to titrate postoperative analgesia to individual requirements.

8.9.1 Patient-controlled epidural analgesia (PCEA)

Patient-controlled epidural analgesia (PCEA) allows the use of local anesthetics, opioids, and multiple combinations for postoperative analgesia. Compared to single bolus epidural morphine, use of opioid-only PCEA with fentanyl or sufentanil provides comparable analgesia, but the high total doses of opioid used by parturients raise the question of whether the analgesic effects are mediated primarily by systemic uptake or a true spinal mechanism. As with intravenous PCA, a basal infusion does not improve the quality of pain relief with PCEA. Background infusions *do* increase sedation. When meperidine is used for PCEA, parturients use approximately 50% less opioid via the PCEA route than the PCA route, and sedation scores are predictably higher in the PCA group (*Figure 8.12*).

Local anesthetics are often added to PCEA for post-cesarean analgesia. The concentration of local anesthetic must be low to avoid significant sensory or motor blockade, as many of these patients are ambulatory within hours of surgery. PCEA with fentanyl or buprenorphine plus 0.03% bupivacaine produces effective analgesia, but motor block interferes with ambulation. With a lower concentration of bupivacaine (0.01%), ambulation is not affected, but the dose of fentanyl consumed is

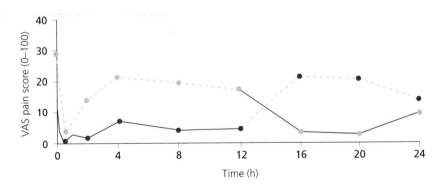

Figure 8.12 A comparison of pain scores between patient-controlled analgesia (intravenous PCA) and patient-controlled epidural analgesia (PCEA) after cesarean delivery. The solid line represents the period parturients received PCEA and the dashed line represents the period they received PCA. From Paech, M.J. *et al.* (1994) Meperidine for patient-controlled analgesia after cesarean section. *Anesthesiology* **80**: 1268–1276.

comparable to that with plain fentanyl PCEA. Thus, it is unclear what benefit including dilute bupivacaine in a PCEA solution provides, if any.

Clonidine and epinephrine (which activate α-2 adrenergic receptors) and neostigmine (which prevents the breakdown of synaptically released Ach) have also been used with PCEA. When combined with sufentanil PCEA, both epinephrine and clonidine significantly reduce epidural opioid use. Unfortunately, clonidine produces significant decreases in blood pressure and heart rate, and neostigmine, even at very low doses, significantly increases nausea and vomiting; both agents, despite their theoretical promise, have significant side effects of their own, which have limited their clinical utility.

Clearly, PCEA can be an effective technique for post-cesarean analgesia. Whether it offers distinct advantages over epidural or intrathecal morphine is a matter of dispute. A disadvantage is the necessity to maintain a functioning epidural catheter in the postoperative period. Further, in many practices cesarean delivery is more likely to be accomplished with spinal than epidural anesthesia, which precludes the technique. It remains a useful technique for selected patients and populations.

8.10 Nonsteroidal agents (NSAIDs)

Nonsteroidal agents (NSAIDs) may be of value in this population in two primary ways. First, most patients who have had a cesarean delivery remain no oral intake (NPO) for some period of time following delivery; during this period, a parenteral alternative to oral medications may be necessary. Second, as noted above, despite the good quality of analgesia available with neuraxial techniques, supplemental analgesia is sometimes necessary and NSAIDs (both oral and parenteral) are a useful adjunct to epidural or intrathecal morphine.

The NSAIDs are not potent enough to provide complete analgesia for most patients after a cesarean delivery. Ketorolac, 30 mg, is roughly comparable to meperidine 75 mg (intramuscular dosing), but ketorolac is somewhat inconsistent and of short duration. When administered via continuous intravenous infusion, diclofenac or ketoprofen decrease postoperative analgesic requirements by about 40% when compared to placebo.

As adjuncts to neuraxial morphine, NSAIDs have shown inconsistent results. While in some situations NSAIDs can decrease postoperative opioid use, at this point it is premature to make a blanket recommendation regarding their use.

8.11 Conclusion

Cesarean delivery is probably the most common major surgical procedure performed in the world today. This huge volume of anesthetics in a remarkably homogeneous population (all being female, relatively young and healthy) has allowed analgesic options to be systematically and carefully evaluated. Given current understanding of analgesic dose–response relationships, planning a cesarean anesthetic should include planning for postoperative analgesia also. The variety of options available means there is an effective technique for every patient.

Further reading

Abouleish, E., Rawal, N., Tobon-Randall, B. *et al.* (1993) A clinical and laboratory study to compare the addition of 0.2 mg of morphine, 0.2 mg of epinephrine, or their combination to hyperbaric bupivacaine for spinal anesthesia in cesarean section. *Anesth. Analg.* 77(3): 457–462.

Behar, M., Magora, F., Olshwang, D. *et al.* (1979) Epidural morphine in treatment of pain. *Lancet* 1: 527–529.

Cohen, S., Amar, D., Pantuck, C.B. *et al.* (1993) Postcesarean delivery epidural patient-controlled analgesia. *Anesthesiology* 78: 486–491.

Cohen, S.E., Desai, J.B., Ratner, E.F. *et al.* (1996) Ketorolac and spinal morphine for postcesarean analgesia. *Int. J. Obstet. Anesth.* 5: 14–18.

Eisenach, J.C., Grice, S.C. and Dewan, D.M. (1988) Patient-controlled analgesia following cesarean section: A comparison with epidural and intramuscular narcotics. *Anesthesiology* **68**: 444–448.

Eisenach, J., Detweiler, D. and Hood, D. (1993) Hemodynamic and analgesic actions of epidurally administered clonidine. *Anesthesiology* **78**: 277–287.

Fuller, J.G., McMorland, G.H., Douglas J. *et al.* (1990) Epidural morphine for postoperative pain after caesarean section: A report of 4880 patients. *Can. J. Anaesth.* **37**: 636–640.

Gambling, D.R., Howell, P., Huber, C. and Kozak, S. (1994) Epidural butorphanol does not reduce side effects from epidural morphine after cesarean birth. *Anesth. Analg.* **78**: 1099–1104.

Gourlay, G.K., Cherry, D.A. and Cousins, M.J. (1985) Cephalad migration of morphine in CSF following lumbar epidural administration in patients with cancer pain. *Pain* **23**: 317–326.

Helbo-Hansen, H.S., Bang, U., Lindholm, P. and Klitgaard, N.A. (1993) Maternal effects of adding epidural fentanyl to 0.5% bupivacaine for caesarean section. *Int. J. Obstet. Anesth.* **2**: 21–26.

Hunt, C.O., Naulty, J.S., Bader, Am. *et al.* (1989) Perioperative analgesia with subarachnoid fentanyl-bupivacaine for cesarean delivery. *Anesthesiology* **71**: 535–540.

Kotelko, D.M., Dailey, P.A., Shnider, S.M. *et al.* (1984) Epidural morphine analgesia after cesarean delivery. *Obstet. Gynecol.* **63**: 409–413.

Kotelko, D.M., Rottman, R.L., Wright, W.C. *et al.* (1989) Transdermal scopolamine decreases nausea and vomiting following cesarean section in patients receiving epidural morphine. *Anesthesiology* **71**: 675–678.

Leicht, C.H., Hughes, S.C., Dailey, P.A. *et al.* (1986) Epidural morphine sulfate for analgesia after cesarean section: A prospective report of 1000 patients. *Anesthesiology* **65**: A366.

Massone, M.L., Lampugnani, E., Calevo, M.G. *et al.* (1998) The effects of a dose of epidural clonidine combined with intrathecal morphine for postoperative analgesia. *Minerva Anestesiologica* **64**: 289–296.

Naulty, J.S., Datta, S., Ostheimer, G.W. *et al.* (1985) Epidural fentanyl for postcesarean delivery pain management. *Anesthesiology* **63**: 694–698.

Paech, M.J., Moore, J.S. and Evans, S.F. (1994) Meperidine for patient-controlled analgesia after cesarean section. *Anesthesiology* **80**: 1268–1276.

Paech, M.J., Pavy, T.J.G., Orlikowski, C.E.P. *et al.* (1997) Postoperative epidural infusion: a randomized, double-blind, dose-finding trial of clonidine in combination with bupivacaine and fentanyl. *Anesth. Analg.* **84**: 1323–1328.

Paech, M.J., Pavy, T.J.G., Orlikowski, C.E.P. *et al.* (2000) Postoperative intraspinal opioid analgesia after caesarean section; a randomised trial of subarachnoid morphine and epidural pethidine. *Int. J. Obstet. Anesth.* **9**: 238–245.

Palmer, C.M. (1999) Post-operative analgesia. In: *Obstetric Anesthesia*, 2nd edn (ed. Norris, M.C.), pp. 697–721. Lippincott, Williams and Wilkins, Philadelphia.

Palmer, C.M. (2001) Continuous intrathecal sufentanil for postoperative analgesia. *Anesth. Analg.* **92**: 244–245.

Palmer, C.M., Voulgaropoulos, D. and Alves, D. (1995) Subarachnoid fentanyl augments lidocaine spinal anesthesia for cesarean delivery. *Reg. Anesth.* **20**(5): 389–394.

Palmer, C.M., Emerson, S., Voulgaropoulos, D. and Alves, D. (1999) Dose-response relationship of intrathecal morphine for post-cesarean analgesia. *Anesthesiology* **90**: 437–444.

Palmer, C.M., Nogami, W.M., Van Maren, G. and Alves, D. (2000) Post-cesarean epidural morphine: a dose response study. *Anesth. Analg.* **90**: 887–891.

Reddy, S.V.R., Maderdrut, J.L. and Yaksh, T.L. (1980) Spinal cord pharmacology of adrenergic agonist-mediated antinociception. *J. Pharmacol. Exp. Ther.* **213**: 525–533.

Robertson, K., Douglas, M.J. and McMorland, G.H. (1985) Epidural fentanyl, with and without epinephrine for post-caesarean section analgesia. *Can. Anaesth. Soc. J.* **32**: 502–505.

Rosen, M.A., Hughes, S.C., Shnider, S.M. *et al.* (1983) Epidural morphine for the relief of postoperative pain after cesarean delivery. *Anesth. Analg.* **62**: 666–672.

Sakura, S., Sumi, M., Morimoto, N.M. and Saito, Y. (1999) The addition of epinephrine increases intensity of sensory block during epidural anesthesia with lidocaine. *Reg. Anesth. Pain Med.* **24**: 541–546.

Sun, H.L., Wu, C.C., Lin, M.S. and Chang, C.F. (1993) Effects of epidural morphine and intramuscular diclofenac combination in postcesarean analgesia: a dose-range study. *Anesth. Analg.* **76**(2): 284–88.

Wang, J.K., Nauss, L.A. and Thomas, J.E. (1979) Pain relief by intrathecally applied morphine in man. *Anesthesiology* **50**: 149–155.

Chapter 9

Pregnancy induced hypertension and preeclampsia

Kenneth E. Nelson, MD and
Robert D'Angelo, MD

Contents

9.1 Introduction

Hypertension during pregnancy is a condition that leads to a marked increase in both maternal and fetal morbidity and mortality. Blood pressure normally decreases somewhat during pregnancy, and any elevation of blood pressure is considered abnormal. 'Hypertensive disorders of pregnancy' includes both pregnancy-induced hypertension (PIH) and chronic hypertension that persists into the puerperium. Although the classic triad of preeclampsia includes hypertension, proteinuria and edema, the American College of Obstetricians and Gynecologists (ACOG) has established specific criteria defining both preeclampsia and severe preeclampsia (*Tables 9.1* and *9.2*). Eclampsia is the condition defined by a seizure that occurs as a complication of preeclampsia. Despite these 'classic' definitions, many clinicians view preeclampsia as a continuous spectrum anchored on one end by mild pregnancy induced hypertension (PIH) and on the other end by eclampsia and HELLP syndrome.

A thorough understanding of the pathophysiology of hypertension in pregnancy is essential in providing safe anesthetic care and decreasing maternal and fetal morbidity. This chapter focuses on the anesthetic implications of preeclampsia, which are outlined briefly in *Table 9.3*.

9.2 Pathophysiology

The exact cause of preeclampsia remains unknown. Early descriptions of 'toxemia' implicated a circulating toxin that was responsible for the pathologic changes seen in preeclampsia. More recent theories have focused on elevated levels of endothelin, reduced levels of nitric oxide, or an imbalance of thromboxane and prostacyclin. In normal pregnancy, both thromboxane and prostacyclin levels increase, but the balance favors prostacyclin and thus vasodilation. In PIH, thromboxane levels increase markedly, while prostacyclin levels are abnormally low. This imbalance favors vasoconstriction. It remains unknown if this imbalance causes PIH, or is the result of other pathophysiologic changes of preeclampsia. Levels of renin, angiotensin

---

Table 9.1 Criteria for the diagnosis of preeclampsia[a]

Hypertension	SBP 140 or DBP 90 mmHg or increase of 15 mmHg DBP or 30 mmHg SBP on two occasions at least 6 hours apart
Proteinuria	24-h collection 300 mg protein or 1g/l in two specimens at least 6 h apart
Edema	> 1+ pitting edema after 12 h bed rest or weight gain ≥ 2.27 kg (5 lbs) in 1 week

[a]Adapted from the ACOG Technical Bulletin. Hypertension in pregnancy. *Int. J. Gynecol. Obstet.* 1996; **53**: 175–183.

Table 9.2 Criteria for severe preeclampsia[a]. The presence of any one of these factors in a patient with preeclampsia is sufficient for classification as severe preeclampsia.

Hypertension	SBP 160 mmHg or DBP 110 mmHg
Proteinuria	5 g in 24-hour collection
	3+ to 4+ on urinalysis

Evidence of end-organ involvement:

Cerebral	Headache, scotomata, altered level of consciousness
Pulmonary	Pulmonary edema, cyanosis
Hepatic	Increased LFTs
Hematologic	Thrombocytopenia
HELLP syndrome	**H**emolysis, **e**levated **l**iver **e**nzymes, **l**ow **p**latelets

[a]Adapted from the ACOG Technical Bulletin. Hypertension in pregnancy. *Int. J. Gynecol. Obstet.* 1996; **53**: 175–183.

Table 9.3 Anesthetic implications of preeclampsia

Blood pressure control	Especially important with general anesthesia to blunt the exaggerated response to laryngoscopy Baseline control with: • Hydralazine 5 mg IV q 20 min up to 20 mg • Labetalol 5 mg IV, double dose q 10 min up to 300 mg total dose • Titrate to DBP 90–100 mmHg • Acute control with nitroglycerin, nitroprusside
Thrombocytopenia	Especially important with regional anesthesia to reduce the risk of epidural hematoma Recent platelet count – within 6 hours of placement • Usually lower threshold of 80 000–100 000/mm^3 (consider lowering when there are contraindications to general anesthesia, or strong indications for regional anesthesia)
Magnesium	>No reduction of succinylcholine dose for rapid sequence induction but expect increased sensitivity >Use nondepolarizing relaxants at reduced doses and titrate to effect; monitor with peripheral nerve stimulator
Airway	Exaggerated edema *Anticipate difficult intubation* • Use smaller ETT • Avoid nasal intubation
Eclampsia	Be aware of the potential for seizure regardless of severity of preeclampsia • Magnesium for prophylaxis • Benzodiazepines or barbiturates for acute management of seizures unresponsive to magnesium

II, and aldosterone also increase during normal pregnancy but vascular responsiveness to exogenous angiotensin II is reduced.

Preeclampsia is a multisystem disorder. In simplistic terms, patients with severe preeclampsia can be thought to have 'total body edema' affecting every major organ system including the brain, lungs, heart, liver and kidneys. Involvement of any of these systems can have significant anesthetic implications, which are discussed below.

9.2.1 Cardiovascular

Increased blood pressure is the hallmark of the disease. Abnormally high blood pressure can be seen as early as the first trimester, yet it is typically progressive starting in the second to third trimester. Preeclamptic parturients may exhibit an increased sensitivity to exogenous catecholamines, so pressors should be used judiciously when necessary. An exaggerated hypertensive response to laryngoscopy should also be expected when general anesthesia is

required, and in extreme cases this acute increase in blood pressure can lead to pulmonary edema and intracranial hemorrhage. Blood volume has been reported to be anywhere from markedly reduced to unchanged from normal pregnant plasma volume. Indeed, measurements of central venous pressure (CVP) and pulmonary capillary wedge (PCWP) suggest that this is a heterogenous disease, with a wide range of individual response.

9.2.2 Coagulation

Thrombocytopenia is common in preeclampsia (up to 30%), yet the platelet count falls below 100 000/mm^3 in less than 10% of patients presenting with severe preeclampsia. Although the exact mechanism of thrombocytopenia in preeclampsia is unknown, it appears that damaged endothelium and serotonin play an important role. Platelets will adhere to the damaged lining of arteries, resulting in the release of thromboxane, serotonin, and other factors from the platelets.

This in turn can cause a cascade of platelet activation, leading to a consumptive thrombocytopenia. The degree of thrombocytopenia is usually related to the severity of disease. Except for this drop in platelet count, other laboratory values may offer evidence of hypercoagulability in preeclamptics, but it does not carry the clinical significance of thrombocytopenia.

9.2.3 Renal
Proteinuria is a marker for renal dysfunction; this proteinuria is due to glomerulopathy which is correlated with the severity of the preeclampsia. Although patients with severe preeclampsia rarely develop chronic renal failure, urine output should be monitored closely. The degree of proteinuria increases with the severity of disease as permeability to proteins goes up. When oliguria occurs in preeclampsia, a balance must be found between providing adequate renal preload and preventing pulmonary edema. If renal output remains below 0.5 ml/kg/h despite intravenous fluid therapy and what is expected to be adequate intravascular volume, it may become necessary to insert a pulmonary arterial pressure monitor to assess preload and cardiac function.

9.3 Complications

9.3.1 Severe preeclampsia
Much of the morbidity and mortality that occurs with preeclampsia is proportional to the severity of disease. The definition of severe preeclampsia includes the objective measures of hypertension and proteinuria described in *Table 9.2*. Additionally, if any of the other complications listed are present a diagnosis of severe preeclampsia is made. Most are related to specific organ dysfunction, such as oliguria, pulmonary edema, impaired hepatic function, thrombocytopenia, and CNS disturbances such as headache and visual changes (*Table 9.2*).

9.3.2 HELLP syndrome
HELLP is an acronym for **h**emolysis, **e**levated **l**iver enzymes, and **l**ow **p**latelet count.

Although usually considered to be a type, or subset, of severe preeclampsia, the syndrome has been described in the absence of hypertension and proteinuria. Most patients will complain of malaise and right upper quadrant pain and experience nausea and vomiting. The platelet count can fall precipitously and maternal morbidity significantly increases as the platelet count falls below 50 000/mm^3. The primary anesthetic implication is awareness of the potential contraindication for regional anesthesia with thrombocytopenia, as discussed below.

9.4 Obstetric management

Obstetric management of patients with preeclampsia will depend on the individual clinical situation, which can change abruptly. Factors used to determine obstetric management include the severity of the hypertension, the presence of complications such as thrombocytopenia and oliguria, and the fetal condition. Fetal distress is a common indication for cesarean section in the preeclamptic. Conservative management of these patients involves controlling the disease until the fetus can be delivered vaginally. More specifically, obstetricians strive to prevent significant hypertension or eclamptic seizures. If the effects of preeclampsia cannot be controlled, or if the intrauterine environment deteriorates despite medical management, cesarean section might become the best option for the well being of both the mother and fetus.

9.4.1 Pharmacologic agents
Magnesium
Although a transient decrease in blood pressure frequently accompanies the use of magnesium, it is not used primarily as an antihypertensive. Instead, magnesium sulfate is used to raise the seizure threshold, and thereby reduce the morbidity associated with eclampsia. Seizure prophylaxis is achieved by different means worldwide, with magnesium being most commonly used in the United States. The recommended dosing schedule for

magnesium sulfate is a 4–6 g loading dose administered over 20 minutes followed by a 1–2 g/h infusion. An additional 2–4 g administered over 10 minutes is recommended for recurrent seizures. The therapeutic index for magnesium is quite narrow, and magnesium levels must be monitored during its use, either with blood levels, or with clinical signs such as patellar deep tendon reflexes (see also Section 12.6.1). Magnesium administration has significant implications for the anesthesiologist, especially when managing a general anesthetic. Via both pre- and post-synaptic mechanisms, magnesium causes skeletal muscle weakness and may potentiate the effects of both depolarizing and nondepolarizing muscle relaxants. Recovery from succinylcholine will be prolonged, which must be kept in mind when performing a rapid sequence induction. The time to return of spontaneous ventilation will be longer in the preeclamptic administered magnesium sulfate, which can be critical in the event of a difficult intubation. Despite this risk, reducing the dose of succinylcholine during induction is not recommended because the primary goal is to rapidly achieve ideal conditions for intubation. In contrast, a 'normal' maintenance dose of a nondepolarizing muscle relaxant could lead to the requirement for prolonged postoperative ventilatory support. Therefore, it is recommended to reduce doses of nondepolarizing muscle relaxants and titrate to effect while closely monitoring with a peripheral nerve stimulator.

Antihypertensives

Blood pressure control is a major goal in the management of preeclampsia, and can be accomplished with many of the same pharmacologic agents that are used to treat hypertension of various other etiologies. Alpha methyldopa (Aldomet®) is an antihypertensive that can be administered orally. It is frequently used as a 'first line' agent in the patient with mild preeclampsia being treated without hospital admission. Parenteral antihypertensives are usually administered for more severe preeclampsia that requires hospitalization. Hydralazine, a direct acting arteriolar vasodilator, and beta-blockers such as labetalol, are examples of drugs used parenterally in the inpatient setting. Since patients with preeclampsia may also have placental insufficiency, the risks of maternal hypertension must be weighed against the risk of reducing placental perfusion and compromising fetal oxygen delivery. Antihypertensive agents are usually titrated to achieve a diastolic blood pressure of 90–100 mmHg. The anesthesiologist must be aware of the frequent use of these drugs, their side effects, and the potential for potentiation of the blood pressure effects of anesthetic agents.

The most important implications for anesthesiologists occur when providing anesthesia for cesarean section. Antihypertensive drugs can potentiate the hypotension due to vasodilatation seen with neuraxial anesthesia, and exaggerate the hypotensive effect of induction agents and volatile agents during induction and maintenance of general anesthesia. In addition, the effect of sympathomimetic drugs such as ephedrine may be diminished in the parturient with a preexisting beta-blockade. Patients with severe preeclampsia usually do not develop significant hypotension following a neuraxial blockade; severe preeclamptics are more likely to require additional antihypertensive medications to blunt the response to laryngoscopy and tracheal intubation during general anesthesia. This is discussed in more detail in the section on the anesthetic management for cesarean section.

9.5 Anesthetic management

9.5.1 General considerations

Volume status

Although the plasma volume can vary significantly in patients with severe preeclampsia, important factors should be kept in mind when caring for these parturients. When using regional anesthesia, the hypotension secondary to sympathectomy can range from profound to nonexistent. It is as if some preeclamptics are 'protected' from hypotension by the toxemia. Crystalloids should be used cautiously in patients with severe preeclampsia due to the risk of volume overload causing pulmonary edema. This risk may be exaggerated in patients administered high doses of labetalol and magnesium sulfate. Rather than administering a routine, fixed volume of intravenous fluid prior to neuraxial anesthesia, a better course is to administer fluid as necessary to support maternal blood pressure should it drop following induction. Vasopressors such as ephedrine must be initially used with caution in anticipation of an exaggerated response. However, many patients will require 'normal' amounts of both intravenous fluids and ephedrine to support blood pressure during regional anesthesia, and appropriate resuscitative therapy should not be withheld.

Coagulation

The maternal platelet count should always be checked for evidence of thrombocytopenia before performing a regional anesthetic in the preeclamptic. The platelet count at which neuraxial anesthesia becomes contraindicated cannot be precisely defined. Trauma to epidural veins is impossible to prevent during epidural or spinal placement, but normally does not present a problem. In the patient with preeclampsia complicated by thrombocytopenia, uncontrolled bleeding from such trauma could result in an expanding epidural hematoma, which if not recognized and treated promptly can lead to permanent neurologic injury. Expert consensus suggests that a spinal needle is less traumatic than an epidural needle, and can be expected to incur a lower risk for an epidural hematoma. Therefore, the platelet count at which a spinal anesthetic is administered might be lower than the threshold for an epidural anesthetic. Since epidural hematomas occur so rarely, the exact platelet count at which a spinal or epidural anesthetic will cause an epidural hematoma will probably never be known with certainty. The anesthesia care provider should weigh the relative risks against the benefits on a case-by-case basis.

In practice, a platelet count of 80 000–100 000/mm^3 serves as a practical cut-off threshold, which may be modified based on each patient's clinical presentation. For example, patients in whom tracheal intubation is anticipated to be difficult, who have relative contraindications to general anesthesia such as malignant hyperthermia or pseudocholinesterase deficiency, or who refuse general anesthesia, it is reasonable to consider a regional anesthetic (particularly for cesarean section) even if the platelet count were as low as 70 000/mm^3. More recently, based on other measures of coagulation such as thromboelastography, some obstetric anesthesiologists have advocated a minimal threshold as low as 50 000/mm^3. Few experts, however, would recommend proceeding with a regional anesthetic in any patient with a platelet count less than 50 000/mm^3.

Airway

The increased danger of general anesthesia in the parturient is well documented. Weight gain, breast engorgement, upper airway edema, and friability of the airway mucosa combine to make endotracheal intubation more problematic. This technical difficulty is further complicated by a decreased functional residual capacity (FRC) and increased oxygen consumption present in all pregnancies. All of these factors are often further exaggerated by preeclampsia, making regional anesthesia a preferable alternative to general anesthesia when feasible. However, when a fetal emergency arises, leaving little time for regional anesthesia, or when regional anesthesia is contraindicated, a general anesthetic may be unavoidable. In these cases, full preparation must be made for a difficult intubation. Suggested equipment for difficult airway management during cesarean section is listed in *Table 9.4* and should be readily available. Ideally, at least one additional skilled assistant should be present. Airway management is further described below under anesthetic management for cesarean section.

Table 9.4 Suggested equipment for difficult airway management during cesarean section[a]

1. Assorted laryngoscopes and blades
2. Assorted endotracheal tubes and stylettes
3. Assorted laryngeal mask airways and/or LMA Fastrach®
4. Endotracheal tube guides (assorted intubating and lighted stylettes)
5. Esophageal-tracheal combitube
6. Cricothyrotomy kit with or without jet ventilation
7. Fiberoptic bronchoscope
8. Jet ventilation capability
9. Ability to perform emergency tracheostomy

[a]Adapted from the practice guidelines for management of the difficult airway: a report by the ASA task force on management of the difficult airway. *Anesthesiology* 1993; **78**: 597–602.

9.6 Anesthetic options

An aggressive approach to providing regional anesthesia in patients presenting with severe preeclampsia likely reduces overall risk in these patients and is outlined in *Table 9.5*.

9.6.1 Labor and vaginal delivery

Regional

Epidural analgesia, in the absence of thrombocytopenia or other contraindication, is widely considered to be ideal for the management of labor pain in the preeclamptic. The physiologic stresses caused by labor pain may exag-

Table 9.5 Strategies for reducing anesthetic risks in patients with severe preeclampsia

1. **Early epidural catheter** placement and testing whenever possible
2. **Spinal anesthesia** can be used for cesarean section when the patient presents without an existing epidural catheter and without contraindications to regional anesthesia
3. **General anesthesia** only when regional anesthesia is contraindicated; maintain an emphasis on blood pressure reduction and blunting the hypertensive response to laryngoscopy

gerate the pathophysiology of preeclampsia, due to the release of catecholamines, and hyperventilation. Perhaps most importantly, however, epidural analgesia allows for the flexibility needed to manage the labor and delivery of the preeclamptic. These parturients frequently have labor induced with oxytocin, and density of epidural block can be titrated in response to varying levels of pain. Further, should cesarean section be required, the epidural can be used to induce anesthesia, thereby avoiding the risks associated with general anesthesia. 'Early' epidural placement in high-risk patients, including the patient with severe preeclampsia, adds to overall safety by reducing the need for general anesthesia in cases of urgent cesarean section. Such patients should be actively identified, and after informed consent is obtained, an epidural catheter should be inserted and tested. Additional local anesthetics can be administered when the patient requests labor analgesia.

Systemic

When regional anesthesia is contraindicated in the patient with preeclampsia, systemic analgesia (see Section 6.3.6) might become the only safe option. However, side effects from analgesics may be more likely in patients administered magnesium sulfate.

9.6.2 Cesarean section

A detailed discussion of anesthetic agents for regional anesthesia for cesarean delivery can be found in Chapter 7. The relative merits of different techniques and their application to the preeclamptic patient are discussed below.

Epidural anesthesia

Epidural anesthesia has been traditionally considered to be the anesthetic of choice for patients with severe preeclampsia requiring cesarean section. Because these patients can present with extreme intravascular volume depletion, a gradual-onset sympathectomy was thought to be necessary. The sympathectomy induced by epidural anesthesia is theoretically of a slower onset than one produced by a spinal anesthetic, making hypotension easier to control. When prolonged surgical times are anticipated, as in coexisting morbid obesity, epidural or CSE anesthetics allow the flexibility to extend the duration of the anesthetic. In many busy obstetric practices, epidural anesthesia is utilized in a large percentage of patients with severe preeclampsia requiring cesarean section, but this reflects the previously described practice of early epidural placement on labor and delivery in anticipation of possible cesarean section rather than *de novo* epidural catheter insertion.

Spinal anesthesia

The theoretical advantage of epidural anesthesia can be weighed against the known benefits of spinal anesthesia, such as greater reliability, less procedural time, and less epidural vascular trauma. Still, the elective use of spinal anesthesia for cesarean section in patients with severe preeclampsia remains controversial. Although it has been assumed that a spinal anesthetic in these potentially hypovolemic patients may produce a rapid sympathectomy and lead to uncontrollable hypotension, more recent data suggest that this is not the case. A retrospective review comparing spinal and epidural anesthesia for cesarean section in patients with severe preeclampsia found no differences in the lowest recorded blood pressure (*Figure 9.1*) or in the amount of ephedrine required between the two groups. Furthermore, a spinal needle may be less likely to cause an epidural hematoma in cases of 'borderline' coagulopathy than an epidural needle. Such data indicate that routine use of spinal anesthesia for cesarean section in the patient with preeclampsia presenting without a pre-existing epidural catheter (and who has no contraindications to regional anesthesia) is justified.

General anesthesia

General anesthesia should be utilized for patients with severe preeclampsia only when regional anesthesia is contraindicated or the use of regional anesthesia is precluded by the

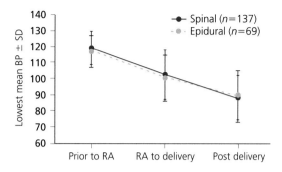

Figure 9.1 A comparison of epidural and spinal anesthesia for cesarean section in parturients with severe preeclampsia. Data points represent lowest mean arterial blood pressure (mmHg) before and during the procedure. There was no difference between groups. 'Prior to RA' is the blood pressure recorded 20 min before induction; 'RA to delivery' is the lowest blood pressure recorded between induction and delivery; and 'Post delivery' is the lowest blood pressure recorded from delivery to the end of surgery. Figure based on internal data and adapted from Hood, D.D. (1999) *Anesthesiology* **90:** 1276–1282.

urgency of the need for delivery. It is well documented that endotracheal intubation is more likely to be difficult in pregnant patients when compared with the nonpregnant population. Preeclampsia can be expected to add to the difficulties encountered during airway management, due to increased extravascular fluid causing engorgement of the upper airway. When general anesthesia cannot be avoided, great care and attention must be paid to airway management. If at all possible, two anesthesia care providers should be present when planning a general anesthetic in the patient with severe preeclampsia; one is dedicated to airway management while the other applies monitors, prepares for induction, administers medications, and provides an extra pair of hands. When time permits, at least three minutes of preoxygenation with a tight mask seal should be accomplished before induction of anesthesia. The time-saving technique of four vital capacity breaths has been suggested as a substitute and can be used in emergency settings when an easy intubation is anticipated, but it does not offer the same margin of safety as five minutes of tidal volume breathing.

An additional important hurdle specific to preeclampsia is preventing a hypertensive response to laryngoscopy. The sympathetic stimulus associated with laryngoscopy, when superimposed on the underlying hypertension, can lead to significant morbid events such as pulmonary edema and intracranial hemorrhage. In this clinical situation, the two primary goals should be reducing the patient's baseline blood pressure and blunting the hypertensive response to laryngoscopy. Reducing the baseline blood pressure at least theoretically increases the margin of safety should the response to laryngoscopy be incompletely controlled. Ideally, blood pressure control should be achieved before induction with longer acting agents, with short acting agents used for perioperative and intraoperative control. Longer acting agents (hydralazine or labetalol) usually need to be administered before the patient is transported to the operating room due to latency of onset. Even in an emergent setting, administering hydralazine and labetalol while transporting the patient to the operating room may slightly reduce the blood pressure before induction. To be most effective, however, hydralazine must be administered at least 20 minutes before surgery; it can result in compensatory tachycardia. Labetalol, on the other hand, acts more acutely than hydralazine, has a long-standing safety record in pregnancy, and is beneficial for its combined alpha- and beta-blocking properties. It reduces systematic vascular resistance (SVR) without increasing heart rate. Recommendations for dosing hydralazine and labetalol are listed in *Table 9.3*. Although esmolol has a faster onset and shorter duration of action than does labetalol, its use in pregnancy remains controversial, as it has rarely been associated with prolonged fetal bradycardia. Nitroglycerin is primarily a venodilator that can be used to control blood pressure during laryngoscopy and intubation due to a rapid onset and short duration of action. It has a wide margin of safety, and can be titrated to

effect with 50–100 µg intravenous boluses administered every 1–2 minutes as needed, or by running an infusion with continuous blood pressure measurement. In contrast to nitroglycerin, sodium nitroprusside is a potent arteriolar vasodilator that can be used with caution. Due to its potency, continuous blood pressure monitoring with an arterial catheter is recommended during its administration. Its use is usually reserved for patients with severe hypertension not responding to the other first line agents.

Although their effectiveness remains controversial, a lipid soluble opioid (fentanyl 100–150 µg, for example) and lidocaine 100 mg can be administered immediately prior to rapid sequence induction to further blunt the hypertensive response to laryngoscopy.

Following intubation, patients with severe preeclampsia should be treated like any other patient undergoing general anesthesia with a special emphasis on blood pressure control and minimizing intravenous fluid administration. Preeclampsia, magnesium sulfate, and labetalol all increase the risk of developing pulmonary edema in the severe preeclamptic. Lastly, additional antihypertensives may be required in preparation for extubation as these patients are likely to develop further hypertension during awakening. A recommended technique for general anesthesia is outlined in *Table 9.6*.

9.7 Summary

Patients with severe preeclampsia usually have multisystemic involvement and are at increased risk for significant obstetric and anesthetic complications. Anesthetic risks can be reduced by early placement of an epidural catheter whenever possible, utilizing spinal anesthesia for urgent cesarean section when patients present without a preexisting epidural catheter, and utilizing general anesthesia only when regional anesthesia is contraindicated. When general anesthesia is required, a potentially difficult airway should be anticipated. In addition, an emphasis should be placed on

Table 9.6 General anesthesia for cesarean section in the preeclamptic: recommended technique

Preparation	Antihypertensive pretreatment prior to OR to achieve DBP 90–100 mmHg if time allows Monitors and left uterine displacement Limit intravenous fluid administration
Airway	Prepare for difficult intubation • Preoxygenate for 3 min and/or 4 vital capacity breaths • 6.5 or 7.0 mm ETT
Induction	Rapid sequence induction[a] • Cricoid pressure until breath sounds identified and positive $ETCO_2$ • 4 mg/kg thiopental; 1–1.5 mg/kg succinylcholine • Consider fentanyl 100–150 mg and lidocaine 100 mg IV, NTG 200 µg (100 µg bolus during induction and 100 µg bolus during laryngoscopy)
Maintenance pre-delivery	50/50 O_2/N_2O prior to delivery 0.5 MAC volatile agent prior to delivery
Maintenance post-delivery	N_2O up to 70% as tolerated by maternal SaO_2 0.2–0.5 MAC inhalational agent Nondepolarizing muscle relaxant titrated to effect Opioids and other agents as needed after delivery Consider additional antihypertensives for extubation

[a]Awake intubation is recommended if difficult intubation is anticipated

preoperative baseline blood pressure reduction and on blunting the hypertensive response to laryngoscopy.

Further reading

American College of Obstetricians and Gynaecologists (1996) ACOG technical bulletin: hypertension in pregnancy. *Int. J. Gynecol. Obstet.* **53**: 175–183.

American Society for Anesthesiologists Task Force on Management of Difficult Airways (1993) Practicee guidelines for management of the difficult airway. *Anesthesiology* **78**: 597–902.

American Society of Regional Anesthesia Consensus Conference (1998) Neuraxial anesthesia and anticoagulation: *Reg. Anesth. Pain Med.* **23** (Suppl.): 2–12.

Ducey, J.P. and Knope, K.G. (1992) Maternal esmolol administration resulting in fetal distress and cesarean section in a term pregnancy. *Anesthesiology* **77**: 829–832.

Hood, D.D. and Curry, R. (1999) Spinal versus epidural anesthesia for cesarean section in severely preeclamptic patients: a retrospective survey. *Anesthesiology* **90**: 1276–1282.

Norris, M.C. and Dewan, D.M. (1985) Preoxygenation for cesarean section: a comparison of two techniques. *Anesthesiology* **62**: 827–829.

Voulgaropoulos, D.S. and Palmer, C.M. (1993) Coagulation studies in the preeclamptic parturient: a survey. *J. Clin. Anesth.* **5**: 99–104.

Chapter 10

Hemorrhage in obstetrics

Craig M. Palmer, MD

Contents

10.1 Introduction

Hemorrhagic complications can arise at almost any point during pregnancy, labor, and delivery, quickly turning an uneventful pregnancy into an emergent situation requiring prompt, aggressive treatment to ensure the health and well-being of mother and infant. Not surprisingly, it is pathology of the uteroplacental unit that is responsible for the majority of hemorrhagic events in the parturient. Understanding the normal anatomy and development of the uterus and placenta facilitates treatment of problems, and aids in the appropriate application of medical or obstetric (interventional) therapy. Finally, recognizing the usual time course of common critical events allows the anesthesiologist to rapidly provide the therapy independent of the obstetrical provider, and can make the difference between a good outcome and a bad one.

10.2 Uteroplacental anatomy and normal delivery

The human uterus is an extremely plastic organ. A nonpregnant, parous uterus weighs only about 70 g; at term, the uterus weighs well over a kilogram. The tremendous increase in size of the myometrium occurs in response to both steroid hormones produced during the pregnant state, and distention due to the developing fetus, placenta, and amniotic fluid volume.

Along with this increase in size and weight, there is a corresponding increase in blood flow to the uterus and placenta. At term, over 15% of maternal cardiac output flows to the uterus and placenta. The primary maternal blood supply to the uterus and placenta is from the uterine arteries, which arise as a branch of the anterior trunk of the internal iliac arteries. The ascending branch of the uterine artery supplies the major portion of the body of the uterus and the placental bed, though with pregnancy a variable portion of the blood supply to these areas may come from the ovarian arteries. In the placental bed, small endometrial (or spiral) arteries supply the actual blood supply to the placenta.

The maternal blood supply to the placenta is unique in that maternal blood actually leaves the maternal circulation, circulates through the intervillous space lined by placental trophoblastic syncytium rather than endothelium, and returns to the maternal circulation (*Figure 10.1*). Maternal arterial pressure provides the driving force that forces maternal blood in spurts into the intervillous space to bathe the chorionic villi, which contain the fetal capillaries. Oxygen and nutrient exchange occurs, and maternal blood is drained back into the maternal circulation through openings in the basal plate of the placenta to the endometrial veins. On the fetal side, deoxygenated blood is delivered to the placenta by the paired umbilical arteries, which branch into capillaries within the chorionic villi. At this level, nutrient and oxygen exchange occurs, and blood returns to the fetus via the umbilical vein.

The decidua is a specialized form of endometrium, which forms the boundary between the maternal and fetal circulations. At delivery, the placenta separates from the placental bed, leaving behind in the uterus the basal zone of the decidua that ultimately gives rise to new endometrium. With separation, the myriad small endometrial arteries that supplied the placenta are torn; in the absence of a mechanism to halt blood loss, they would continue to spurt blood into the now empty uterine cavity. Two mechanisms normally prevent on-going blood loss: the elasticity of the arterioles allows them to retract and constrict, and contraction of the myometrium physically compresses the disrupted vessels. Obstetric hemorrhage most often results from impaired myometrial contraction

The causes of obstetric hemorrhage can be generally classified as occurring pre-, intra-, or post-partum, although there is some overlap between these categories.

10.3 Maternal hemorrhage: prepartum

10.3.1 Placental abruption
Placental abruption refers to the partial premature separation of a normally implanted

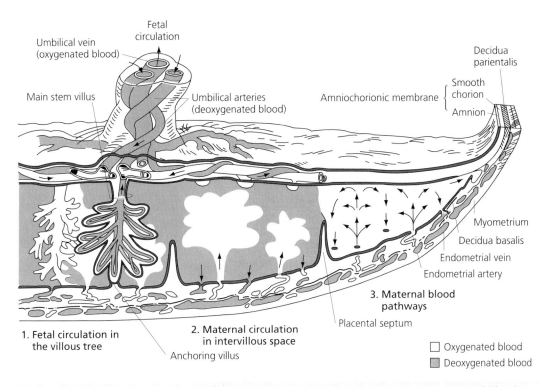

Figure 10.1 Schematic cross-section of the anatomy of a normal human placenta. Deoxygenated blood from the fetus enters the placenta and flows through capillaries in the villi where oxygen and nutrient exchange occurs, before returning to the fetal circulation via the umbilical vein. Maternal blood enters via the endometrial arteries, circulates through the intervillous space and returns to the maternal circulation through the endometrial veins. From *Willam's Obstetrics*, 19th edition (eds Cunningham, F.G., Macdonald, P.C., Gant, N.F., *et al.*) Appleton and Lange, Norwalk, CT.

placenta; in rare instances, the separation may be complete. This may occur either pre- or intrapartum. The reported frequency of occurrence of abruption depends on the criteria used for diagnosis, but the incidence has been estimated to be between 1 in 77 and 1 in 86 deliveries. While there is no single cause for abruption, a number of conditions have been associated with a higher incidence of abruption (*Table 10.1*). Hypertension, both chronic and pregnancy-induced, is a clearly implicated etiologic factor. External trauma (particularly motor vehicle accidents), preterm rupture of membranes, and uterine abnormalities such as leiomyoma increase risk. Lifestyle factors (smoking, ethanol abuse, and particularly cocaine abuse) increase the incidence of abruption.

Abruption has both maternal and fetal implications. Uterine bleeding associated with delivery is usually limited by myometrial contraction as discussed above; in abruption, placental separation is not followed by myometrial contraction. The uterus does not empty, therefore effective myometrial

Table 10.1 Factors associated with placental abruption

Pregnancy-induced hypertension (PIH)

Chronic hypertension

Premature rupture of membranes

External trauma

Cigarette smoking

Cocaine abuse

Uterine leiomyoma

Increased parity

Increased age

contraction cannot occur, and on-going maternal blood loss usually results. For the fetus, the decrease in placental surface area may result in asphyxia. Abruption is severe enough to be fatal to the fetus in about 1 in 750 deliveries, and accounts for about 15% of third trimester stillbirths. Additionally, severe neurologic damage may occur in surviving neonates.

The most common symptom of abruption is vaginal bleeding, usually associated with uterine tenderness or back pain. Other signs include fetal heart rate abnormalities, preterm labor or uterine hypertonus, and infrequently, fetal demise (*Table 10.2*). Up to 90% of abruptions will be either mild or moderate, without fetal distress, maternal hypotension or coagulopathy. It is important to note that the amount of visible vaginal blood loss usually markedly underestimates the actual maternal blood loss. While some vaginal bleeding is usually apparent, up to 3000 ml of blood can be sequestered behind the placenta in a 'concealed' hemorrhage without external bleeding. This may occur when the placenta remains circumferentially adherent around a central area of abruption (*Figure 10.2*).

In severe cases, maternal coagulopathy can occur; abruption is the most common cause of disseminated intravascular coagulation (DIC) during pregnancy. This is manifested as thrombocytopenia, hypofibrinogenemia, and decreased levels of factors V and VIII; fibrin-split products appear in the maternal circulation, and clinical oozing may become apparent. Two possible mechanisms for the

Table 10.2 Signs and symptoms of placental abruption

Sign/symptom	Frequency (percent of cases)
Vaginal bleeding	78
Uterine tenderness or back pain	66
Fetal distress	60
Increased uterine tone/contractions	34
Preterm labor	22
Fetal demise	17

After Hurd, W.W., Miodovnik, M., Hertzberg, V., and Lavin, J.P. (1983) *Obstet. Gynecol.* **61**: 467–473.

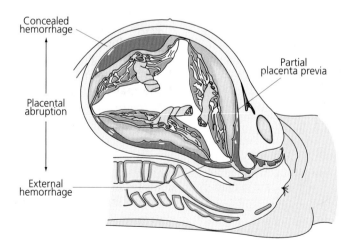

Figure 10.2 Hemorrhage from placental abruption and placenta previa. External (vaginal) bleeding is usually apparent in both conditions, although up to 3 liters of blood may be lost in a concealed hemorrhage without evidence of external blood loss. From *Willam's Obstetrics*, 19th edn (eds. Cunningham, F.G., Macdonald, P.C., Gant, N.F., *et al.*) Appleton and Lange, Norwalk, CT.

development of this coagulopathy have been proposed: it may result from activation of circulating plasminogen, or alternatively, placental thromboplastin may trigger activation of the extrinsic clotting pathway.

10.3.2 Anesthetic management: placental abruption

If abruption is suspected, blood should be drawn immediately to check hemoglobin and hematocrit, platelet count, fibrinogen, and fibrin-split products, as well as for type and crossmatch. Subsequent management depends on the severity of the situation (*Figure 10.3*). Without on-going blood loss, maternal hypovolemia, or coagulopathy (and in the presence of a reassuring fetal heart rate), labor may be induced with continuous fetal monitoring. Regional anesthesia can be safely employed in these patients, assuming there is no evidence of uncorrected maternal hypovolemia, and the platelet count is stable at 100 000 or higher.

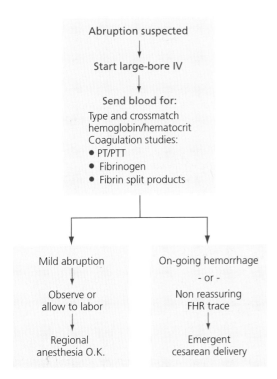

Figure 10.3 Management of the parturient with suspected placental abruption.

Most obstetric anesthesiologists will accept a platelet count as low as 70 000 if there are strong maternal indications for using a regional anesthetic. Regional anesthesia should be avoided if the mother is hypo-volemic, there is on-going hemorrhage, or there are significant fetal heart rate abnormalities.

With a severe abruption (i.e. with on-going blood loss, coagulopathy, or a nonreassuring fetal heart rate), emergent cesarean delivery may be necessary, with general anesthesia usually indicated. Once the decision to proceed to cesarean delivery has been made, the first anesthetic consideration should be the maternal volume status. A healthy term parturient can lose 10–15% of circulating blood volume without any change in vital signs; if a parturient is tachycardic, hypotensive, or oliguric, she is likely to be severely volume depleted (*Table 10.3*). Adequate intravenous access is essential; at least one (ideally two) large-bore IV catheters (16 gauge or larger) should be in place. In addition to routine precautions for cesarean delivery (Chapter 7), the hypovolemic parturient presents additional considerations (*Table 10.4*). Because sodium thiopental is a vasodilator, it is not an appropriate induction agent. Ketamine, which supports blood pressure through sympathetic stimulation, is the agent of choice. After induction, but before delivery, support of the fetus is critical – delivery of 100% oxygen will maximize oxygen delivery to the fetus. After delivery, up to 70% nitrous oxide may be used if the maternal SaO_2 remains adequate, and conversion to a 'nitrous/narcotic' anesthetic allows use of minimal concentrations of inhaled anesthetic; all the inhaled anesthetic agents cause dose-related uterine relaxation which can contribute to blood loss. If aggressive fluid resuscitation fails to restore adequate maternal blood pressure, additional 'stat' labs should be sent to check hematocrit, coagulation status, and acid–base balance (arterial blood gas analysis). In the unstable parturient, serious consideration should be given to placement of an arterial line for continuous blood pressure monitoring and repeated blood draws for laboratory work.

Table 10.3 Clinical signs and symptoms of blood loss and hypovolemia in the term parturient

Amount of blood loss		Clinical finding
Mild bleeding	15% of blood volume (up to 1000 ml)	Mild tachycardia Normal blood pressure and respiration Negative tilt test Normal urine output
Moderate bleeding	20%–25% of blood volume (up to 1600 ml)	Tachycardia (heart rate 110–130) Decreased pulse pressure Moderate tachypnea Positive capillary blanching test Positive tilt test Urine output <1 ml/kg/h
Severe bleeding	30%–35% of blood volume (up to 2400 ml)	Marked tachycardia (heart rate 120–160) Cold, clammy, pallid skin Hypotension Tachypnea (respirations >30/min) Oliguria
Massive bleeding	40% of blood volume (over 2400 ml)	Profound shock Mental status changes/disorientation Systolic blood pressure <80 mmHg Peripheral pulses absent Marked tachycardia Oliguria or anuria

After Ferouz, F. (1998) Peripartum hemorrhage and maternal resuscitation. In: *Obstetric Anesthesia,* 2nd edn (ed. Norris, M.C.), p. 564. Lippincott, Williams & Wilkins, Philadelphia.

Even following delivery, be prepared for massive blood loss. Blood infiltrating the myometrium may result in a 'Couvelaire' uterus, preventing adequate uterine contraction and inhibiting hemostasis. In addition to oxytocin, other uterotonic agents may be necessary for adequate uterine contraction (see Section 10.6). In rare situations, internal iliac artery ligation or hysterectomy may be necessary to stop hemorrhage. Once hemorrhage is controlled, coagulation should return to normal within several hours, but getting control of the bleeding may require aggressive treatment of the coagulopathy, utilizing not only packed red blood cells (PRBCs), but also fresh-frozen plasma, platelet concentrates, and even cryoprecipitate. Use of these blood products is ideally based on laboratory evidence of derangements, but clinical judgement may be the only tool available in a rapidly changing, emergent situation.

10.3.3 Placenta previa

Placenta previa refers to an abnormal implantation of the placenta, over or close to the cervical os. It can be classified as complete, partial, or marginal (*Figure 10.4*). The incidence of placenta previa at term is about 1 in 200 to 250 deliveries. Routine prenatal ultrasonography generally identifies a higher percentage of previa in early gestation, but most of these resolve by the third trimester as enlargement of the gravid uterus carries the implantation site away from the cervical os. Previa is more common in the multipara, particularly those with prior cesarean delivery (see Section 10.5.3), or a history of prior previa.

The problem with placenta previa is that as the cervical os begins to dilate with the onset of labor, the placenta over the os will detach and maternal hemorrhage will ensue. The detachment occurs as in a normal delivery, but as with abruption, the bleeding will continue

Adequate IV access

Routine precautions
- Aspiration prophylaxis – oral sodium citrate
- Denitrogenation
- Assistance available

Anesthetic agents
- Induction: Ketamine, 1–1.5 mg/kg
- Relaxation: Succinylcholine relaxant of choice

Maintenance (pre-delivery)
- Nitrous oxide (with on-going fetal stress, 100% O_2 indicated for fetal oxygenation)
- Inhalational agents: 0.5 MAC or less if maternal blood pressure tolerates

Maintenance (post-delivery)
- Continue relaxation (follow train-of-four)
- Inhalational agent: isoflurane 0.2% or sevoflurane 0.5% for amnesia
- Nitrous oxide (up to 70%) if tolerated
- Opioid – fentanyl

Monitoring
- Routine: ECG, BP, PO, ET-CO_2 and Foley
- Invasive? Consider arterial line

until the uterus can contract effectively (i.e. after delivery). Because neither the mother nor the fetus can tolerate the blood loss or the loss of placental surface area, respectively, once diagnosed, delivery will always be via cesarean section.

The undiagnosed placenta previa usually presents as painless vaginal bleeding in the third trimester; for this reason, *all vaginal bleeding in the third trimester should be considered placenta previa until proven otherwise.* Bleeding due to previa may stop spontaneously, or it may be sudden and severe. In the past, the definitive diagnosis of placenta previa was made by direct examination of the cervical os with a vaginal speculum exam. Because such an exam can provoke brisk, even torrential hemorrhage, the exam was performed as a 'double set-up' – the parturient was placed in lithotomy position for the speculum exam in the operating room, but with her abdomen prepped and draped in preparation for an immediate cesarean delivery. Today, the wide-spread use and availability of ultrasonography, and its excellent accuracy in diagnosis, have all but eliminated the need for the double set-up.

10.3.4 Anesthetic management: placenta previa

Management of the diagnosed previa depends on the stage of gestation and clinical presentation. In the face of on-going bleeding, expeditious cesarean delivery is indicated. With rapid or massive blood loss, general anesthesia is usually necessary, as it is the most rapid way to deliver the infant and stabilize the mother – blood loss will continue until infant and

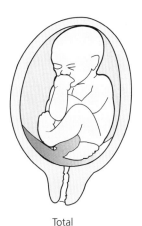 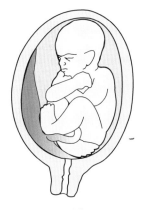 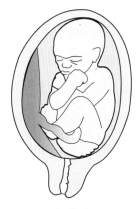

Total   Partial   Marginal

Figure 10.4 Classification of placenta previa.

placenta are delivered. If the initial bleeding episode has stopped spontaneously, regional anesthesia can be employed following careful assessment of maternal volume status (heart rate, blood pressure, urine output); maternal hypovolemia is a strong relative contraindication to the use of regional anesthesia.

When diagnosed prior to about 32 weeks' gestation, obstetric management is 'expectant' – primarily bed rest and hope (that the patient will not start bleeding). Due to the increased risk of bleeding near term, after about 32 weeks' gestation, fetal maturity is assessed (usually by amniocentesis), and elective cesarean delivery undertaken once maturity is confirmed.

10.4 Maternal hemorrhage: intrapartum

10.4.1 Uterine rupture

Uterine rupture may occur pre-, intra-, or even postpartum, but is most commonly an intrapartum event, as uterine contractions increase in force. While the associated mortality is usually low (about 0.1% in the US), it can be catastrophic for both the mother and infant. By far the major cause of uterine rupture is separation of a previous uterine scar, from a prior cesarean section. A scar from a classical (vertical) uterine incision is more likely to dehisce during labor than a low-transverse segment scar. The classical incision extends well into the myometrium, whereas the low-transverse segment incision is primarily through connective tissue; this lower incision heals much more solidly than an incision through uterine muscle. Other, less frequent causes are listed in *Table 10.5*. Maternal mortality is higher if there is no prior uterine scar, or the rupture is traumatic.

Symptoms of rupture include vaginal bleeding, severe uterine or abdominal pain, shoulder pain, the disappearance of fetal heart tones, and/or hypotension. In a parturient with obvious hypotension or shock, general anesthesia is indicated to rapidly deliver the infant and explore the abdomen to control hemorrhage.

Table 10.5 Conditions associated with uterine rupture

Previous uterine scar (prior cesarean section: 'VBAC')

External trauma

Excessive oxytocin stimulation

Grand multiparity

Fetal malpresentation

Uterine distention (macrosomia, hydramnios)

Internal trauma :
- forceps, vacuum use
- curettage
- internal version
- manual exploration

10.4.2 Anesthetic considerations: vaginal birth after cesarean delivery

The American College of Obstetricians and Gynecologists has determined that almost all parturients with a prior low-uterine-segment cesarean delivery can safely undergo a trial of labor and subsequent vaginal delivery. When this practice first began to be widely employed in the 1980s, many obstetricians believed regional anesthesia was contraindicated, fearing that epidural block would mask the pain associated with uterine rupture and delay diagnosis. However, experience has shown that pain is not the only, or even most prominent, symptom of intrapartum rupture in 'VBAC' (vaginal birth after cesarean) patients (*Table 10.6*). Several large series have indicated that regional anesthesia *can* be safely employed, and can actually increase the chance of successful vaginal delivery by allaying maternal pain and anxiety (*Table 10.7*).

Table 10.6 Signs and symptoms of intrapartum uterine rupture

Fetal heart rate abnormalities/fetal stress

Vaginal bleeding

Abnormal labor pattern or uterine hypertonus

Hypotension

Atypical abdominal pain (not associated with uterine contractions)

Abdominal tenderness

Table 10.7 Epidural anesthesia for labor and success of VBAC

Mode of delivery	Epidural anesthesia (n = 60)	No anesthesia (n = 172)	Total (n = 242)
Vaginal	66 (94.2%)	118 (68.6%)	184
Cesarean	4 (5.8%)	54 (31.4%)	58

Data from Nguyen, T.V, *et al.* (1992) Vaginal birth after cesarean section at the University of Texas. *J. Reprod. Med.* **37**: 880–882.

Prudence still dictates that the lowest concentration of local anesthetics that provide adequate analgesia should be used in these patients; combination techniques using opioids and epinephrine can allow very low concentrations (bupivacaine 0.0625% or lower) to be used.

10.5 Maternal hemorrhage: postpartum

While technically any bleeding within 6 weeks after delivery is considered postpartum hemorrhage, truly significant blood loss usually occurs immediately after delivery, or within 1–2 hours. Postpartum hemorrhage is the most common cause of serious blood loss in obstetrics.

10.5.1 Retained placenta
Retained placenta occurs in about 1% of deliveries, and usually requires manual exploration of the uterus. If the uterus does not empty completely after delivery, it will not be able to fully contract, and arteries of the decidua basalis will continue to bleed. Anesthetic management of retained placenta must take into account two factors: uterine relaxation and analgesia. In order to manually explore the uterus, it is often necessary to relax the uterus; traditionally, the inhalational agents (halothane, isoflurane) have been used for this – at inhaled concentrations well over 1 MAC, they are very effective uterine relaxants. Use at these concentrations means inducing a general anesthetic, however, with all the associated concerns of aspiration risk, airway management, maternal volume status, etc. Nitroglycerin has been shown to be an effective alternative for uterine relaxation, and has the

advantage of not being an anesthetic agent. Bolus intravenous administration of 100–200 μg nitroglycerin will produce uterine relaxation within 30–45 seconds that lasts only 60–90 seconds due to its short half-life (*Table 10.8*). Due to systemic vasodilatation, maternal hypotension can be significant, but this should be a short-lived side effect. Nitroglycerin does not provide analgesia, however, so other measures may need to be taken. If a parturient has an epidural catheter in place from labor, this can be used for analgesia, but again, careful consideration must be paid to maternal volume status before dosing the epidural and potentially vasodilating the patient.

10.5.2 Uterine atony
Uterine atony occurs in varying degrees following 2–5% of deliveries, and is the most common cause of serious blood loss in obstetrics. With 15% or more of maternal cardiac output at term going to the gravid uterus, a completely atonic uterus can easily lose 2 l of

Table 10.8 Clinical use of nitroglycerin for uterine relaxation

Prepare appropriate dilution
- NTG supplied as 50 mg/10 ml vial (5 mg/ml)
- Add to 500 ml normal saline
- Result: 100 μg/ml

Administration: bolus dosing
- Begin with 100 μg bolus
- Increase by increments of 100 μg until desired effect (i.e. uterine relaxation)

Action
- Onset 30–45 seconds
- Duration 60–90 seconds

Side effects: hypotension
- R_x with phenylephrine bolus IV as necessary

blood in 5 minutes. A number of factors have been shown to increase the risk of uterine atony (*Table 10.9*).

Initial management is medical – fluid resuscitation of the parturient is critical to restore blood volume, and can be life-saving. Oxygen supplementation (high flows via face mask), uterine massage, and use of uterotonics may allow avoidance of operative intervention (see Section 10.5.4).

10.5.3 Placenta accreta

Placenta accreta (and variants, placenta increta and percreta) refers to abnormal development and implantation of the placenta without the decidua basalis layer. The decidua basalis forms the normal interface and cleavage plane between the placenta and the uterus; in its absence, the placenta implants directly onto (placenta accreta) the myometrium. Placenta increta refers to a placenta that invades into the myometrium, and with placenta percreta, the placenta actually invades through the myometrium and may implant on other intra-abdominal structures. With any of the variations, separation of the placenta after delivery disrupts the myometrium and can result in severe bleeding; complete separation of the placenta is not possible, and continuing blood loss results.

The overall incidence of placenta accreta is 1 in 2000 deliveries or less, but it is not usually diagnosed until after delivery, when prompt action becomes necessary. One patient population has been found to have a predictably higher incidence of placenta accreta however: patients with known placenta previa and a prior cesarean section. As the number of prior cesareans increases, the risk of a placenta accreta also increases: with a previa and four prior cesaream sections, the incidence has been reported as over 50% (*Table 10.10*).

10.5.4 Anesthetic management: 'gravid' hysterectomy

While on infrequent occasions hemorrhage can be controlled with curettage, more often surgical intervention is necessary, usually hysterectomy. As noted above, maternal blood flow to the uterus at term is substantial, and the major vessels are located deep in the pelvis; control of these vessels is the major obstacle facing the obstetrician, and is rarely accomplished without substantial blood loss.

Table 10.9 Conditions associated with uterine atony

High parity

Dysfunctional labor

Uterine distention
- Multiple gestation
- Polyhydramnios
- Macrosomia

Retained placenta

Infection
- Chorioamnionitis

Medications
- Prolonged oxytocin use during labor
- Tocolytic agents
- Inhalational anesthetics

Table 10.10 Association of placenta accreta in parturients with placenta previa and prior cesarean delivery

Number of prior cesarean sections	Number of parturients with placenta accreta (*n* = 236)	Placenta previa and accreta (*n* = 29)	%
0	238	12	5
1	25	6	24
2	15	7	47
3	5	2	40
4	3	2	67

Data from Clark, S.L. *et al.* (1985) Placenta previa/accreta and prior cesarean section. *Obstet. Gynecol.* 66: 89–92.

Once the decision to perform a 'gravid' hysterectomy is made (or even considered), the anesthesiologist should anticipate a difficult case with major on-going blood loss (*Table 10.11*). The first priority should be to establish large-bore intravenous access for fluid resuscitation. It is important to try to do this before major blood loss has occurred, because once the patient has become hypovolemic, vasoconstricted, and cold, it becomes very difficult to place peripheral IV lines. With regard to monitoring, an arterial cannula is extremely useful, as blood pressure swings can be rapid and frequent; the arterial line also provides a convenient method to draw blood for serial determinations of hemoglobin, hematocrit, and coagulation profile. Anticipating the likelihood of the need for transfusion, type- and cross-matched blood should be brought to the operating room; if cross-matched blood is not available, 'emergency release' type O-negative blood should be requested. Finally, even if the delivery has been performed with an adequate regional anesthetic, if the maternal airway can be easily secured, conversion to a general, endotracheal anesthetic should be strongly considered. The wide swings in blood pressure which often occur usually make for a very uncomfortable, nauseous patient, and it is difficult to attend to the patient and aggressively volume resuscitate her at the same time. A second pair of hands to help in these cases is almost essential.

The primary goal during a gravid hysterectomy is to maintain circulating blood volume. Depending on the degree of blood loss, transfusion with packed red blood cells is usually necessary. The degree of blood loss will

also dictate the need to support maternal coagulation status: with substantial blood loss, fresh-frozen plasma and platelet transfusion are often necessary.

10.6 Uterotonics

The initial management of uterine atony is medical; uterotonics are used to increase uterine contraction and tone, to allow the normal process of post-delivery hemostasis to occur. Three classes of uterotonics are currently available for clinical use: oxytocin, ergot alkaloids, and prostaglandins (*Table 10.12*).

Among the uterotonics, oxytocin is usually the initial therapy – up to 40 Iμ/l may be infused as rapidly as possible; increasing the dose beyond this does not offer any benefit. Oxytocin is a naturally occurring neurohypophyseal hormone for which specific receptors exist in the myometrium. Systemically, it is a vasodilator, and may aggravate hypotension if administered rapidly; if both rapid volume infusion and rapid oxytocin infusion are necessary concurrently, consider using two intravenous lines.

The ergot alkaloids have been used in obstetrics for over 400 years; they are derived from a fungus that grows upon grain, particularly rye. Methylergonovine (Methergine®), a commercially available ergot alkaloid, is a second line agent for the treatment of uterine atony, and is particularly effective for producing a sustained increase in uterine tone. Because it has a relatively long half-life, it does not need to be given via continuous infusion, as does oxytocin. Methylergonovine is administered intramuscularly at a dose of 0.4 mg; if two doses do not result in appropriate uterine tone, other therapy should be instituted. Systemically, methylergonovine can cause hypertension, likely due to α-adrenergic stimulation; systemic hypertension is a relative contraindication to its use.

Carboprost tromethamine is a third uterotonic option. Carboprost is a stable analog of the naturally occurring prostaglandin, PGF$_{2\alpha}$. It is given at a 0.25 mg dose IM, or can be injected directly intramyometrially. Total dose

Table 10.11 Anesthetic considerations for 'gravid' hysterectomy

Expect major blood loss
- Call for blood in the room
- Place large-bore IVs early before the patient is symptomatic

Strongly consider arterial line

Convert to general anesthesia

Table 10.12 Uterotonics

Medication	Class	Administration	Dosing	Side effects	Comments
Oxytocin	Neurohypophyseal hormone	Infusion	Up to 40 IU/l	Hypotension with rapid infusion	Initial therapy
Methylergonovine	Ergot alkaloid	Intramuscular	0.4 mg IM; repeat once	Hypertension	Sustained increase in uterine tone
Carboprost	Prostaglandin	Intramuscular Intramyometrial	0.25 mg IM repeat up to 1.0 mg total	Systemic and pulmonary hypertension, bronchospasm	Never administer intravenously

should probably not exceed 0.75–1.0 mg. Carboprost is an extremely effective uterotonic, but it has significant systemic side effects; it should never be administered intravenously. Carboprost is a potent systemic and pulmonary vasoconstrictor, and bronchoconstrictor. Intravenous administration can be associated with severe bronchospasm, and systemic and pulmonary hypertension. Intramyometrial administration should also be used with caution, as rapid uptake by uterine venous sinuses can have the same effect as intravenous administration. Due to its propensity to cause bronchospasm, carboprost should be used with caution in asthmatics; the urgency of the need to increase uterine tone should be weighed against the severity of the patient's asthma.

10.7 Transfusion in obstetrics

The need for transfusion in the obstetric population is not uncommon, but there is often reluctance on the part of anesthesiologists to employ it, due to the perceived risks. A considered decision to employ transfusion therapy must take into account not only the risks, but also the benefits of the therapy.

10.7.1 Risks of transfusion

The risks associated with transfusion can be classified as infectious and noninfectious. Noninfectious risk is most often due to human error, and can occur at many points in the transfusion process. An ABO incompatible transfusion occurs about 1:12 000 transfused units, but is fatal in only a small number of cases (estimated at 19 per year in the US). Acute lung injury and circulatory overload occurs in about 1 in 2000 patients requiring transfusion overall, but should be less frequent and carry lower morbidity in the obstetric population.

Infectious risks are about twice as common. Fear of acquiring HIV is common, but the risk of acquiring HIV via transfusion is actually quite low: about 1:450 000 units or less. Hepatitis B is more common, at 1:63 000 units, but only about 1 in 10 patients infected develop long-term sequelae. Most problematic is hepatitis C; about 1:125 000 units are potentially infectious. Though our understanding of this disease is still evolving, the current best estimates indicate that almost all patients infected will eventually develop chronic disease, either cirrhosis or chronic active hepatitis. It can take decades to develop clinically apparent disease after infection with hepatitis C, but the young age of the obstetric population means that once infected, most will live long enough to become symptomatic.

10.7.2 Benefits of transfusion

The obvious benefits of transfusion include increased oxygen-carrying capacity of the blood (resulting in increased tissue delivery of oxygen), restoration of circulating blood volume, and elevation of clotting factors. The critical level of oxygen delivery is probably in the range of 300–330 ml/min/m of body surface area (BSA). In an average parturient with a BSA of 1.7 m^2, cardiac output of 6 l/min, and hemoglobin of 6.0 g/dl, oxygen delivery will be only 277 ml/min/m. Such a situation should be unusual however: the normal response to blood loss is to increase cardiac output to compensate, increasing oxygen delivery proportionately. Increasing cardiac output to 12 l/min (within reason for almost all parturients) will increase oxygen delivery to over 550 ml/min/m. In practice, few parturients will require transfusion with a hemoglobin level of 7.0 g/dl or greater, assuming appropriate volume replacement has been provided. Complete (albeit slow) recovery in parturients who refused transfusion despite hemoglobin levels below 3.0 g/dl has been reported.

Use of blood products other than PRBCs is most common in the setting of massive blood loss (≥150 ml/min, or loss of over 50% of circulating blood volume in 3 hours). The most common (earliest) derangement in this setting is thrombocytopenia. Platelet transfusion should infrequently be necessary with a platelet count over 50 000 /μl. In the average (70–80 kg) parturient, each unit of platelets should raise the platelet count by 5–10 000 /μl; a unit of plasmapherized platelets is equivalent to 5–8 single donor units. Acutely, massive blood loss and rapid replacement is also likely to require replacement of circulating clotting factors with FFP; cryoprecipitate should be used to specifically raise fibrinogen levels.

10.7.3 Blood storage and salvage

In recent years, new strategies to reduce the need for homologous transfusion have been applied to the obstetric population; these include autologous donation of blood, and intraoperative blood salvage. Autologous donation has been found to be safe for pregnant patients and their fetuses, assuming the parturient does not have a preexisting anemia (hgb < 11g/dl). The limitation of autologous donation is in identifying appropriate candidates; the low incidence of the need for transfusion in the overall obstetric population does not make autologous donation practical or cost-effective for routine use. It may have a place in the management of certain high-risk patients, such as those with placenta previa or accreta, women with known abnormal antibodies, or those undergoing scheduled cesarean hysterectomy.

Blood salvage has recently been shown to be a viable option in the obstetric population. Initial fears that autologous transfusion during cesarean delivery might induce amniotic fluid embolism have proven unfounded, using published salvage protocols. As with autologous donation, the low incidence of the need for transfusion at cesarean delivery does not make it cost-effective for routine use. In those settings where major blood loss can be anticipated, it is certainly worth consideration.

Further reading

Clark, S.L., Koonings, P.P. and Phelan, J.P. (1985) Placenta previa/accreta and prior cesarean section. *Obstet. Gynecol.* **66**: 89–92.

Douglas, W.J. and Ward, M.E. (1994) Current pharmacology and the obstetric anesthesiologist. *Int. Anesth. Clin.* **32**: 1–10.

Iyasu, S., Saftlas, A.P., Rowley, D.L. *et al.* (1993) The epidemiology of placenta previa in the United States, 1979 through 1987. *Am. J. Obstet. Gynecol.* **168**: 1424–1429.

Lynch, J.C., and Pardy, J.P. (1996) Uterine rupture and scar dehiscence. A five-year survey. *Anaesth. Intens. Care* **24**: 699–704.

Nguyen, T.V., Dinh, T.V., Suresh, M.S. *et al.* (1992) Vaginal birth after cesarean section at the University of Texas. *J. Reprod. Med.* **37**: 880–882.

Nunn, J.F. and Freeman, J. (1964) Problems of oxygenation and oxygen transport during anaesthesia (I). *Anaesthesia* **19**: 120–121.

Nunn, J.F. and Freeman, J. (1964) Problems of oxygenation and oxygen transport during haemorrhage (II). *Anaesthesia* **19**: 206–216.

Rainaldi, M.P., Tazzari, P.L., Scagliarini, G. *et al.* (1998) Blood salvage during caesarean section. *Br. J. Anaesth.* **80**: 195–198.

Rall, T.W. (1993) Oxytocin, prostaglandins, ergot alkaloids, and other drugs: tocolytic agents. In: *Goodman's and Gilman's Pharmacology*, 8th edn (ed. Gilman, A), pp. 933–953. McGraw Hill, New York.

Rasanayagam, S.R. and Cooper, G.M. (1996) Two cases of severe postpartum anaemia in Jehovah's witnesses. *Int. J. Obstet. Anesth.* **5**: 202–205.

Rasmussen, S., Irgens, L.M., Bersjo, P. and Dalaker, K. (1996) The occurrence of placental abruption in Norway 1967–1991. *Acta Obstet. Gynecol. Scand.* **75**: 222–228.

Rasmussen, S., Irgens, L.M., Bersjo, P. and Dalaker, K. (1996) Perinatal mortality and case fatality after placental abruption in Norway 1967–1991. *Acta Obstet. Gynecol. Scand.* **75**: 229–234.

Riley, E.T., Flanagan, B., Cohen, S.E. and Chitkara, U. (1996) Intravenous nitroglycerin: a potent uterine relaxant for emergency obstetric procedures. Review of literature and report of three cases. *Int. J. Obstet. Anesth.* **5**: 264–268.

Saftlas, A.F., Olson, D.R., Atrash, H.K. *et al.* (1991) National trends in the incidence of abruption placentae, 1979–1987. *Obstet. Gynecol.* **78**: 1081–1086.

Schreiber, G.B., Busch, M.P., Kleinman, S.H. *et al.* (1996) The risk of transfusion-transmitted viral infections. *NEJM* **33**: 1686–1690.

United States General Accounting Office (1997) Blood Supply: Transfusion-associated risk. GAO/PEMD-97-2. Washington, DC.

Chapter 11

Obesity

Medge Owen, MD and
Robert D'Angelo, MD

Contents

11.1 Introduction

Obesity is a worldwide public health problem reaching epidemic proportions. Throughout Europe and the United States obesity affects 20–25% of the population. Interestingly, the prevalence of obesity varies with socioeconomic status. In developed countries, poverty is associated with obesity whereas in developing countries, affluence carries a higher risk. In obstetric patients, obesity may be the most common high-risk problem seen by the anesthesiologist. Roughly, 8–10% of obstetric patients are obese and the incidence is increasing, as is the incidence of extreme obesity (>100 kg). Obesity is a condition of excess body fat. Many criteria have been used to define obesity, without agreement. Most commonly, body mass index (BMI) is used to define obesity (Table 11.1), but a simpler definition of morbid obesity is twice ideal body weight. In addition, many consider any patient weighing more than about 140 kg to be morbidly obese.

11.2 Pathophysiology

Obesity during pregnancy increases the risk of maternal and fetal morbidity and mortality. Obesity exaggerates the normal physiological changes of pregnancy creating more work for an already stressed cardiorespiratory system. Obesity creates strain on the body's most vital organ systems. The most significant pathophysiological changes with anesthetic implications occur in the pulmonary, cardiovascular and gastrointestinal systems (Table 11.2).

11.2.1 Pulmonary

Increased body size increases energy requirements, causing oxygen consumption and carbon dioxide production to increase in proportion to weight. To meet the added energy demands, minute ventilation must also increase, but a large body habitus makes this difficult. Increased chest wall weight decreases lung compliance requiring even greater energy expenditure to lift the chest during inspiration. Abdominal weight also restricts diaphragmatic movement, especially in the supine or Trendelenburg position, making breathing more difficult. Lung volumes and capacities are reduced and functional residual capacity (FRC) may become less than closing capacity resulting in airway closure during tidal ventilation. Abdominal and chest wall weight also promotes airway closure in dependent parts of the lung shifting ventilation to the more compliant, nondependent lung areas. Since pulmonary blood flow preferentially occurs in the dependent lung segments, ventilation/perfusion mismatch and hypoxemia can result. Despite all the pulmonary alterations with obesity, airway resistance and diffusion capacity usually remain normal.

11.2.2 Cardiovascular

Pulmonary hypertension is relatively common in the morbidly obese patient and can develop from increased pulmonary blood flow, chronic hypoxemia, or both. Obesity is associated with a three-fold increase in hypertension that can

Table 11.1 Weight classification by BMI[a]

Weight	BMI
Normal	18.5–24.9
Overweight	25.0–29.9
Obesity I	30.0–34.9
Obesity II	35.0–39.9
Obesity III	> 40

[a]BMI = Body mass index = $\dfrac{\text{Weight (kg)}}{\text{Height (m)}^2}$

Table 11.2 Pathophysiologic changes associated with obesity

Pathophysiological changes

↑ Energy requirements	↑ Cardiac output
↑ O_2 consumption	Pulmonary hypertension
↑ CO_2 production	Chronic hypertension
↓ FRC	Hiatal hernia
V/Q mismatch	Delayed gastric emptying
Chronic hypoxemia	Diabetes mellitus

lead to left ventricular hypertrophy and abnormal diastolic function. There is a clear relationship between obesity and death due to cardiovascular causes including ischemic heart disease, coronary artery disease, and cardiac arrhythmias. In obese young adults 25–34 years of age, a 12-fold increase in the risk of death from cardiovascular disease has been reported. This includes women of childbearing potential.

11.2.3 Gastrointestinal
Obese patients have an increased prevalence of hiatal hernia and delayed gastric emptying. In a fasting state, most obese patients will have a gastric volume more than 25 ml with a gastric pH less than 2.5, putting them at risk of aspiration pneumonitis. During pregnancy the risk of aspiration is particularly high. Therefore, all obese parturients should be considered to have a full stomach even when fasting and receive a nonparticulate oral antacid prior to surgery.

11.3 Pregnancy and obesity

In some instances, pregnancy may offer a degree of protection to the obese patient. Frequent shallow respirations are more efficient for obese patients, but during pregnancy, hormone-induced increases in tidal volume produce higher PaO_2 levels compared with nonpregnant obese patients. This increased ventilation accounts for similar $PaCO_2$ values seen in both obese and nonobese pregnant patients. Although FRC is decreased in both

pregnancy and obesity, the conditions are not additive.

11.4 Obstetric complications

Obstetric problems associated with obesity are listed in *Table 11.3* and can occur throughout the puerperium.

11.4.1 Antepartum
Obese mothers tend to be older and more parous than nonobese mothers, which may account for some of the coexisting medical problems. Independent of medical problems, obesity alone places the parturient in a 'high risk' category and can complicate the obstetric course. Obesity prior to pregnancy, weight gain during pregnancy, and the higher incidence of gestational diabetes in the obese parturient can lead to fetal macrosomia, a problem that can dramatically alter the course of labor and delivery.

11.4.2 Intrapartum
Obese parturients are at lower risk for premature labor compared with nonobese controls, but are at greater risk for late or failed spontaneous onset of labor. For this reason, medical induction of labor frequently occurs. Fetal macrosomia may lead to complicated vaginal delivery, but more likely results in cephalopelvic disproportion (CPD) and arrest of labor necessitating cesarean section. Induction of labor, fetal macrosomia, and obesity are independent risk factors for cesarean section. In fact, the incidence of cesarean section in

Table 11.3 Obstetric complications associated with obesity

Hypertension	Thrombophlebitis
Preeclampsia	Pulmonary embolus
Gestational diabetes	Pneumonia
Failed spontaneous onset of labor	Urinary tract infection
Failed induction of labor	Wound infection
↑ Instrumental delivery	Wound dehiscence
↑ Cesarean section	Prolonged hospitalization
Prolonged surgery time	↑ Cost of medical care
↑ Operative blood loss	Sudden death
Postpartum hemorrhage	

patients weighing over 137 kg (300 lb) is as high as 60%, with half of these surgeries for urgent or emergent indications. If cesarean section is required, a prolonged surgical duration and increased blood loss should be anticipated.

11.4.3 Postpartum

Obesity increases the risk of postoperative complications. Post-surgical wound infection is related to larger incisions, protracted surgery times, excess operative traction causing tissue trauma and the inability of adipose tissue to resist infection secondary to decreased blood flow. In addition, the presence of diabetes mellitus increases the risk of wound infection. Restoration of normal pulmonary function may take several days following abdominal surgery and atelectasis may lead to pneumonia. With the obesity-related increase in deep vein thrombosis and the pregnancy-related hypercoagulability, these patients are at an increased risk for pulmonary thromboembolism.

11.5 Fetal complications

Fetal complications associated with obesity are listed in *Table 11.4*. Newborns of obese parturients are at increased risk for complications, admission to the neonatal intensive care unit, and death. Prenatal fetal anomalies may be undiagnosed because ultrasonographic visualization is impaired with morbid obesity. Macrosomia, the biggest threat, is correlated with birth trauma, shoulder dystocia, and asphyxia. Neonatal hypoglycemia can alter newborn thermoregulation and decrease cardiac output.

Table 11.4 Fetal complications associated with obesity

Fetal complications	
Macrosomia	Birth asphyxia
Multiple gestation	Birth trauma
Breech presentation	Neonatal hypoglycemia
Shoulder dystocia	↑ NICU admission

11.6 Anesthetic considerations

In obese parturients, the lack of an anesthetic plan can be disastrous. As previously discussed, women weighing more than 137 kg (300 lb) have an approximate 30% chance of requiring an urgent or emergent cesarean section. An anesthetic plan is essential for optimizing medical management, which should include early consultation by the anesthesiologist. Of paramount importance is evaluation of the airway, followed by consideration of coexisting medical problems. Keep in mind that a previous uneventful anesthetic may be irrelevant when changes such as further weight gain and pregnancy occur. A history of obstructive sleep apnea may suggest the potential for mechanical airway obstruction when the level of consciousness is decreased. It is important to discuss anesthetic interventions in advance, particularly regional anesthesia techniques and awake fiberoptic intubation.

11.6.1 Equipment

Equipment must be available to accommodate the patient's size and weight. Standard hospital beds are usually adequate, but the operating table may have a weight limit. Know the weight limit and keep in mind that left uterine displacement may create an unstable situation. The patient must be well secured to the operating table because the abdomen may shift markedly when the patient is tilted leftward. In rare cases it may be necessary to use the labor bed as an operating table. It is important to have extra personnel available to safely transport the patient, especially if she is immobilized due to regional anesthesia.

Other related problems include monitoring and the possibility of difficult intravenous access. A standard blood pressure cuff will give falsely high measurements when placed on a large, funnel-shaped arm. The width of the blood pressure cuff should cover at least half the length of the upper arm. As an alternative, a standard-sized cuff may also be placed on the forearm. Despite increased amounts of subcutaneous fat, establishing intravenous access is generally not difficult due to an expanded blood volume.

11.6.2 Positioning

With an obese parturient, the semi-recumbent or lateral position through labor and delivery improves lung expansion and minimizes cardiovascular stress. In this position, the panniculus is displaced off the abdomen, reducing intraabdominal pressure and allowing greater diaphragmatic excursion during respiration. Head elevation also reduces premature airway closure, thus reducing hypoxemia. Oxygen administration is helpful and provides a margin of safety to the mother and fetus throughout labor and delivery. The supine position should be avoided because aortocaval compression may be exacerbated by the weight of a large panniculus. Airway obstruction and circulatory changes such as hypotension and elevated pulmonary arterial pressures can occur and cardiac arrest has been reported when morbidly obese patients have been placed in the supine position.

11.7 Analgesia for labor and delivery

Although parenteral analgesics during labor, supplemented with pudendal block and perineal local infiltration at delivery, may be appropriate for some obese patients, they are more often ineffective and increase the risk of complications, including opioid-induced respiratory depression. Additionally, since the potential for complicated vaginal or surgical delivery requiring profound anesthesia is higher in obese patients, regional anesthesia is preferred whenever possible.

11.7.1 Epidural analgesia

In obese parturients, the most appropriate anesthetic technique for labor pain relief is epidural analgesia. Benefits of epidural analgesia include decreased oxygen consumption, decreased work of breathing, improved oxygenation, and decreased catecholamine secretion that may increase blood pressure and cardiac output during labor and delivery. Most importantly, an epidural allows for controlled drug administration that can be utilized for surgical anesthesia should cesarean section be required.

Ideally, morbidly obese parturients should be identified and seen by an anesthesiologist upon admission; informed consent should be obtained, and an epidural catheter inserted and tested even before the onset of active labor. Later, when the patient requests labor analgesia, additional local anesthetics can be administered. Early epidural catheter placement is important for several reasons. First, it usually takes longer to position the patient and to place the block. Catheter placement before active labor will minimize patient movement and improve cooperation, thus increasing the chance for success. In obese parturients, block placement can be technically challenging due to obscured anatomical landmarks. Most importantly, this technique minimizes overall risk by maximizing the likelihood of a successful regional anesthetic should an urgent cesarean section be required. Patients invariably consent to early epidural catheter placement when these risks and benefits are presented in clearly understandable terms.

The sitting position usually provides easier identification of midline, although locating an interspace is not guaranteed. When other landmarks cannot be identified, the epidural needle is inserted in the midline, perpendicular to the skin at an imaginary point anchored horizontally by the first skin crease above the gluteal fold and vertically by an imaginary line drawn from the C_7 spinous process to the gluteal fold (*Figure 11.1*). The increased depth to the epidural space contributes to a high failure rate by exaggerating minor directional errors and increasing the chance of identifying the lateral epidural space (*Figure 11.2*). In cases of difficult placement, the patient can assist by reporting any left or right-sided discomfort. Directing the epidural needle hub towards the discomfort will direct the needle tip in the opposite direction and back towards the midline. Even in the morbidly obese patient, the inability to identify the epidural space is more likely misdirection rather than inadequate needle length. Although a standard 3.5 inch epidural needle is almost always sufficient, a longer needle may occasionally be required. For this reason, a stock of 5-inch disposable epidural needles should be kept readily available. Once the epidural space is identified, the epidural catheter should be inserted at least 6 cm within the epidural space to minimize the risk of subsequent catheter dislodgement because of the potential for increased movement of the tissues between the skin and the epidural space. It may be prudent to secure the catheter in the lateral position since merely moving the patient from the sitting to lateral position can dislodge the catheter from the epidural space. Enough local anesthetic (usually 10 ml of 1–2% lidocaine) is administered to fully test the catheter. If the patient develops bilateral analgesia, no additional local anesthetics are administered until the patient requests pain relief. Otherwise, the catheter is manipulated or replaced until a well-functioning epidural catheter is established. Although initial epidural catheter failure may be as high as 42% in obese parturients, success rates comparable to nonobese parturients can be obtained in patients weighing more than 137 kg (300 lb) with this aggressive management. A recommended technique for epidural catheter placement is listed in *Table 11.5*.

When initiating labor analgesia, local anesthetics alone should be used to establish catheter function. Opioid administration by

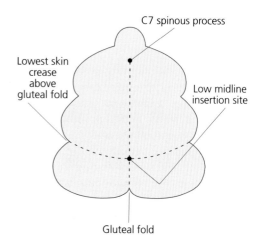

Figure 11.1 Approach to epidural catheter insertion in the morbidly obese parturient. With the patient in the sitting position, insert the epidural needle in the midline perpendicular to the skin at a point anchored horizontally by the first skin crease above the gluteal fold and vertically by an imaginary line drawn from the C_7 spinous process to the gluteal fold.

any route produces some degree of pain relief and may theoretically mask a malpositioned catheter. Once the catheter function is proven and a bilateral block has been established, epidural opioids can be safely administered. Although local anesthetic requirements may be reduced with obesity due to a reduction in epidural volume by fatty infiltration or engorged epidural veins, epidural analgesic requirements generally remain similar to those of nonobese parturients.

Table 11.5 Recommended technique for epidural catheter placement in the morbidly obese parturient

1. Early epidural catheter placement
2. Sitting position
3. Low midline approach (see *Figure 11.1*)
4. > 6 cm catheter insertion length
5. Secure catheter with patient in lateral position
6. Test catheter with 10 ml 2% lidocaine (2 + 5 + 3 ml)
7. For
   - adequate analgesia: administer additional local anesthetics when patient requests analgesia
   - inadequate analgesia: withdraw catheter 2–3 cm and administer additional lidocaine 5 ml
   - persistent inadequate analgesia: remove epidural catheter and replace

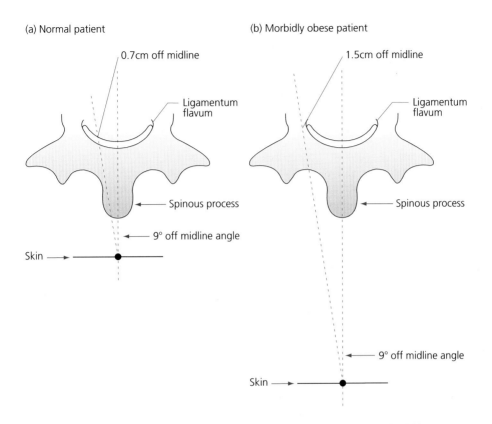

(a) Normal patient

0.7cm off midline

Ligamentum flavum

Spinous process

9° off midline angle

Skin

(b) Morbidly obese patient

1.5cm off midline

Ligamentum flavum

Spinous process

9° off midline angle

Skin

Figure 11.2 The increased skin-to-epidural space depth in obese patients can exaggerate minor directional errors during epidural needle insertion and increase the failure rate. As drawn, a 9° off-midline angle at the skin translates into an approximate 0.7 cm deviation from the midline when entering the epidural space in the normal patient (a) versus an approximate 1.5 cm deviation from midline in the morbidly obese patient (b). The distance from skin to epidural space in this example is 4 cm and 9 cm for the normal and morbidly obese patient, respectively.

11.7.2 Combined spinal epidural (CSE) analgesia

The routine use of CSE anesthetics in obese parturients cannot be recommended. The CSE technique theoretically delays recognition of a poorly functioning epidural catheter that may become problematic should an emergency cesarean section be required. The incidence of epidural catheter failure with CSE in the obese patient population remains unknown. Although it has been suggested that a successful CSE improves subsequent catheter function since obtaining cerebrospinal fluid likely indicates a midline epidural needle position, adequate epidural anesthesia cannot be guaranteed. The benefit of faster onset labor analgesia does not outweigh the risk of epidural catheter failure in the event of an emergency cesarean section.

11.7.3 Continuous spinal analgesia

A subarachnoid catheter can be dosed incrementally or by continuous infusion for labor analgesia. As with epidural analgesia, the block can be quickly augmented in the event of cesarean section, but unilateral blockade is less likely. However, at least theoretically, problems may exist with this technique. First, during a long course of labor, tachyphylaxis may develop to intrathecal local anesthetics making assessment difficult. Second, catheter lengths inserted more than 4 cm into the spinal space theoretically increase the risk of spinal cord penetration or spinal nerve root compression. Third, with 4 cm or less of subarachnoid catheter, patient movement may be more likely to dislodge the spinal catheter. Finally, in a setting where multiple individuals are involved in the care of the patient, a spinal catheter may be mistaken for an epidural catheter and increase the risk of high spinal blockade should epidural doses of local anesthetic be administered intrathecally.

Though these concerns are theoretical (no large series are available to accurately quantify these risks), it is probably prudent to limit this technique to urgent situations when a difficult tracheal intubation is anticipated or when a patient has experienced an inadvertent wet tap during difficult epidural catheter placement. In these situations, the catheter can be threaded into the subarachnoid space and managed as in Table 8.5.

11.8 Anesthesia for cesarean section

During cesarean section, obesity increases the risk of maternal mortality. Most anesthesia-related maternal deaths occur due to airway related problems encountered during general anesthesia. For this reason, general anesthesia should be avoided if at all possible.

11.8.1 Epidural anesthesia

Epidural anesthesia is an excellent choice for cesarean section in morbidly obese patients whether presenting for elective surgery or coming from the labor ward. If a preexisting epidural catheter is in place, epidural local anesthetics may be administered in the labor room, obviating failure should the catheter become dislodged during transport to the operating room. However, if anesthesia appears to be inadequate for a surgical incision, it is best to move the patient to the operating room table, withdraw the epidural catheter so that 3–4 cm remains within the epidural space, and then administer additional local anesthetics.

Although some have suggested that epidural local anesthetic requirements are reduced by approximately 20% in obese parturients, individual patients have varying requirements. Nevertheless, if the block exceeds the desired sensory level, then a slight head-flexion of the operating table lessens patient complaints without adversely affecting the surgery. Other benefits of epidural anesthesia include potentially better hemodynamic control compared to spinal anesthesia and the flexibility to administer opioid and local anesthetic solutions for postoperative analgesia. In an emergency, a well-functioning labor epidural can usually be quickly extended for surgical anesthesia, but establishing a block *de novo* may take too long and a spinal technique may be preferable.

11.8.2 Spinal anesthesia

Spinal anesthesia is an option for cesarean section, but as with other regional techniques in obese patients, placement can be difficult. Fatty deposits about the hips can lead to false identification of the superior iliac crests with subsequent unintended high placement, which raises the possibility of spinal cord damage if the needle is inserted above the L_2 spinous process. Some reports indicate that customary cesarean section doses of local anesthetics may produce higher than expected spinal blockade in obese patients. Reasons for this exaggerated anesthetic spread may include higher than anticipated block placement, decreased cerebral spinal fluid volume and large buttocks placing the vertebral column in a relative Trendelenburg position. Accordingly, when administering spinal anesthesia in obese patients, it is prudent to slightly elevate the *head* of the operating table (as opposed to reverse Trendelenburg position) to minimize high block cephalad spread. Because of excessive abdominal and chest wall mass, even the usual midthoracic sensory levels required for cesarean section may cause inadequate ventilation in obese patients. When prolonged surgical duration is anticipated, a continuous spinal or CSE anesthetic may be more appropriate choices than a one-shot spinal. These techniques similarly provide rapid anesthesia but allow for subsequent dosing if necessary.

11.8.3 General anesthesia

Any discussion of general anesthesia in the obese parturient must begin with special emphasis on airway evaluation. In obese parturients, general anesthesia for cesarean section should be used only in patients with contraindications to regional anesthesia. Difficult intubation has been reported in 33% of obese parturients having cesarean section, compared to 13% in obese patients undergoing abdominal surgery. Whenever possible, two anesthesia providers should be present for induction since maintaining the airway may be complicated and the primary anesthesia provider can fatigue quickly. In the obese patient, the complexity of intubation coupled with the propensity for rapid desaturation can be disastrous. Assorted laryngoscope blades, a variety of endotracheal tubes, a gum elastic bougie, standard and intubating laryngeal mask airways, and equipment for transtracheal ventilation should be immediately available (see also *Table 9.4*). A short-handled laryngoscope is also useful because limited extension of a short, thick neck and pendulous breasts often hamper insertion with a standard length handle. A large tongue and airway soft tissue engorgement can further complicate the process. When preparing for general anesthesia in an obese patient, proper positioning is vitally important. When supine, adipose tissue on the upper back ('buffalo hump') can elevate the chest in relation to the skull. This may impair the alignment of the oro-glottic axis and make vocal cord visualization difficult. It may be necessary to elevate the head more than usual to obtain the proper 'sniffing' position. Be aware that if the head is positioned midline and the body tilted leftward, visualization may be obscured.

In obese parturients, swift intubation is important because rapid desaturation may occur despite adequate preoxygenation, due to the decreased FRC and increased oxygen requirements. Hypoxemia and hypercarbia can precipitate sudden pulmonary hypertension and cardiac arrhythmias. If mask ventilation becomes necessary, airway obstruction and high abdominal pressure can impede ventilation. In this scenario insufflation of the stomach may occur and increase the risk of aspiration. Obesity impairs identification of the cricoid ring making it difficult to properly apply cricoid pressure and to perform cricothyrotomy in an emergency. If a difficult intubation is anticipated, and regional anesthesia cannot be used, an awake intubation is recommended. Topical anesthesia consumes time, and in the presence of fetal distress, an anesthesiologist may feel compelled to proceed with rapid sequence induction. In this situation, the risk of a failed intubation and potential catastrophic maternal outcome must be weighed against the risk of fetal compromise by delaying surgery to secure the airway.

Within 30 minutes of surgery, 30 ml of a nonparticulate antacid should be administered. Preoxygenation is recommended using a tight fitting mask for at least 3 minutes with 4 vital capacity breaths administered just before induction. Sodium thiopental 500 mg and succinylcholine 1–2 mg/kg of actual body weight up to 200 mg are recommended for rapid sequence induction. This dose of sodium thiopental is less than the usual 4 mg/kg recommended dose because larger doses may prolong awakening in case of failed intubation.

Once the airway is secured, a balanced anesthetic technique is recommended. Atracurium, mivacurium and cisatracurium are recommended nondepolarizing agents because their metabolism is not organ dependent. Fentanyl is the preferred opioid as elimination is similar in obese and nonobese patients whereas sufentanil and alfentanil may have longer elimination times in the obese patient. Isoflurane is the least significantly metabolized volatile anesthetic agent, which theoretically minimizes the risk of serum fluoride accumulation. While no single anesthetic regimen has been shown to be superior in obese patients, it is logical that these recommended agents may lessen any residual postoperative anesthetic affects.

Intraoperatively, tidal volumes of 10–12 ml/kg ideal body weight are recommended. PEEP is rarely indicated and can actually worsen hypoxemia in obese patients. Large tidal volumes coupled with low chest wall compliance can produce high peak inspiratory pressures. High-inspired oxygen fractions may be required, thus limiting the use of nitrous oxide and possibly increasing the risk of intraoperative awareness. End-tidal capnography may be a poor guide to the adequacy of ventilation due to a large alveolar-to-arterial difference in carbon dioxide. During pregnancy, it is important to maintain $PaCO_2$ levels in the low to mid 30s and arterial blood gas analysis may be required.

Following surgery, residual anesthetic effects, increased sensitivity to opioid analgesics, and neuromuscular blocking agents may delay tracheal extubation. Prior to extubation, gastric contents should be suctioned. Postoperatively, the morbidly obese patient remains at increased risk for postoperative respiratory insufficiency and supplemental oxygen may be required for several days. Finally, the obese patient should be closely monitored for cardiopulmonary complications during the postoperative period. Pain control is important to encourage deep breathing. Patient-controlled analgesia and patient-controlled epidural analgesia are recommended because these techniques probably reduce the likelihood of side effects, improve respiratory function, and lead to earlier mobilization than intermittent p.r.n. dosing. Subcutaneous and intramuscular injection routes should be avoided since absorption may be less reliable in obese patients.

11.9 Summary

Obesity during pregnancy increases the risk of maternal and fetal morbidity and mortality and poses significant anesthetic challenges. Anesthetic risks may be reduced by early aggressive intervention. Epidural catheter insertion and testing as early in labor as possible will increase the likelihood of a successful regional anesthetic should an emergency cesarean section be required. General anesthesia should be utilized in obese parturients only when regional anesthesia is contraindicated, and only after careful evaluation of the airway.

Further reading

Adams, J.P. and Murphy, P.G. (2000) Obesity in anaesthesia and intensive care. *Br. J. Anaesth.* **85**: 91–108.

Cooper, J.R. and Brodsky, J.B. (1987) Anesthetic management of the morbidly obese patient. *Seminars in Anethesia* **4**: 260–270.

Dewan, D.M. (1999) Obesity. In: *Obstetric Anesthesia: Principles and Practice* (ed. Chestnut, D.H.), pp. 986–999. Mosby, New York.

Hogan, Q.H., Prost, R., Kulier, A., Taylor, M.L., Liu, S. and Leighton, M. (1996) Magnetic resonance imaging of cerebrospinal fluid volume and the influence of body habitus and abdominal pressure. *Anesthesiology* **84**: 1341–1349.

Honor, M.W. and Gross, T.L. (1994) Obesity in pregnancy. *Clin. Obstet. Gynecol.* **37**: 596–604.

Hood, D.D. and Dewan, D.M. (1993) Anesthetic and obstetrical outcome in morbidly obese parturients. *Anesthesiology* **79**: 1210–1218.

Narang, V.P.S. and Linter, S.P.K. (1988) Failure of extradural blockade in obstetrics. *Br. J. Anaesth.* **60**: 402–404.

Perlow, J.H. and Morgan, M.M. (1994) Massive maternal obesity and perioperative cesarean morbidity. *Am. J. Obstet. Gynecol.* **170**: 560–565.

Shenkman, Z., Shir, Y. and Brodsky, J.B. (1993) Perioperative management of the obese patient. *Br. J. Anaesth.* **70**: 349–359.

Chapter 12

Complications
of labor

Craig M. Palmer, MD

Contents

12.1 **Introduction**

Despite the best efforts and intentions of obstetricians in caring for the parturient, complications can arise which impact the management of labor and delivery and have implications for the anesthesiologist caring for the patient. As with complications such as hemorrhage (Chapter 10), understanding the underlying pathophysiology improves our approach to anesthetic management.

12.2 **Prematurity and preterm labor**

12.2.1 Definitions

Preterm labor is defined as regular uterine contractions occurring at least once every 10 minutes and resulting in cervical change prior to 37 weeks' gestation. A preterm infant is any infant delivered before 37 weeks of gestation. Any infant weighing less than 2500 g at birth is a low birth weight (LBW) infant and any infant below 1500 g at birth is a very low birth weight (VLBW) infant, regardless of gestational age. At 29 weeks' gestation, over 90% of estimated fetal weights are below 1500 g.

12.2.2 Incidence

Prematurity is the leading cause of perinatal morbidity and mortality in the United States. The high incidence of preterm delivery is one of the major reasons the US ranks so low (23rd in 1988) among developed nations in infant mortality. The overall incidence of preterm delivery in the US was 10.7% in 1989, but there was a significant disparity between racial groups – the incidence was 8.8% in white parturients and 18.9% in black parturients.

12.2.3 Neonatal morbidity and mortality

Perinatal mortality approaches 90% for infants born before 24 weeks gestation; by 30 weeks gestation, survival exceeds 90%. Within this 6-week time frame, even minimal delays in delivery can have a significant impact on neonatal survival. Between 25 and 26 weeks gestation, each *day* that delivery can be delayed improves survival rate by up to 5 percentage points. By 34 weeks gestation, neonatal survival should exceed 98% (*Figure 12.1*). Delay of delivery from a gestational age of 25 weeks to 31 weeks improves neonatal survival rate from just over 15% to almost 95%.

Neonatal mortality figures only tell a small part of the story, however. While advances in neonatology have decreased mortality for very low birth weight infants, such neonates still usually encounter a stormy course following delivery. Very low birth weight infants are at risk of significant morbidity from a number of complications, including respiratory distress syndrome (RDS), necrotizing enterocolitis, sepsis, and intraventricular hemorrhage (IVH) (*Figure 12.2*). The incidence of RDS is almost 90% in infants born before 27 weeks gestation,

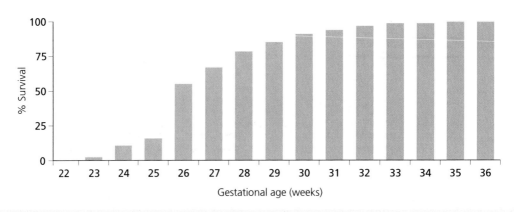

Figure 12.1 Predicted survival by gestational age derived from logistic regression equation.

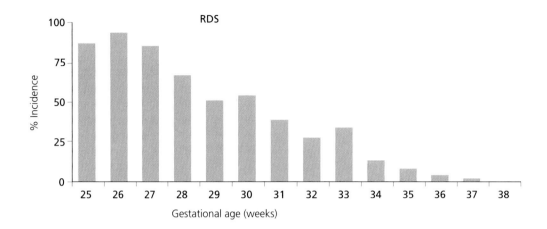

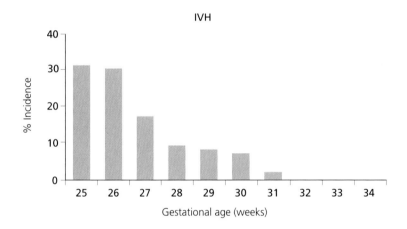

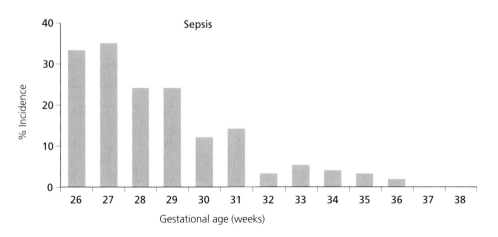

Figure 12.2 The incidence of respiratory distress syndrome (RDS), intraventricular hemorrhage (IVH), sepsis, and necrotizing enterocolitis (NEC) related to gestational age at birth. After Robertson, P.A. *et al.* (1992) Neonatal morbidity according to gestational age and birth weight from five tertiary care centers in the United States, 1983–1986. *Am. J. Obstet. Gynecol.* **166**: 1629–1645.

and declines almost linearly to near 0% by 36 weeks. The incidence of serious (grade III and IV) IVH exceeds 30% at 26 weeks gestation, but declines rapidly to near 0% by 31 weeks. Both sepsis and necrotizing enterocolitis follow gestational age-related incidences. Treatment of these problems is tremendously expensive, often requiring stays of months in a neonatal intensive care unit setting. It has been estimated that for infants of 900 g, about 26 weeks gestational age, the total cost per survivor exceeds the expected lifetime earnings per survivor.

Even beyond the immediate perinatal period, survivors are often left with neurologic abnormalities, chronic pulmonary problems, and visual disturbances (*Figure 12.3*). Because of this overwhelming impact on the infants, their families, and the healthcare system, it becomes imperative for all involved to do whatever is possible to avoid preterm delivery.

12.2.4 Obstetric management

Current obstetrical practice focuses on delaying delivery in patients who develop preterm labor (PTL). The initial assessment of a patient with PTL consists of a thorough physical examination to eliminate treatable medical conditions that may have precipitated labor, and a pelvic exam to rule out premature rupture of membranes. Bed rest, intravenous hydration, continuous fetal heart rate monitoring, and tocography are almost universally indicated. Bed rest and hydration alone are effective in a substantial portion of patients. If these conservative measures are ineffective, ultrasonography is undertaken to establish gestational age; on occasion, amniocentesis will be used to assess fetal lung maturity and rule out infection.

Once the diagnosis is established, the obstetrician must decide whether to institute pharmacologic tocolytic therapy. This decision is based on the estimated gestational age, fetal weight, and the presence or absence of fetal distress and infection. In general, a gestational age between 20 and 34 weeks with a fetal weight less than 2500 g in the absence of fetal distress are indications for tocolytic therapy.

12.2.5 Physiology of preterm labor

While the processes that initiate labor are incompletely understood, the physiology of uterine contraction is well understood. Like all smooth muscle, the myometrium contains myosin and actin filaments that generate the contractile force. Pacemaker cells within the myometrium are capable of initiating spontaneous contractile activity, which spreads throughout the myometrium via gap junctions between cells.

Calcium plays a critical role in uterine contractility. Prior to contraction, the intracellular calcium concentration increases, due to release of calcium from the sarcoplasmic reticulum and/or flux across the sarcolemma (*Figure 12.4*). Calcium interacts with calmodulin (a regulatory enzyme), which in turn activates myosin light-chain kinase (MLK). Activated MLK phosphorylates myosin, which then binds with actin. Adenosine triphosphate (ATP) is hydrolyzed by myosin ATPase, releasing the energy that causes movement of the actin–myosin elements and myometrial contraction. A reduction in intracellular calcium concentration, or

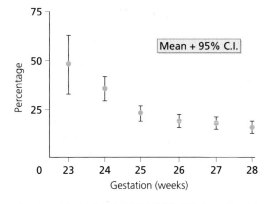

Figure 12.3 Estimated rates of major permanent disability versus gestational age at birth in preterm infants. After Wood, N. and Marlow, N. (1999) The contribution of preterm birth to outcomes in children. In: *Fetal Medicine: Basic Science and Clinical Practice* (eds Rodeck, C.H. and Whittle, M.J.), pp. 1071–1086. Churchill Livingstone, London.

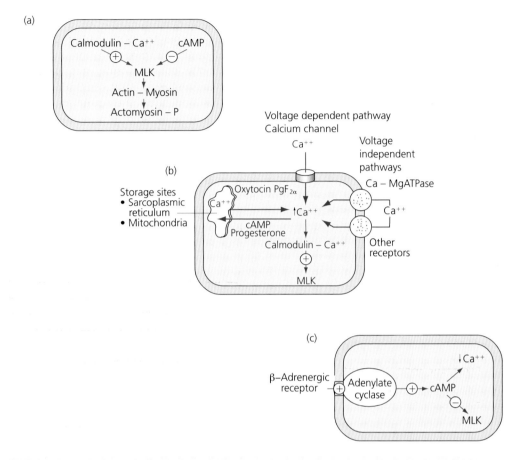

Figure 12.4 Control of myometrial contractility. (a) Calcium interacts with calmodulin, which in turn activates myosin light-chain kinase (MLK), leading to myometrial contraction via a sequence of events. See text for full explanation. (b) Intracelluar calcium (Ca^{2+}) concentration can be affected by both intracellular and extracellular sites and mechanisms. (c) Increasing cyclic AMP (cAMP) concentration decreases intracellular Ca^{2+} concentration. After Main, D.M. and Main, E.K. (1986) Management of preterm labor and delivery. In: *Obstetrics: Normal and Problem Pregnancies* (eds. Gabbe, S.G., Niebyl, J.R. and Simpsom, J.L.). Churchill Livingstone, New York.

dephosphorylation of myosin, inhibits the actin–myosin interaction causing relaxation.

This cascade offers several opportunities for pharmacologic intervention. Activation of β_2-adrenergic receptors within the myometrium activates adenylate cyclase, converting ATP to cyclic AMP. Increased cyclic AMP decreases intracellular calcium, inhibiting MLK and decreasing contractile activity. Magnesium sulfate decreases uterine activity, probably by decreasing intracellular free calcium concentration, and competitively inhibiting calcium through competition for binding sites. It may also acti-

vate adenylate cyclase, increasing synthesis of cyclic AMP. By blocking voltage-dependent calcium channels in the cell membrane (or altering intracellular uptake and release mechanisms), calcium channel blocking agents decrease the concentration of free calcium within the myometrium. Prostaglandins $F_{2\alpha}$ and $E_{2\alpha}$ are potent stimulators of uterine activity. During labor, their concentration increases in maternal blood and amniotic fluid. The non-steroidal anti-inflammatory agents that inhibit prostaglandin synthetase can inhibit the production of these prostaglandins (*Table 12.1*).

Table 12.1 Pharmacological agents for control of preterm labor

Agent	Site of action	Mechanism
Magnesium sulfate	Intracellular Ca^{2+} binding sites ?Adenylate cyclase	Direct competition for binding sites Increases cAMP synthesis
β-agonist agents Terbutaline Ritodrine	β$_2$-Adrenergic receptors	Activates adenylate cyclase, increases cAMP
Calcium channel blockers	Voltage-dependent calcium channels	Decrease intracellular Ca^{2+} concentration
Nonsteroidal anti-inflammatory agents (NSAIDs)	Prostaglandin synthetase	Inhibit production of prostaglandins F$_{2\alpha}$ and E$_{2\alpha}$

12.2.6 Management and anesthetic implications

No single agent is uniformly successful as tocolytic therapy for all patients, and each agent possesses side effects that can limit its usefulness. Further, because of the high stakes and long-term consequences involved in the care of the preterm infant, it has proven difficult to compare the efficacy of agents in randomized clinical trials. Each of the tocolytic agents currently in use has the potential for significant interactions with commonly used anesthetic agents. In addition, the prematurity of the infant itself may have implications for the route of delivery (i.e. vaginal or abdominal).

Magnesium sulfate

Magnesium is the intravenous tocolytic agent of choice in many centers, probably because of a relatively low incidence of serious side effects. The normal serum magnesium level ranges from 1.4 to 2.2 mEq/l. Therapy for termination of preterm labor is initiated with an intravenous bolus of 4–6 g, followed by a continuous infusion. The infusion is titrated to maintain a serum concentration of 5–8 mg/dl; while often sufficient to inhibit uterine activity, even at this concentration, magnesium is not always successful. Increasing the serum concentration is not usually more effective, and increases side effects.

Magnesium causes peripheral vasodilatation, and parturients often experience warmth, flushing, and nausea. Maternal tachycardia and hypotension may result, but are transient. At higher serum concentrations, other effects are seen. Widening of the QRS complex and prolongation of the PR interval are uncommon below concentrations of 10 mEq/l, but can be seen at therapeutic levels. At concentrations of 10 to 12 mEq/l, deep tendon reflexes are lost (deep tendon reflexes can be followed as a rough clinical measure of serum concentration). A concentration of 15 to 18 mEq/l can result in respiratory arrest, and at 25 mEq/l cardiac arrest may occur. Fetal effects are infrequent; decreased fetal heart rate variability has been reported, as has a reduced biophysical profile score (see Chapter 3). Respiratory depression, hyporeflexia, and decreased tone have been reported in neonates following prolonged maternal magnesium therapy (Table 12.2).

Due to vasodilatation, hypotension tends to occur more often in these patients during regional anesthetics. Careful attention to maternal blood pressure allows the use of either epidural or spinal anesthesia. The slower onset of epidural techniques may make them preferable to spinal anesthetics, as intravenous fluids can be titrated to maintain maternal blood pressure. Parturients receiving magnesium are more susceptible to muscle relaxants. At the neuromuscular junction, magnesium

Table 12.2 Clinical effects of magnesium sulfate therapy

Serum concentration (mEq/l)	Clinical effects
1.4–2.2	Normal serum concentrations
5–8	Therapeutic concentration for inhibition of preterm labor
6–10	Widening of QRS complex and PR interval on ECG
10–12	Loss of deep tendon reflexes
15–18	Respiratory arrest; S-A and A-V block on ECG
25	Cardiac arrest

inhibits release of acetylcholine and decreases sensitivity of the postsynaptic endplate to acetylcholine. This increased sensitivity is especially important when general anesthesia is necessary. Following the use of succinylcholine, the train-of-four response must be closely followed with a peripheral nerve stimulator to guide further use of relaxants. When necessary, further relaxants should be administered in very small doses because of their exaggerated effect. While magnesium has been shown to decrease the MAC of halothane at therapeutic levels, this is not a clinically significant effect.

β₂-Adrenergic agents

Both ritodrine and terbutaline (by virtue of their β₂-receptor activity) are tocolytic, but only ritodrine is FDA-approved for tocolysis. Both are usually administered by continuous intravenous infusion, titrated in response to the uterine contraction pattern. Terbutaline is sometimes administered as a single intravenous or subcutaneous dose for prompt but temporary inhibition of uterine activity.

Both drugs have significant β₁-receptor effects, accounting for the majority of their side effects. This β₁ activity can cause vasodilatation (resulting in hypotension) and hyperglycemia. Direct β₁ activity increases myocardial contractility and heart rate, leading to increased cardiac output.

The most significant side effects of β-agonist therapy are due to these cardiac effects. Pulmonary edema occurs in up to 1% of patients, and may be either cardiogenic or noncardiogenic in nature. It requires discontinuation of therapy, but, fortunately, discontinuation usually leads to resolution of the pulmonary edema. Likewise, myocardial ischemia has also been reported, manifesting as chest pain and ECG change; this also resolves with discontinuation of therapy. Finally, hyperglycemia (often requiring insulin therapy in diabetic patients) and hypokalemia are frequently seen in these patients, as is tremulousness (*Table 12.3*).

When anesthesia is required, a period of 60–90 minutes between discontinuation of therapy and the anesthetic is ideal; because of the short half-life of these agents, this allows their acute effects to subside. Unfortunately, a delay of this magnitude may jeopardize the fetus. The vasodilatation accompanying β-agonist therapy can aggravate hypotension when regional techniques are used. For this reason, epidural anesthesia with its slower onset is probably preferable to spinal anesthesia. Intravenous fluids can be used to support maternal blood pressure, but aggressive hydration may exacerbate pulmonary edema if present. Vasopressor therapy (i.e. ephedrine) may need to be used more aggressively to maintain maternal blood pressure; if ephedrine exacerbates maternal tachycardia,

Table 12.3 Side effects of β-agonist therapy

Side effect	Reported incidence (approx.)
Hypokalemia[a]	50
Hyperglycemia[a]	30
Shortness of breath or chest pain	10
'Ischemic' ECG change	5
Cardiac arrhythmias	3
Hypotension	3
Pulmonary edema	<2

[a]Transient (less than 24 hours).

phenylephrine may be cautiously used as long as the fetal heart rate is continuously monitored.

Prostaglandin synthetase inhibitors

Prostaglandins $E_{2\alpha}$ and $F_{2\alpha}$ are potent stimulators of uterine activity and also cause softening of the cervix near term. Prostaglandin synthetase inhibitors (PSIs) prevent the conversion of arachidonic acid into the active prostaglandins. While all drugs in this class possess this capacity, only indomethacin is widely used in the treatment of preterm labor. It can be administered both orally and rectally, but fetal side effects (below) usually limit the duration of therapy. Therapy can be continued for several weeks.

In contrast to magnesium and β-agonists, indomethacin has few maternal side effects. All PSIS may affect maternal coagulation, but despite the widespread use by parturients, this does not seem to be of major clinical importance. In an otherwise healthy parturient without clinical evidence of impaired hemostasis, further evaluation of maternal coagulation status is generally not indicated.

These agents may have significant fetal effects, however. PSIs may result in premature closure of the fetal ductus arteriosus in utero; this effect appears related to gestational age, and is less of a problem prior to 32 weeks gestation. Indomethacin may cause decreased fetal urine excretion, leading to oligohydramnios and, rarely, neonatal renal failure. Finally, an increased incidence of necrotizing enterocolitis, intracranial hemorrhage, and bronchopulmonary dysplasia has been noted in neonates following in utero indomethacin therapy (Table 12.4). Because of these side effects, the total recommended dose of indomethacin is 400 mg; this limitation means indomethacin therapy is usually limited to 48 h or less.

Calcium channel blockers

By inhibiting transmembrane calcium flux, the calcium channel blockers reduce myometrial contractility. Nifedipine is most widely used for tocolysis. The drug has a rapid onset

Table 12.4 Reported fetal effects of indomethacin therapy for preterm labor

Premature closure of fetal ductus arterious

Pulmonary hypertension

Oligohydramnios

Neonatal renal failure

Increased neonatal incidence of:
- necrotizing enterocolitis
- intracranial hemorrhage
- bronchopulmonary dysplasia

following sublingual administration, and therapy is maintained via the oral route.

Maternal side effects of nifedipine therapy are generally mild. Nifedipine has few cardiac effects, but vasodilatation and decreased blood pressure are often seen. This may be associated with a reflex tachycardia, headache, and nausea. It has few clinically significant fetal effects.

12.2.7 Management of delivery

It is important to remember that the uterine relaxant properties of all these agents do not stop with delivery. Depending on the duration of therapy and the half-life of the agent, all may contribute to uterine hypotonia. Vigorous pharmacologic therapy may be necessary to restore uterine tone and prevent significant maternal blood loss (see Chapter 10).

Despite aggressive therapy, tocolysis often fails and labor progresses. When delivery becomes inevitable, a choice as to the best route of delivery must be made. Currently, the lower limit of viability hovers around 24–25 weeks gestational age.

Some obstetricians have advocated routine cesarean delivery for all infants with an estimated gestational weight below 1500 g to reduce head trauma and subsequent intracranial hemorrhage, but there is little evidence to support this position. No difference has been shown in the incidence of intracranial hemorrhage in infants under 1500 g with vertex presentation and vaginal delivery, compared with cesarean delivery. Likewise, there is no evidence to suggest the routine use of outlet forceps provides protection against head trauma. In the preterm infant with breech presentation, however, there is evidence to indicate that a cesarean delivery is safer than a vaginal delivery; the advantages of surgical delivery for the infant must be weighed against the increased maternal morbidity of cesarean delivery.

For vaginal delivery, epidural anesthesia has several theoretical advantages. When the vaginal delivery of a preterm infant is planned, it is important to avoid a precipitous delivery that may increase the risk of intracranial hemorrhage. Further, 'pushing' efforts by the mother before full cervical dilatation must be avoided, and a well-relaxed perineum allows for controlled delivery of the infant's head. Each of these goals can be achieved with solid epidural blockade. Likewise, if delivery is known to be imminent, spinal anesthesia can be used to the same ends.

It is probably most important when planning for the delivery of a very premature infant, to ensure the presence of trained neonatal personnel for resuscitation and ready access to a neonatal intensive care unit for subsequent care. Such neonatal expertise and facilities are responsible for lowering the gestational age of viability to the point where it is today.

12.3 **Multiple gestation**

12.3.1 Incidence

The incidence of multiple gestation has been increasing over the last 15 years due to the proliferation of assisted reproduction technology and increased use of ovulation inducing drugs. Currently in the US, 3% of all pregnancies are multiple. Ordinarily, about 1 in 90 pregnancies is a twin gestation, about 1 in 9800 is triplet, and only about 1 in 70 000 are higher order gestations. Considerable geographic and ethnic variation exists – the rate of twin pregnancies is 50 per 1000 pregnancies in Nigeria, while only 4 per 1000 in Japan. Multiple gestation is more common in older parturients and those of higher parity.

12.3.2 Maternal and fetal risks

A number of physiological changes are associated with multiple gestation, which can increase maternal risk (*Table 12.5*). Cardiac output increases more in multiple gestation than singleton pregnancies, and the increase occurs earlier in gestation. There is an increased incidence of anemia due to a greater increase in blood volume, but a relatively smaller increase in red cell volume. The size of the uterus is larger, and the increase in size

Table 12.5 Maternal consequences of multiple gestation (compared with singleton pregnancies)

System	Consequence	Comments
Cardiovascular	Increased cardiac output	Occurs earlier in gestation
Hemotologic	Increased incidence of anemia	Increase in blood volume relatively greater than increase in RBC mass
Respiratory	↓ Total lung capacity ↓ Functional residual capacity ↑ Closing volume	All increase risk of hypoxemia or induction of general anesthesia
Metabolic	↑ O_2 consumption ↑ Metabolic rate	
Reproductive	Larger uterus	Increased incidence of aorta compression when supine Contributes to lower total lung capacity and FRC. Greater risk of aspiration

occurs earlier in gestation, placing the parturient at greater risk of supine-hypotension syndrome and aortocaval compression. The larger size of the uterus contributes to a lower total lung capacity (TLC), a decreased functional residual capacity (FRC), and an elevated closing volume. Together with an increased metabolic rate and greater oxygen consumption, these factors contribute to an increased risk of hypoxemia during apnea (as occurs during induction of general anesthesia). Finally, the larger size of the uterus increases cephalad pressure on the stomach, placing parturients at greater risk of aspiration.

Fetal mortality is increased in multiple gestation; the risk of fetal mortality is 5–6-times higher in twin pregnancies than singleton pregnancies. Most of this risk is due to a greater incidence of prematurity. Mortality of the second twin is also increased over that of the first twin, due to intrapartum events including placental abruption, cord prolapse or entrapment, and malpresentation.

12.3.3 Obstetric risks

Preterm labor complicates 40–50% of multiple gestations. The requirement for tocolytic therapy is likewise increased, increasing the risk of tocolytic interactions with anesthetic agents noted above. The inherent risks of tocolytic therapy for the parturient, such as pulmonary edema, are also likely increased in this population. The risk of uterine atony and postpartum hemorrhage after delivery are increased by both the use of tocolytic agents and the increased distention of the uterus at term.

Pregnancy-induced hypertension is as much as five-times more common in multiple gestation than single gestation. The risk of placental abruption, placenta previa, and malpresentation are all increased with multiple gestation.

12.3.4 Obstetric management

The course of obstetric management depends upon the intrauterine presentation of the fetuses. Ultrasonography is used to determine as precisely as possible their orientation. The route and method of delivery are also highly dependent on the expertise of the individual obstetrician attending the delivery. With triplet or higher gestations, delivery will almost always be via cesarean section.

Vaginal delivery is possible for most twin gestations. Several combinations of presentation are possible with twins: twin A vertex/twin B vertex (occurring in about 42% of cases); twin A vertex/twin B nonvertex (about 38%); and twin A nonvertex (about 19%). In the first two cases, vaginal delivery is usually feasible, while in the last case, cesarean delivery is usually performed. In the case of twin A vertex/twin B nonvertex, the second twin (twin B) must be smaller than twin A, but over 1500 g estimated fetal weight. Twin B may be delivered from either a vertex or breech presentation. Maneuvers including external cephalic version or internal podalic version may be used to turn twin B after delivery of twin A; delivery of twin B may be accomplished with either partial or complete breech extraction (see Section 12.3.5). The time interval between deliveries is not critical, although continuous fetal heart rate monitoring of twin B is necessary until delivery is accomplished. On occasion, surgical delivery (i.e. cesarean section) is necessary for delivery of the second twin.

12.3.5 Anesthetic considerations

The anticipated vaginal delivery of a parturient with a twin gestation is a very strong indication for epidural anesthesia. Effective epidural anesthesia will facilitate the manipulations mentioned above, as well as providing a method of inducing surgical anesthesia if cesarean delivery becomes necessary. The epidural catheter should be placed as early in labor as practical, and its function assured; if any doubt as to the reliability of the catheter exists, it should be replaced. Additionally, due to the increased risk of postpartum hemorrhage, large bore (16 gauge or larger) intravenous access should be established, and blood sent for type and crossmatch. Finally, because of the relatively greater size of the uterus, aortocaval compression must be carefully avoided.

Delivery should take place in an operating room where everything necessary for surgical intervention (both from an obstetric and anesthetic standpoint) is readily available. Upon moving to the OR, the parturient should receive an oral antacid in anticipation of the possible need to induce general anesthesia. Routine monitors should be applied to the parturient, and oxygen, via simple face mask, should be administered; this may improve fetal oxygenation, and provides an increased margin of safety against desaturation if general anesthesia must be induced.

Communication with the obstetrician is of vital importance: the obstetric plan can change quickly and dramatically depending on the course of the delivery, and anticipating obstetric interventions can save valuable moments. During labor and through the delivery of twin A, the nature of the epidural block should not differ greatly from epidural analgesia supplied in any other routine vaginal delivery. After delivery of twin A, however, it may be necessary to rapidly increase density of the block to allow obstetric manipulations as noted above. 2-Chloroprocaine, 3%, is the local anesthetic of choice when rapid establishment of a surgical block is necessary. It can be used for perineal anesthesia for episiotomy or application of forceps, for internal version of twin B, or for cesarean delivery. In cases of dire fetal distress, it may be necessary to induce general anesthesia.

For internal manipulations, uterine relaxation may be necessary. Intravenous nitroglycerin is an effective agent for this purpose; an initial dose of 100 µg should be used, and can be increased as necessary, up to 500 µg. It should rarely be necessary to use inhalational agents solely for uterine relaxation, although they are effective at high concentrations. Following delivery, be alert for excessive bleeding due to uterine atony; aggressive therapy including methergine and prostaglandin $F_{2\alpha}$ may be necessary.

For elective cesarean delivery of multiple gestations, regional anesthesia, either epidural or spinal, is preferable to general anesthesia, partly to decrease the risk of neonatal depression. From a maternal perspective, greater weight gain associated with multiple gestation can contribute to a higher incidence of difficult intubation in these patients, and together with the propensity for rapid desaturation and increased aspiration risk, makes avoidance of general anesthesia preferable.

12.4 Abnormal presentation

12.4.1 Definitions

The 'presentation' of the infant refers to the most dependent (or 'presenting') part of the infant. The 'lie' refers to the long axis of the infant; longitudinal lies are by far the most common, but they may be either vertex (cephalic) or breech (caudal). Vertex presentation, with infant's head delivering first is the most common presentation, but depending on the flexion, extension and rotation of the fetal head, may still constitute a malpresentation. In normal labor, the fetal head presents with a flexed cervical spine (the fetal chin on its chest) and the fetal face turned posteriorly ('occiput anterior'). This presentation gives the greatest chance of a successful spontaneous vaginal delivery.

12.4.2 Breech presentation

Breech presentation is the most common malpresentation. It may be further classified as complete, frank, or incomplete (footling), depending on the position of the lower extremities (*Figure 12.5*). At term, about 3% of singleton fetuses are in breech presentation. It has long been known that the fetus is at increased risk when vaginal delivery is attempted with breech presentation. The risk of fetal death is 16-times greater than vertex presentation, the risk of asphyxia is over three-times greater, and birth trauma is 13-times more common. The risk of cord prolapse is increased 15-times with incomplete breech presentation, and five times with complete breech

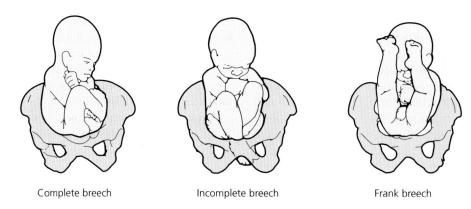

Complete breech   Incomplete breech   Frank breech

Figure 12.5 Classification of breech presentation. After Seeds, J.W. (1986) Malpresentations. In: *Obstetrics: Normal and Problem Pregnancies* (eds. Gabbe, S.G., Niebyl, J.R. and Simpsom, J.L.). Churchill Livingstone, New York.

presentation. Maternal risk is also increased: infectious risk increases due to the intrauterine manipulations that are often necessary with vaginal delivery. The likelihood of perineal trauma is increased, as are uterine atony and postpartum bleeding resulting from use of tocolytic agents.

These increased risks have led some to advocate cesarean delivery for all cases of breech presentation, but this does not completely eliminate fetal risk; delivery of the fetus can be difficult even with surgery. This stance also does not take into account the increased maternal morbidity of a surgical delivery. Regardless, over 90% of breech presentations are delivered by cesarean section in the US at present.

12.4.3 Obstetric considerations

External cephalic version (ECV) is the rotation of the fetus from breech to vertex presentation by manipulation of the uterus through the abdominal wall. Near term (over 36 weeks gestation) the maneuver is successful in 50–80% of cases, and the reversion rate (back to breech presentation) is as low as 2%. Complications are rare, but include placental abruption, hemorrhage, and preterm labor. A tocolytic is often administered to facilitate the procedure.

The use of regional anesthesia for ECV is controversial. Epidural or spinal anesthesia

certainly increases maternal comfort during the procedure, and some recent series have shown an increased success rate without increased morbidity when regional anesthesia is used. Use of anesthesia is resisted by some obstetricians who feel that maternal discomfort is an important gauge of the amount of force which can be applied during the procedure.

12.4.4 Anesthetic considerations

There are three main methods to accomplish a breech delivery: spontaneous delivery, partial breech extraction, or total breech extraction. With a spontaneous delivery, there is no obstetric intervention or manipulation involved. With partial breech extraction, the infant is allowed to deliver to the level of the umbilicus, and then the obstetrician assists with the delivery of the thorax and head, either manually or with Piper forceps. With total breech extraction, the obstetrician begins with traction on the fetal legs and feet, and delivers the entire fetal body; this maneuver is rarely used except in the delivery of a second twin in breech presentation.

The attempted vaginal delivery of a breech presentation is a very strong indication for epidural anesthesia. Epidural anesthesia has several advantages: it provides excellent maternal pain control; it can inhibit the maternal urge to push until full cervical dilation is achieved; and it provides excellent perineal relaxation to facilitate a controlled delivery. Additionally, an *in situ* epidural catheter provides a quick and effective route to rapidly increase the density of blockade to facilitate the obstetric maneuvers noted above, or to convert to anesthesia for cesarean delivery if necessary.

During labor (until full cervical dilation), standard regimens of epidural analgesia (see Chapter 5) should prove adequate, unless a deeper block is necessary to inhibit maternal pushing urges. During the actual delivery, a deeper block, such as obtained with bupivacaine, 0.25%, is usually helpful. A surgical block (as obtained with 2-chloroprocaine, 3%, or lidocaine, 2%) is helpful for forceps-assisted deliveries, although the level of the block should not need to exceed T_8. As with twin deliveries, clear communication with the obstetrician is essential. Ideally, the obstetrical plan of management should be discussed beforehand. A means of rapidly providing uterine relaxation, such as intravenous nitroglycerin, should be readily at hand (see Section 12.2.5).

For an elective cesarean delivery, regional techniques (either spinal or epidural) are equally efficacious.

12.4.5 Other abnormal presentations

Vertex malpresentations include face and brow presentations, and persistent occiput posterior presentation. Face and brow presentations result when the fetal cervical spine fails to flex with descent to the pelvic brim; in a face presentation, the cervical spine is in an extended position, and in brow presentation it is usually neutral. Either of these presentations poses problems because a larger diameter is presented to the pelvic inlet. With a face presentation, a successful vaginal delivery is most likely if the fetus is in a mentum anterior (chin anterior) position. Brow presentations usually convert spontaneously during the course of labor to either a face or occiput anterior presentation. Vaginal delivery with a persistent occiput posterior presentation can usually be expected, though the parturient may experience more discomfort than usual and have a longer labor. Generally speaking, management of labor analgesia in these situations will be the same as for a routine occiput anterior presentation and labor.

A transverse lie or shoulder presentation usually mandate a cesarean delivery.

12.5 Summary

When abnormalities occur in the process of labor and delivery, a more aggressive anesthetic approach is necessary to ensure an optimal outcome. Familiarity with the medications associated with preterm labor is essential, as most have the potential for interaction with common anesthetic agents and techniques; the anesthesiologist must be aware of the medications the parturient may be taking, must understand these interactions, and prepare or alter the anesthetic plan accordingly. Finally, during delivery of the patient with a multiple gestation or abnormal presentation, communication with the obstetrician can be the key to ensuring a successful outcome. Anticipating what the obstetrician will do, and knowing what is necessary in terms of anesthesia to accomplish it, can save valuable time in an urgent situation. Communication, anticipation, and understanding separate the average obstetric anesthesiologist from the excellent one.

Further reading

Benedetti, T.J. (1983) Maternal complications of parenteral beta-sympathomimetic therapy for preterm labor. *Am. J. Obstet. Gynecol.* **154**: 1–6.

Bottoms, S.F., Paul, R.H., Mercer, B.M. *et al.* (1999) Obstetric determinants of neonatal survival: antenatal predictors of neonatal survival and morbidity in extremely low birth weight infants. *Am. J. Obstet. Gynecol.* **180**: 665–669.

Carlan, S.J., Marshall, J.D., Huckaby, T. *et al.* (1994) The effect of epidural anesthesia on safety and success of external cephalic version at term. *Anesth. Analg.* **79**: 525–528.

Chestnut, D.H., Pollack, K.L., Thompsom, C.S. *et al.* (1990) Does nifedipine worsen maternal hypotension during epidural anesthesia in gravid ewes? *Anesthesiology* **72**: 315–312.

Childress, C.H. and Katz, V.L. (1994) Nifedipine and its indications in obstetrics and gynecology. *Obstet. Gynecol.* **83**: 616–624.

Copper, R.L., Goldenberg, R.L., Creasy, R.K. *et al.* (1993) A multicenter study of preterm birth weight and gestational age-specific neonatal mortality. *Am. J. Obstet. Gynecol.* **168**: 78–84.

Hill, W.C. (1995) Risks and complications of tocolysis. *Clin. Obstet. Gynecol.* **38**: 725–745.

Main, D.M. and Main, E.K. (1986) Management of preterm labor and delivery. In: *Obstetrics: Normal and Problem Pregnancies* (eds. Gabbe, S.G., Niebyl, J.R., and Simpson, J.L.), pp. 689–737. Churchill Livingstone, New York.

Malloy, M.H. *et al.* (1991) The effect of cesarean delivery on birth outcome in very low birth weight infants. *Obstet. Gynecol.* **77**: 498–503.

Mcgrath, J.M. and Chestnut, D.H. (1994) Preterm labor and delivery. In: *Obstetric Anesthesia: Principles and Practice* (ed. Chestnut, D.H.), pp. 643–668. Mosby-Year Book, Inc., St. Louis, MO.

McIntire, D.D., Bloom, S.L., Casey, B.M. and Leveno, K.J. (1999) Birth weight in relation to morbidity and mortality among newborn infants. *New Engl. J. Med.* **340**: 1234–1238. Q2

Palmer, C.M. (1999) Preterm labor. In: *Complications in Anesthesia* (ed. Atlee, J.L.), pp. 802–805. W.B. Saunders Company, Philadelphia, PA.

Pisani, J. and Rosenow, E.C. (1989) Pulmonary edema associated with tocolytic therapy. *Ann. Intern. Med.* **110**: 714–718.

Ramanathan, S., Gandhi, S., Arismendy, J., Chalon, J. and Turndorf, H. (1982) Oxygen transfer from mother to fetus during cesarean section under epidural anesthesia. *Anesth. Analg.* **61**: 576–581.

Robertson, P.A., Sniderman, S.H., Laros, R.K. *et al.* (1992) Neonatal morbidity according to gestational age and birth weight from five tertiary care centers in the United States, 1983 through 1986. *Am. J. Obstet. Gynecol.* **166**: 1629–1645.

Van Zundert, A., Vaes, L., Soetens, M. *et al.* (1991) Are breech deliveries an indication for epidural analgesia? *Anesth. Analg.* **72**: 399–403.

Walker, D.B., Feldman, A., Vohr, B.R. and Oh, W. (1984) Cost–benefit analysis of neonatal intensive care for infants weighing less than 1000 grams at birth. *Pediatrics* **74**: 20–25.

Wilkins, I.A. *et al.* (1988) Efficacy and side effects of magnesium sulfate and ritodrine as tocolytic agents. *Am. J. Obstet. Gynecol.* **159**: 685–689.

Wood, N. and Marlow, N. (1999) The contribution of preterm birth to outcomes in children. In: *Fetal Medicine: Basic Science and Clinical Practice* (eds Rodeck, C.H. and Whittle, M.J.), pp. 1071–1086. Churchill Livingstone, London.

Chapter 13

Coexisting disease

Michael Paech, FANZCA,
Craig M. Palmer, MD,
Laura S. Dean, MD and
Robert D'Angelo, MD

Contents

13.1 Introduction

Obstetric anesthesiologists are often called upon to care for parturients with other significant medical problems in addition to their pregnancies. In such cases, management of the patient's labor anesthetic will often be based as much on the patient's disease as their pregnancy. It is essential to understand the natural course of the disease process, and its interaction with various anesthetic techniques in order to provide optimal care.

13.2 Diabetes

Before the ready availability of insulin, few diabetic patients carried successful pregnancies to term because of the high maternal and fetal mortality associated with the untreated disease. Currently, however, with good blood glucose control and careful monitoring during gestation, maternal mortality should be very rare and the perinatal mortality rate should approach that of the nondiabetic population.

Pregnancy has sometimes been termed a 'diabetogenic' state because the diagnosis is often first made in parturients during their pregnancies. During the first trimester, estrogen and progesterone induce hyperplasia of pancreatic β cells, which actually increases insulin production; this usually results in lower blood glucose values in both diabetic and nondiabetic pregnancies. It is during the second and third trimesters that increased levels of human placental lactogen, an insulin antagonist, along with increased levels of prolactin, cortisol, estrogen, and progesterone, tend to increase blood glucose levels.

In a normal pregnancy, insulin production increases about 30% to compensate for these metabolic changes. Patients with pre-existing diabetes cannot increase their insulin production, and will require more exogenous insulin. Patients with marginal function may be fine when not pregnant, but cannot increase their insulin production enough to meet this demand. These patients are called gestational diabetics, and are the diabetic parturients most commonly encountered. Gestational diabetics are also called class A diabetics (see *Table 13.1*); class A1 diabetics can be managed throughout pregnancy with dietary modifications, while class A2 require insulin. The severity of disease correlates with maternal and fetal outcome.

In the US, virtually all parturients are screened for diabetes. The standard test is a nonfasting, 50 g oral glucose load with blood glucose sampling performed one hour later at 24 to 28 weeks gestation. If this test is abnormal, a fasting 100 g oral glucose tolerance test is performed.

In most cases, the fetal risks far outweigh maternal risks. Pre-existing diabetics have a significantly higher rate of fetal congenital anomalies than nondiabetics or even gestational diabetics, indicating a first trimester metabolic teratogenic effect. This risk can be minimized with strict preconceptual blood glucose control. Growth disturbances are

Table 13.1 Classification of diabetes in pregnancy

Class	Age of onset (years)	Duration (years)	Vascular disease	Therapy
A	Any	Any	0	A-1, diet only A-2, insulin
B	>20	<10	0	Insulin
C	10–19	10–19	0	Insulin
D	<10	>20	Benign retinopathy	Insulin
F	Any	Any	Nephropathy	Insulin
R	Any	Any	Proliferative retinopathy	Insulin
H	Any	Any	Heart disease	Insulin

common, both macrosomia and intrauterine growth retardation (IUGR). Macrosomia is likely due to fetal hyperglycemia, secondary to maternal hyperglycemia (glucose crosses the placenta via active transport, and maternal and fetal levels are closely correlated). IUGR is likely secondary to decreased utero-placental perfusion, due either to existing vascular disease or developmental compromise. Preterm delivery is twice as common as in nondiabetic parturients, often the result of maternal complications such as hypertension and preeclampsia. Pulmonary maturation is delayed in the fetus of the diabetic mother, compounding the problem of preterm delivery. Finally, neonatal hypoglycemia is common following delivery.

Diabetic mothers face an increased risk of urgent or emergent delivery; due to decreased utero-placental perfusion in many diabetics, the fetus may be unable to tolerate the stress of labor. The high incidence of macrosomia increases the likelihood of shoulder dystocia or cephalopelvic disproportion, and the need for operative intervention or cesarean delivery. Following delivery, diabetics are at increased risk of uterine hypotonia and significant hemorrhage.

The usual preoperative evaluation of the diabetic should include a very careful evaluation of the airway due to the increased risk of urgent delivery; gestational diabetics are often obese, which can complicate airway management. During labor, continuous maternal blood glucose control is important. Elevated intrapartum maternal glucose levels can produce fetal hyperglycemia and hyperinsulinemia, which can in turn lead to fetal hypercarbia and acidemia. In class A1 parturients, blood glucose should be checked every 2 to 4 hours during labor. In insulin-dependent diabetics, an intravenous insulin drip and dextrose infusion should be started (*Table 13.2*). Blood glucose should be checked via fingerstick hourly, and the rate of the infusions adjusted to maintain maternal glucose between 90 and 110 mg dl^{-1}. After delivery, insulin requirements drop quickly, so contin-

ued monitoring is necessary. Class A1 and A2 diabetics usually do not need insulin after delivery.

Diabetes in the parturient is a strong relative indication for regional analgesia/anesthesia during labor. Epidural analgesia has been shown to decrease circulating catecholamines, which can decrease uteroplacental perfusion and increase insulin requirements. Further, a functional epidural catheter provides a route for rapid induction of surgical anesthesia if necessary urgently. If a fluid load is felt necessary before institution of regional anesthesia, only nonglucose-containing fluids should be used.

For scheduled cesarean deliveries, an early morning start time is best, as this minimizes the NPO period, making management of insulin requirements easier. Blood glucose should be checked upon patient arrival, and insulin and dextrose infusions begun if necessary. Both spinal and epidural anesthesia are suitable for cesarean delivery. After delivery, it is important to make sure the individual responsible for neonatal evaluation and resuscitation is aware of the mother's diabetes, so the infant can be observed for signs of hypoglycemia.

13.3 **Cardiac disease**

13.3.1 Implications of cardiac disease during pregnancy

Although maternal cardiac disease occurs in only 1–2% of pregnancies and is now less common, its importance has become disproportionately high in terms of maternal mortality,

Table 3.2 Suggested insulin and glucose infusion rates based on finger-stick glucose measurements

Glucose (mg/100 ml)	Insulin dose (units/h)	Intravenous fluids (125 ml/h)
<100	0	D$_5$LR
100–140	1.0	D$_5$LR
141–180	1.5	Normal saline
181–220	2.0	Normal saline
>220	2.5	Normal saline

with increasing numbers of such deaths over recent times. In the Confidential Enquiry into Maternal Death (CEMD) in the UK 1994–96, the number of cardiac deaths surpassed those from hypertension. Cardiac disease was the leading cause of indirect maternal death, constituting half of all such deaths. These changes appear a consequence of several trends.

Maternal age at first pregnancy has risen, so ischemic heart disease is more prevalent (*Table 13.3*). An increasing number of women with severe congenital heart disease or respiratory disease now achieve reproductive age; rheumatic heart disease remains prevalent in poorer countries; and more women with severe cardiac disease appear willing to confront the risks of pregnancy.

Despite advances in the anesthetic management of cardiac disease in pregnancy, substandard care remains an issue and the CEMD highlights areas of potential improvement (*Table 13.4*). The earlier a consultative team approach and regular review is initiated, the better. This team may involve obstetricians and midwives, cardiologists and obstetric physicians, anesthesiologists and intensivists, neonatologists, psychologists and community health care workers. Members must seek a diagnosis; appreciate the pathophysiology and severity of the disease; the effects induced by the physiological changes of pregnancy, labor and delivery; and the impact of the disease on pregnancy outcome (*Table 13.5*).

Table 13.3 Reasons for the increased prevalence of myocardial ischemia during pregnancy

Increased maternal age of nullipara

Extension of the reproductive age range by application of infertility procedures

Increased prevalence of associated medical conditions such as diabetes and hypertension

Increased cigarette smoking among young women

Increased recreational cocaine use

Table 13.4 Areas for potential improvement in the obstetric care of women with cardiac disease

Failure to identify women at risk (assessment may be difficult)

Inadequate pre-conception and early pregnancy counseling of women with cardiac disease (How high is the risk? Should the pregnancy continue? Is corrective surgery feasible before pregnancy?)

Delayed referral to specialist multidisciplinary care and tertiary obstetric care

Poor communication and planning among health care specialists (decisions regarding drug therapy including anticoagulants; mode of delivery; analgesia and anesthesia; monitoring; contingency plan for urgent delivery; antibiotic prophylaxis)

Over-concern about some investigative technologies, even chest X-ray

Failure to optimize the woman's medical condition

Relevant physiological changes in pregnancy

Physiological changes in pregnancy (see Chapter 2) have an adverse impact on the compromised heart and women with cardiac disease often deteriorate symptomatically as gestation increases. The New York Heart Association (NYHA) classification based on exercise tolerance (*Table 13.6*) typically deteriorates at least one level and the worse the pre-pregnancy state, the more likely further deterioration ensues and the higher the mortality (class 3 and 4 mortality 75% or more). Blood volume increases by about 40%, mainly in early pregnancy, with plasma volume increasing more than red cell mass. Pulse rate increases 10–20 beats per minute in the first trimester and in response to increased oxygen demand cardiac output continues to rise, by 40% at about 30 weeks gestation, after which it stabilizes until an early postpartum peak. Systemic vascular resistance falls, but central venous and pulmonary artery pressure remain similar. Oxygen consumption increases slightly, then rises significantly during labor.

Even more dramatic changes in the peripartum period maximize cardiac stress and the

Table 13.5 General principles of management of parturients with cardiac disease

Antenatal

Pre-pregnancy consultation and planning (What is the risk of pregnancy?)

Regular antenatal review by a cardiologist or obstetric physician
- Echocardiography, electrocardiography with special emphasis on rhythm, ventricular function and pulmonary vascular resistance

Multidisciplinary review and planning
- Delivery time and mode; analgesia and anesthesia; concurrent drug therapy

Correction of anemia and infection

Fetal surveillance

Aim for (assisted) vaginal delivery in most cases

Labor and delivery

Provide appropriate antibiotic prophylaxis

Avoid aortocaval compression in labor, transfer for cesarean delivery and anesthesia

Appropriate monitoring
- Korotkoff sounds, automated noninvasive blood pressure, pulse oximetry
- Consider direct arterial BP and blood gas monitoring; central venous or pulmonary artery catheter
- Fetal heart rate monitoring

Appropriate medical management
- Supplemental oxygen; fluid balance; drug therapy

Appropriate obstetric management
- Senior obstetric and midwifery staff involvement
- Usually avoid pushing in the second stage of labor
- Avoid ergometrine at delivery

Appropriate anesthetic management
- Epidural or combined spinal-epidural analgesia in labor, avoiding falls in systemic vascular resistance
- Senior staff involvement in determining anesthetic method for cesarean delivery

Postpartum

Good postpartum care, at least a high-dependency unit
- Avoid fluid overload; monitor for cardiac failure; discuss contraception

risk of cardiac decompensation. Cardiac output rises during labor secondary to sympathetic stimulation, autotransfusion of 500 ml of blood from the contracted uterus and the relief of aortocaval compression. Cardiac output peaks at 200–300% above pre-pregnancy level in the first hour after delivery, then rapidly falls after 24 hours, tapering to normal after 10 days postpartum. Symptoms of breathlessness, fatigue, decreased exercise tolerance and edema may be normal responses, but may also be pathophysiological and should not be dismissed. A hyperdynamic circulation is reflected in the physical examination by flow murmurs, but further investigation is often warranted as less severe congenital lesions may present for the first time in teenage or young adult pregnancy.

General considerations

The anesthesiologist has a range of questions and issues to consider, related to medical, obstetric and anesthetic management and risk-benefit in relation to cardiac disease during

Table **13.6** New York Heart Association classification (NYHA)	
Class	**Definition**
Class I	No undue symptoms associated with ordinary activity and no limitations of physical activity
Class II	Slight limitation of physical activity, ordinary physical activity results in fatigue, palpitation, dyspnea or angina; patient comfortable at rest
Class III	Marked limitation of physical activity with less than ordinary activity causing fatigue, palpitation, dyspnea; patient comfortable at rest
Class IV	Inability to carry on any physical activity without discomfort; symptoms of cardiac insufficiency or angina possible, even at rest

Table 13.7 Anesthetic questions related to the parturient with cardiac disease

- What are the anatomical changes and pathophysiology of this cardiac disease?
- What was the pre-pregnancy status and what is the current maternal and fetal condition?
- What investigations have and need to be performed?
- What antenatal treatment must be instituted now?
- Where is the parturient best delivered?
- What is the plan for delivery, management of delivery and the puerperium?
- Where is the best location for postpartum care?
- What method of labor analgesia is advisable?
- What method of anesthesia for CS should be recommended?
- What are the special considerations for the above?
- What monitoring should be used?
- How should hemodynamic or other emergencies be managed?

pregnancy (*Tables 13.7* and *13.8*). In some high-risk conditions and end-stage disease (*Table 13.9*), successful outcomes are reported, but the risk of mortality mandates sensitive discussion as to whether the pregnancy should continue. Rarely, severe deterioration during pregnancy and failure of medical management may necessitate cardiac surgery during pregnancy (for example, mitral commissurotomy or replacement for severe mitral stenosis). This is normally performed during the late second trimester when organogenesis is complete and potential fetal viability has been reached.

Antibiotic prophylaxis against bacterial endocarditis may be warranted (*Table 13.10*) and the risks of terato- and organogenesis from drug therapy must be weighed against those of deteriorating medical status. A good example is anticoagulant therapy, which is indicated for atrial fibrillation, mechanical prosthetic heart valves, pulmonary hypertension or a previous thromboembolic event. Warfarin is avoided during organogenesis, with many units also continuing with heparin in the second and third trimesters in preference, because of warfarin-induced embryopathy. When regional block is planned in conjunction with doses of unfractionated heparin or the use of long-acting low molecular weight heparins, attention to timing of insertion and catheter removal is needed to reduce the risk of epidural hematoma. The anesthetic implications, should premature labor or urgent delivery for maternal or fetal reasons occur, need consideration. When regional analgesia is considered an unacceptable risk, intramuscular injection should also be avoided. Intravenous opioid patient-controlled analgesia (PCA) in labor is a good option, and general anesthesia (GA) is likely for operative delivery.

13.3.2 Specific cardiac conditions

Rheumatic valvular disease
Mitral stenosis (isolated or as part of mixed valvular disease) is the most common lesion, whereas aortic stenosis is rare. Mortality is low (1%), rising to 5% with New York Heart Asso-

Table 13.8 Principles of general anesthesia for cardiac disease

General anesthesia is occasionally preferable to regional anesthesia
- e.g., for severe aortic stenosis; poorly controlled cardiac failure, but always perform an individual risk-benefit assessment

Remember hemodynamic changes tend to be greater than with regional anesthesia

Obtund the sympatho-adrenal 'stress response' to laryngoscopy and intubation
- e.g., with appropriate doses of opioid, membrane stabilizing agents and vasodilatory drugs

Nitrous oxide increases pulmonary vascular resistance

Choose the inhalational anesthetic with the least adverse cardiac and vascular effects on the condition

Use neuromuscular blocking drugs free of cardiovascular side effects

Provide good postoperative analgesia
- e.g., patient-controlled intravenous analgesia with morphine; adjuncts such as acetoaminophen (paracetamol); nonsteroidal anti-inflammatory drugs if no renal impairment or cardiac failure

ciation (NYHA) class III or IV classification and 15% with atrial fibrillation. As mitral stenosis develops, a gradient across the valve is established and with increased flow atrial pressure rises. Severe stenosis (valve area < 1 cm^2) is most likely to be associated with large left atrial size and secondary pulmonary hypertension leading to right ventricular failure. Control of arrhythmia and heart rate is very important, because increased rate reduces diastolic filling time and increases left atrial pressure, while atrial fibrillation reduces preload from loss of atrial contraction. Many women will benefit from β-blockers, digoxin and anticoagulation in the presence of atrial fibrillation, and other antiarrhythmic drugs or cardioversion may be necessary. By far the most common complication is pulmonary edema, which may also complicate moderate or mild disease (*Figure 13.1*). Physiological changes and cardiovascular stress in labor are usually well tolerated despite tachycardia, and careful epidural anesthesia (*Table 13.11*) is suitable for cesarean delivery.

In aortic stenosis, pain and labor-induced tachycardia predispose to myocardial ischemia or heart failure due to inadequate coronary

Table 13.9 Obstetric and anesthetic mortality risk classification

Very high risk (mortality 25–50%)	High risk (mortality 5–15%)	Lower risk (mortality ,1%)
Pulmonary hypertension (primary and secondary, especially Eisenmenger's syndrome)	Severe aortic stenosis	Mild to moderate aortic or mitral stenosis
Complicated aortic coarctation	Mitral stenosis with atrial fibrillation or NYHA class III or IV	Aortic or mitral incompetence and mitral valve prolapse
Marfan's syndrome with aortic involvement	Severe cardiomyopathy	Corrected congenital heart disease (e.g. tetralogy of Fallot, atrial and ventricular septal defect)
Aortic aneurysm and acute aortic dissection	Uncorrected congenital heart disease	Cardiac arrhythmia
	Uncomplicated coarctation of aorta	Prosthetic heart valve
	Myocardial ischemia or previous myocardial infarction	Post-cardiac surgery or transplant
	Marfan's with normal aorta	

Table 13.10 Antibiotic prophylaxis against endocarditis in cardiac disease[a]

Prophylaxis recommended (high-risk)	Prophylaxis optional (for high-risk patients)	Prophylaxis not recommended
Prosthetic heart valves	Vaginal delivery	Surgically repaired atrial or ventricular septal defect, patent ductus arteriosus
Previous bacterial endocarditis	*Regimen:* Ampicillin 2 g IV/IM + gentamicin 1.5 mg/kg (max. 120 mg) within 30 min + 6 h later Ampicillin 1 g IV/IM or amoxycillin 1 g PO	Isolated secundum atrial septal defect
Complex cyanotic congenital disease		Mitral valve prolapse without regurgitation
Surgically constructed systemic-pulmonary shunts or conduits (moderate-risk)	*Regimen for penicillin allergy:* Vancomycin 1 g IV over 1–2 h + gentamicin 1.5 mg/kg (max. 120 mg) once only within 30 min	Previous coronary artery surgery
Most other congenital cardiac malformations other than minor (see below)		Cardiac pacemakers and implanted defibrillators
		Other diseases, without valvular dysfunction
Acquired valvular disease or for Mitral valve prolapse with regurgitation		Cesarean section
		Genitourinary surgery
		Vaginal hysterectomy
		Procedures in uninfected tissue

[a]Based on recommendations of the American Heart Association 1997.

diastolic filling and inadequate oxygen supply to the thickened left ventricle. Bradycardia may reduce cardiac output and cause heart failure. Provided calcification has not developed, balloon valvuloplasty is an option in severe mitral or aortic stenosis during the second trimester after medical therapy has failed, but may create significant regurgitation. Valve replacement is associated with high fetal loss.

In contrast, regurgitant lesions such as mitral and aortic incompetence often improve during pregnancy, due to mild afterload reduction and increased blood volume. Atrial fibrillation is common with severe mitral regurgitation and a plan of anticoagulation management for all contingencies is important. Mitral valve prolapse is a common condition and regurgitation is usually trivial. In significant cases, hypo-volemia and tachycardia may decrease left ventricular volume and increase regurgitation.

Anesthetic management. In rheumatic valvular disease, good pain relief with epidural or spinal analgesia during labor (using opioids or low concentration local anesthetic/opioid combinations delivered slowly by infusion) is ideal. This minimizes sudden reduction in peripheral vascular resistance, while maintaining normal maternal heart rate and allowing controlled delivery without Valsalva maneuver. If epidural analgesia is contraindicated, parenteral meperidine is unsatisfactory and may cause tachycardia. Intravenous PCA with fentanyl or remifentanil and control of heart rate with a β-blocker is advisable for NYHA class III or IV patients. Monitoring of fluid balance to

full, fast, & loose

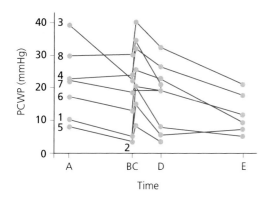

Figure 13.1 Intrapartum changes in pulmonary capillary wedge pressure (PCWP) in eight parturients with mitral stenosis. (A) First stage of labor; (B) second stage of labor, 15–30 min before delivery; (C) 5–15 min postpartum; (D) 4–6 hours postpartum; (E) 18–25 hours postpartum. Reproduced with permission of Harcourt Brace, Orlando from Clark, S. L. *et al.* (1985) Labor and delivery in the presence of mitral stenosis: central hemodynamic observations. *Am. J. Obstet. Gynecol.* **152**: 986.

maintain normovolemia, judicious intravenous fluid and vasoactive drug administration with α-agonists (e.g. phenylephrine) rather than ephedrine for vasoconstriction (to avoid its undesirable chronotropic effects) are

recommended. Oxytocin should be infused slowly, to avoid peripheral vasodilatation and reflex tachycardia, ergot preparations avoided, and in severe mitral stenosis, furosemide should be considered to reduce the risk of post-partum pulmonary edema.

Cesarean section is used on obstetric grounds only, and in the absence of sound evidence, the merits of regional versus GA can be debated. Both single-shot spinal anesthesia (SA) and rapid epidural anesthesia (EA) can cause sudden cardiovascular collapse. Titrated regional techniques are preferred and are usually beneficial, provided volume overload and bradycardia are avoided. In an elective setting, the slow establishment of EA with nonepinephrine (adrenaline) containing solution provides optimal hemodynamic stability (see *Table 13.11*). Direct arterial blood pressure monitoring and even continuous venous oximetry to assess adequacy of oxygen delivery may be indicated. During GA, nitrous oxide increases pulmonary vascular resistance and isoflurane reduces systemic vascular resistance. The intubation response and myocardial depression should be attenuated, because sudden increases in heart rate and afterload may precipitate pulmonary edema in mitral

---

Table 13.11 Principles of regional analgesia and anesthesia for cardiac disease

The benefits of regional analgesia in labor almost always outweigh disadvantages
- Spinal or epidural opioid analgesia in labor initially, with subsequent epidural infusion using low doses of local anesthetic and opioid
- Avoid epinephrine (adrenaline) containing epidural local anesthetic
- Fluid restriction; no intravenous fluid preloading; left uterine displacement; appropriate monitoring; no ergometrine

Establish regional anesthesia slowly
- Poorly managed regional anesthesia with rapid changes in peripheral or pulmonary vascular resistance or high block is particularly dangerous in right-to-left shunt, severe valvular stenosis and cardiomyopathy

Maintain systolic blood pressure close to baseline values
- Use prophylactic and therapeutic IV vasopressor
- Use ephedrine if bradycardia is a concern (severe regurgitant valvular disease, poor ventricular function)
- Use metaraminol or phenylephrine to avoid β-agonist activity of ephedrine when tachycardia is deleterious (e.g., hypertrophic obstructive cardiomyopathy, severe valvular stenosis)

Use postoperative epidural analgesia including local anesthetic
- Avoid the deleterious effects of pain and use vasodilatation to counteract the increase in circulating blood volume in the early postpartum period

stenosis or ischemia in aortic stenosis (see *Table 13.8*) and inotropic drugs must be available.

Severe congenital heart disease and pulmonary hypertension

Congenital disease is now the leading cause of cardiac maternal death, followed by ischemic heart disease and other conditions, such as aortic dissection. There are a large number of congenital disorders of varying complexity, some cyanotic (e.g., tetralogy of Fallot) and others left-to-right shunts (patent ductus arteriosis, ostium secundum atrial septal defect, ventricular septal defects). These vary in significance and require individual assessment, some needing only antibiotic prophylaxis and others aggressive control of physiological variables and management of hyperviscosity. Those of most concern often involve pulmonary hypertension (*Figure13.2*) (pulmonary artery pressure >30/15 mmHg and right ventricular hypertrophy) or reversal of left-to-right shunt (Eisenmenger's syndrome).

Primary pulmonary hypertension is a rare disorder that presents in women of reproductive age, whereas secondary pulmonary hypertension with right ventricular hypertrophy and/or right heart failure may develop with congenital left-to-right shunts, prolonged mitral stenosis or severe hypoxemia from various respiratory diseases (e.g. cystic fibrosis).

Pregnancy-induced physiological changes tend to increase cardiac work and right-to-left shunting, predisposing to right heart failure. Mortality is between 30 and 50%. Increases in pulmonary and reduction in systemic vascular resistance (e.g. hypovolemia and hypoxemia) are generally poorly tolerated, so regional analgesia and anesthesia have traditionally been considered contraindicated. However, GA for cesarean section is associated with significant morbidity and mortality from hemorrhage, infection and thromboembolism. Hypoxia, hypercarbia and acidosis increase pulmonary artery pressure and resistance, making prolonged labor, severe pain, the respiratory depressant effect of systemic opioids and inadequate hydration potential hazards (*Figure 13.3*). Pre-pregnancy polycythemia or oxygen saturation <85% on air are poor prognostic indicators for the fetus in cyanotic heart disease without Eisenmenger's syndrome.

Anesthetic management. In the presence of a shunt, the loss-of-resistance to air technique for epidural placement is contraindicated due to the possibility of paradoxical embolism in the cerebral circulation. Anticoagulation, avoiding air in intravenous infusion lines and prophylaxis against bacterial endocarditis are other considerations. Successful outcomes are achieved using epidural opioids followed

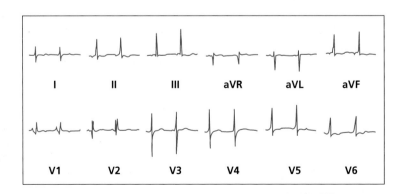

Figure 13.2 Electrocardiograph of a parturient with pulmonary hypertension, showing sinus rhythm with right atrial P waves (V1), an inferior axis and evidence of right ventricular pressure overload (V1–2).

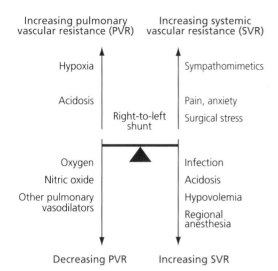

Figure 13.3 Factors affecting cardiac shunt.

by opioid/local anesthetic (e.g. an infusion of bupivacaine 0.0625%), or a combined spinal-epidural approach using subarachnoid opioid alone. Recent small prospective series indicate cautious EA (see *Table 13.11*), balancing factors affecting pulmonary and systemic resistance (*Figure 13.3*), is associated with minimal hemodynamic change (*Figure 13.4*) and good outcome. Given that randomized trials of anesthetic technique are not feasible, this is reassuring. Monitoring of changes in arterial oxyhemoglobin saturation is a valuable noninvasive tool for the detection of hypoxemia from shunt reversal or increased pulmonary pressure. Thermodilution pulmonary artery catheters and echocardiography are used in some units, but, if in doubt, it may be wisest to manage without, particularly in view of the problems of the former (arrhythmias, pulmonary artery rupture and accuracy issues). Inhaled pulmonary vasodilators such as nitric oxide, 100% oxygen, aerosolized or intravenous prostaglandins (epoprostenol, iloprost or PGI_2) may be tested to determine patient response, bearing in mind that platelet dysfunction may be induced, with implications for central neuraxial block. Intensive postpartum care is warranted, as deaths may occur after an apparently uncomplicated intra- and early postpartum course, possible related to declining pulmonary prostaglandin levels.

Acyanotic congenital heart disease
There are a variety of cardiac structural and developmental abnormalities that have a good prognosis. Complex disease, if satisfactorily corrected in early childhood, or conditions such as Ebstein's anomaly, which may not present until late childhood, are generally suitable for epidural analgesia and regional anesthesia. Ebstein's anomaly (downward displacement of the triscuspid valve with atrialized proximal portion of the right ventricle) has a good prognosis in pregnancy, despite paroxysmal arrhythmias and possible right-to-left shunting. The secundum atrial septal defect is one of the most common defects first diagnosed in pregnancy. Supraventricular arrhythmias are poorly tolerated as shunt is increased, and blood loss may cause abrupt fall in cardiac output, but like corrected ventricular septal defect, patent ductus and aortic coarctation, these abnormalities usually pose few problems.

Myocardial ischemia
Although uncommon in pregnancy, this problem seems likely to increase (see *Table 13.3*). Most cases of acute myocardial infarction occur in the third trimester in women more than 35 years of age and mortality is high (30%, rising the closer the infarct occurs to term gestation). During pregnancy and under regional anesthesia for cesarean section, changes in the electrocardiogram (ECG) such as sinus tachycardia, left axis deviation and ST-T changes may make interpretation more difficult. However, unlike the muscle-brain isoenzyme of creatinine kinase (CK-MB), maternal troponin I levels are unchanged during pregnancy. A rise within 4 hours lasting several days is specific for myocardial injury. Usual medical therapies such as nitrates, β-blockers and calcium-channel antagonists should be continued during pregnancy and heparin thromboprophylaxis is often instituted.

187

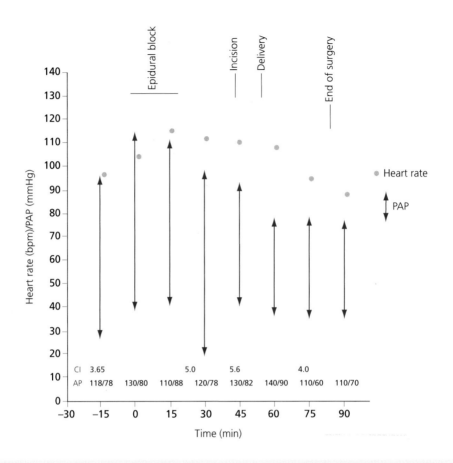

Figure 13.4 Hemodynamic changes during cesarean section in a parturient with primary pulmonary hypertension. CI, cardiac index (l/min); AP, arterial pressure (mmHg); PAP, pulmonary artery pressure (mmHg); bpm, beats per minute. Reproduced from Khan, M.J. *et al.* (1996) Anesthetic considerations for parturients with primary pulmonary hypertension: review of the literature and clinical presentation. *Int. J. Obstet. Anesth.* **5**: 38, with permission of the publisher Churchill Livingstone.

With unstable angina or acute infarction, aspirin is appropriate but fibrinolytic therapy is associated with a very high risk of maternal hemorrhage and premature labor. Emergency coronary angioplasty and full anticoagulation for severe ventricular hypokinesis or mural thrombus may be required. Vaginal delivery appears safer than CS after myocardial infarction during pregnancy.

Anesthetic management In the presence of adequate myocardial function, regional analgesia is recommended for labor and delivery. Supplemental oxygen, avoiding increased oxygen demand from shivering (warm fluids and surface warming, spinal opioid with local anesthetic, treatment with intravenous clonidine 30 µg) and monitoring of temperature, oxygenation, blood pressure and ECG are prudent. Regional anesthesia (incremental epidural, sequential spinal-epidural or continuous spinal anesthesia) for operative delivery and α-agonist vasocontrictors (phenylephrine, metaraminol) are preferred management options. Spinal anesthesia or rapid EA are probably best avoided due to the cardiovascular consequences of uncompensated sympathectomy and a modified approach to GA should be used (see *Table 13.8*). High thoracic epidural analgesia for postoperative analgesia has been shown to favorably influence the endocardial to epicardial blood flow ratio in the heart.

Arrhythmias

Benign arrhythmias are common and serious arrhythmias rare during pregnancy. Drug therapy requires consideration of safety in pregnancy, because some anti-arrhythmics such as phenytoin and amiodarone are associated with fetal effects (*Figure 13.5*). Atrial fibrillation of onset during pregnancy is worrying and often associated with mitral valvular disease, though thyrotoxicosis and other heart disease should also be excluded. Management includes rate control with digoxin and anticoagulation. When hemodynamic compromise accompanies the sudden onset of any supraventricular arrhythmia, direct-current cardioversion (50 joules under appropriate GA) is safe and fetal heart rate changes transient and benign.

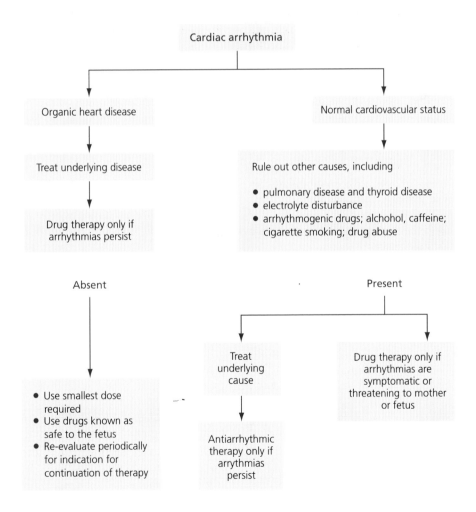

Figure 13.5 Management of cardiac arrhythmias during pregnancy. Reproduced with permission of Adis International, Auckland from Rotmensch, H.H. *et al.* (1987) Management of cardiac arrhythmias during pregnancy. *Drugs* **33**: 628.

Hypertrophic obstructive cardiomyopathy

This autosomal dominant disorder with variable penetrance, involving a mutation on the myosin heavy chain gene, usually presents in young adulthood and is commonly termed HOCM (also idiopathic hypertrophic subaortic stenosis). It has some similarities to aortic stenosis in that an asymmetric hypertrophy of the interventricular septum produces left ventricular outflow obstruction that is worsened by low ventricular volume, increased ventricular ejection velocity or low arterial pressure. Management is directed toward avoidance of hypovolemia and arrhythmias (especially the loss of atrial 'kick' with atrial fibrillation), and rapid additional β-blockade for tachycardia (thus increasing end-diastolic ventricular filling and reducing myocardial oxygen demand and ventricular velocity). Direct-acting vasoconstrictors are preferred to ephedrine (see *Table 13.11*) and epidural or CSE analgesia in labor with arterial blood pressure monitoring is of benefit, by reducing catecholamines released in response to pain, but an individual risk-benefit assessment is necessary for operative delivery. Both careful, slowly titrated EA and GA have been used successfully for CS, and although pregnancy outcome is usually good, sudden death due to ventricular arrhythmia or pulmonary edema may occur.

Peripartum cardiomyopathy and heart-lung transplantation

Although cardiomyopathy has various etiologies (viral myocarditis, drug-induced etc.), in about 1 in 2000–4000 pregnancies low-output cardiac failure arises without apparent cause during the third trimester or more commonly (60%) in the postpartum period. Peripartum cardiomyopathy has first presented as unexpected hypotension, bradycardia and cardiac arrest at induction of anesthesia for CS, but problems usually relate to management of a failing heart and anticoagulation to prevent mural thrombus. Mild reduction of afterload using appropriate regional analgesia is of benefit in labor, and well-managed EA for CS (avoiding SA) appears safe. An epidural

technique that minimizes cardiac work and hypotension (see *Table 13.11*) with no, or minimal, intravenous fluid loading avoids the adverse effects of the stress response to intubation and the myocardial depressant effects associated with GA. However, in dyspneic patients, supine positioning may not be possible and invasive monitoring, including pulmonary artery catheterization, is indicated with vasodilators, inotropes and intensive care support available. When GA is used, a technique based on moderate to high-dose opioid is recommended (see *Table 13.8*). The prognosis is variable and cardiac transplantation offers an alternative for those with persistent dysfunction.

In the rare case of successful pregnancy after transplantation, high rates of hypertension, preeclampsia and premature labor increase the likelihood of anesthetic involvement, although obstetric and maternal outcome is generally good. A balance must be struck between graft rejection and infection risk and immunosuppressive therapy may require adjustment (for example, an increased dose of cyclosporin due to the pharmacokinetic changes). The denervated heart has higher resting heart rate due to loss of vagal tone. This is unaffected by indirect-acting drugs like atropine and ephedrine, but the effects of direct-acting drugs may be exaggerated by β-adrenoreceptor up-regulation, and the myocardial depressant effects of anesthetic agents predominate. Preload must be maintained and epinephrine-containing local anesthetic avoided.

Other conditions

Systemic disorders may also present with cardiac disease: for example, autoimmune diseases such as scleroderma and rheumatoid arthritis (myocardial fibrosis, pericarditis, arrhythmias) or connective tissue diseases such as Marfan's syndrome. Features of the latter autosomal dominant disease of connective tissue (fibrillin gene mutations) include mitral valve prolapse or regurgitation, aortic root dilatation and regurgitation and aortic dissection. The latter is the most common cause of death and more likely in late pregnancy. Patients with aortic diameter greater than 4 cm or progressive dilatation warrant frequent transthoracic echocardiography, aggressive control of hypertension and epidural techniques for labor or operative delivery.

13.4 Pulmonary disease

Profound changes in respiratory physiology and anatomy occur during pregnancy. Underlying pulmonary disease should be recognized and treated early in gestation to prevent complications.

13.4.1 Asthma

Asthma is the most common pulmonary disease in women of childbearing age. Complicating 1–5% of all pregnancies, asthma follows a rule of thirds. It is unchanged in one third, worsened in one third and improved in one third of patients. Severe asthmatics are likely to have exacerbations of their disease during pregnancy and any woman who has had worsening of her asthma during a previous pregnancy is likely to have a similar experience in subsequent pregnancies. Hyperresponsive airways lead to hypersecretion of mucus, edema and contraction of smooth muscle, which intermittently obstructs the airway. An allergen–antibody complex binds to mast cells that release mediators that further attract inflammatory cells. This cascade results in capillary and airway damage that stimulates edema and bronchoconstriction. Clinically, asthmatics present with wheezing and decreased FEV_1. An asthma 'attack' results in hyperinflation of lung volumes. Air trapping increases the work of breathing and decreases perfusion to overdistended alveoli leading to V/Q mismatch. This imbalance will manifest as hypoxemia and hypercarbia.

The obstetric complications associated with asthma are summarized in *Table 13.12*. Asthma is a risk factor for maternal as well as neonatal complications. The etiology for these complications is probably multifactorial. Poor control

Table 13.12 Obstetric complications associated with asthma

Spontaneous abortions
Prematurity
Low birthweight babies
Premature rupture of membranes
Chorioamnionitis
Hyperemesis
Hemorrhage
Chronic hypertension
Preeclampsia
Gestational diabetes mellitus
↑ Operative delivery

of bronchospasm with resultant hypoxia may contribute to complications and there may be deleterious effects of the medications used to treat asthma.

The differential diagnoses for an acute asthmatic episode are listed in *Table 13.13*. When evaluating the pregnant asthma patient it is important to obtain a pertinent history. A patient who has previously been intubated and mechanically ventilated or who has had a prolonged duration of symptoms is likely to be difficult to manage. A complete list of medications should be obtained. On physical exam, respiratory rate, speech pattern, wheezing and accessory muscle use are important to evaluate. Pulse oximetry, peak flows and an arterial blood gas should be obtained when indicated. Management of asthmatics during pregnancy is directed towards prevention, monitoring and pharmacotherapy when necessary. Inhaled β-agonists, cromolyn sulfate, theophylline and beclomethasone are the preferred methods of treatment during pregnancy. Oral corticosteroid therapy may also be indicated. A pulmonary consult should be considered to assist with severe cases.

Table 13.13 Differential diagnosis of acute asthma

Airway obstruction: tumor, laryngeal edema, foreign body
Bronchitis
Emphysema
Pulmonary embolism
Congestive heart failure

13.4.2 Pneumonia

Pneumonia is a common cause of morbidity in pregnancy and remains a potentially fatal infection in otherwise healthy females. There is an associated increased rate of prematurity, abortion and fetal death. Aggressive management is warranted. Nearly half of all cases of pneumonia in pregnancy are preceded by upper respiratory infection (URI). The incidence of URI in pregnancy is the same as in the nonpregnant state but should be evaluated and treated promptly.

13.4.3 Pulmonary edema

The etiologies of pulmonary edema in pregnancy are listed in *Table 13.14*. Treatment includes diagnosis and therapy of the underlying disease, fluid restriction, diuresis, and supportive care.

13.4.4 Pulmonary embolus

Normal physiological changes of pregnancy (including increased clotting factors and altered venous compliance) increase the risk of deep venous thrombosis. This translates into a propensity for pulmonary emboli during pregnancy. Additional risk factors include age >35, cesarean section, bedrest and obesity. Recognition of risk factors and early postoperative ambulation are important prophylactic measures.

13.4.5 Aspiration

Mendelson described the effects of acid aspiration and pneumonitis in 1946. Prevention is the paramount therapy. Administration of an oral nonparticulate antacid within 30–45 minutes of surgery is prudent. Thirty milliliters of

Table 13.14 Etiologies of pulmonary edema during pregnancy

Aspiration	See Section 13.3.6
Preeclampsia	See Chapter 12
Sepsis	
Tocolytic therapy	See Section 12.1.6
Underlying cardiac disease	See Section 13.2
Iatrogenic fluid overload	

sodium citrate can neutralize in excess of 250 ml of hydrochloric acid to a pH of 7.0. All parturients should be considered to have a full stomach and rapid sequence induction with cricoid pressure should be performed when general anesthesia is indicated. While other agents, such as H_2 antagonists and metoclopramide, have been recommended they have not been shown to reduce morbidity and mortality and are expensive. Therefore, 30 ml of sodium citrate should be routinely administered before any operative intervention. Attempt to administer the nonparticulate antacid before transporting the patient to the operating room as this may help with mixing of the antacid with the stomach contents.

13.4.6 Cigarette smoking

Cigarettes remain one of the most abused legal substances in our society that cause significant preventable morbidity and mortality. More than 20% of pregnant women smoke and 80% of smokers continue to do so during pregnancy. Heavy smokers are less likely to quit during pregnancy than those who smoke only occasionally. Although cigarette smoke contains in excess of 1000 compounds, carbon monoxide and nicotine are the two compounds believed to cause most of the smoking-related problems associated with pregnancy. Carbon monoxide binds to the oxygen receptor on hemoglobin much more tightly than oxygen, which can result in significant carboxyhemoglobin levels. This produces a left shift in the maternal oxyhemoglobin dissociation curve causing an increased infinity of hemoglobin for oxygen. The net result is a decreased availability of oxygen for the mother and fetus. Nicotine, on the other hand, potentially decreases uteroplacental perfusion by directly increasing uterine vascular resistance. *Table 13.15* lists the obstetric complications associated with cigarettes. The adverse affects of cigarette smoking on the fetus may be subtle and long lasting since neonates of mothers who smoke cigarettes during pregnancy may be at increased risk for a number of long-term disorders (*Table 13.16*). Pregnant smokers

Table 13.15 Obstetric complications of cigarette smoking

Ectopic pregnancy
Spontaneous abortion
Preterm delivery
Placenta previa
Low birthweight babies/intrauterine growth retardation
↓ Uteroplacental perfusion

Table 13.16 Neonatal risks associated with smoking cigarettes during pregnancy

Impaired suckling
Learning disorders
Sleep disturbances
Sudden infant death syndrome (SIDS)
Childhood cancers

Table 13.17 Adverse physiologic affects of cigarettes

↑ Mucus secretion
↓ Mucociliary transport
Airway hyperreactivity
Small airway narrowing
↑ Carboxyhemoglobin levels
Impaired immune response
Hepatic enzyme induction

should be educated about these risks and encouraged to quit whenever possible.

In addition to the aforementioned risks, cigarette smoking produces a number of additional adverse physiological changes that can have anesthetic implications (*Table 13.17*). Since nearly all smokers have hyperreactive airways, it is advisable to avoid airway instrumentation whenever possible. Although regional anesthesia is preferable over general anesthesia in all pregnant patients, the pregnant patient who smokes cigarettes theoretically derives even greater benefits from regional anesthesia.

13.5 Neurologic and neuromuscular disease

The anesthetic approach to the parturient with neurologic or neuromuscular disease must be individualized; because of the dominance of regional anesthesia and central administration of medications in modern obstetric practice, potential interaction with the disease process becomes a primary issue. Some anesthesiologists have advocated avoidance of regional techniques in this population, due to the perception that any exacerbation of the disease will inevitably be blamed on the anesthetic. It

is unfair to deprive these patients of the major benefits of regional anesthesia and analgesia because of theoretical concerns, however. A better approach is to discuss options with the patient, along with potential advantages and drawbacks, and jointly decide upon an anesthetic plan.

13.5.1 Multiple sclerosis

Multiple sclerosis is a demyelinating disease of the central nervous system, characterized by periodic remissions and exacerbations. While there is no definitive treatment, most patients with the disease maintain a high level of function for years or decades. It is not uncommon in women of childbearing age. While many theoretical concerns about regional anesthesia in these patients have been raised, there is little scientific or clinical information available. For example, some local anesthetics have been shown to be neurotoxic in some situations, and there is controversy regarding whether they may have deleterious effects on demyelinated neurons.

Retrospective reports indicate that regional anesthesia can be safely used for labor analgesia. Some weak evidence associates high concentrations of local anesthetics (i.e. bupivacaine over 0.25%) used for epidural anesthesia with a higher postpartum relapse rate than lower concentrations, but a number of confounding variables could also account for this association. It should be noted that the relapse rate in the 3 months after delivery is higher than would be expected in a nonpregnant population in the first place. Other factors that are known to predispose to relapse include increased temperature, stress (both physical and emotional), and fatigue, all common in the postpartum population.

From a practical standpoint, when administering epidural analgesia to a parturient with multiple sclerosis, it is probably prudent to avoid the use of high concentrations of local anesthetics. Current techniques rely on relatively dilute local anesthetics (bupivacaine 0.125% or lower) in combination with opioids for routine labor analgesia, and these mixtures should cause little if any problem in this population. Due to the association of epidural labor analgesia and increased maternal temperature, maternal and labor room temperature should be closely monitored. For cesarean delivery, epidural anesthesia can be used following discussion of the theoretical risks with the patient; otherwise, general anesthesia would be the only option for routine procedures. Spinal anesthesia is best avoided except in urgent circumstances where there are strong indications for use of a regional technique (an urgent cesarean section in a patient with a poor airway, for example).

13.5.2 Myasthenia gravis

Myasthenia gravis is a disease affecting the acetylcholine receptors at the neuromuscular junction. It is characterized by weakness and easy fatigability of voluntary muscles. The underlying cause is not known, but patients usually have antibodies to muscular acetylcholine receptors that interfere with the action of this neurotransmitter. Therapy usually consists of oral anticholinesterase agents, such as pyridostigmine.

In the preanesthetic evaluation of patients with myasthenia gravis, the patient's symptoms and the affected muscles should be elicited. Of major concern is the involvement of the respiratory muscles and difficulties in ventilation; fortunately, such problems should be uncommon in the pregnant population. If there is concern of respiratory involvement, it can be readily evaluated with spirometry.

For labor analgesia, regional techniques are effective, although some care should be given to avoiding high anesthetic levels if pulmonary problems are suspected. For cesarean delivery, the choice of anesthetic technique is dependent on ventilatory status. Some patients may not be able to lie flat due to respiratory weakness. Regional techniques can markedly impair respiratory muscle function and ventilation. If a patient cannot tolerate the respiratory demands of labor, it is unlikely she will be able to tolerate a regional anesthetic for cesarean delivery; epidural anesthesia is preferable to spinal anesthesia because it can be titrated more carefully to minimize respiratory effects.

With general anesthesia, the response to muscle relaxants will most likely be altered. Succinylcholine usually produces prolonged blockade, and patients are very sensitive to nondepolarizing relaxants. If it is necessary to use nondepolarizers, the shortest acting agents (mivacurium, rocuronium, or rapacuronium) are the best choice. Regardless of agent, careful monitoring of the block and its reversal are necessary using a twitch monitor. Lingering effects of other anesthetic agents (inhalation or induction agents) that are benign in normal populations may result in respiratory compromise in myasthenics; postoperative ventilation may be necessary.

13.5.3 Spinal cord injury

While patients with paraplegia or quadriplegia are at risk for a number of medical complications, the major concern during labor and delivery is autonomic hyperreflexia (AH). Autonomic hyperreflexia affects primarily those patients with spinal cord injuries at or above T_6, although it has been reported in patients with lower injuries. It results from reflex sympathetic discharge in response to a visceral stimulus in the absence of inhibition from higher supraspinal centers. This unopposed reflex sympathetic discharge provokes both a neural and humoral response, causing severe vasoconstriction. This vasoconstriction causes severe hypertension, leading to bradycardia, as carotid and aortic baroreceptor reflexes are activated (*Figure 13.6*). Consequences of AH can include intracranial

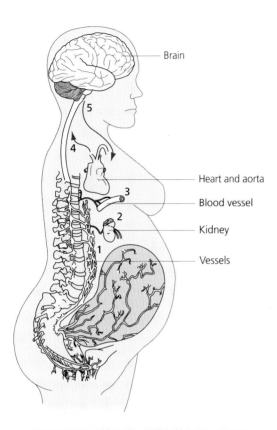

Brain

5

4

3 — Heart and aorta

— Blood vessel

2 — Kidney

1 — Vessels

Figure 13.6 Mechanism of cardiovascular response to labor in autonomic hyperreflexia. Sensory afferents enter the cord below the level of the spinal cord lesion (1), eliciting reflex sympathetic outflow to (2) the adrenal medulla (T_5-T_9) and (3) the peripheral vasculature (T_1–L_1). These two responses provoke severe hypertension. Carotid and aortic baroreceptors (4) respond to the hypertension with afferent outflow to the brainstem, which in turn stimulates parasympathetic efferents to the sinus node via the vagus nerve (5), resulting in bradycardia.

hemorrhage and cerebral edema in the patient, and can have deleterious fetal consequences as well (abruption, bradycardia, etc.). Labor appears to be a very strong stimulus for AH, and it has been reported in parturients during labor who have had no prior history of the problem. On occasion, presentation with AH signals the onset of labor. In some patients, it may not become clinically apparent until after delivery.

In anesthetic management of the spinal cord injured patient, particular attention should be paid to the level of injury – with a lesion above T_6, autonomic hyperreflexia during labor should be anticipated. Regional anesthesia can effectively block AH. In parturients with a history of AH, labor probably should be electively induced and prophylactic regional anesthesia undertaken to avoid the problem. Even in the absence of prior symptoms or episodes of AH, most perinatologists feel regional anesthesia for labor and delivery is indicated in these patients.

Epidural placement may be difficult in the spinal cord injured patient due to prior back surgery for stabilization, fusion, or instrumentation. In these patients, continuous spinal anesthesia should be considered a viable option (see Chapter 5). Following placement of the epidural catheter, the usual test dosing should be performed (there is no evidence epinephrine-containing test doses are deleterious). Unlike the majority of parturients, the density of anesthetic block is not an issue – a solid regional block is indicated (bupivacaine 0.25% or the equivalent should be used to institute the block, and an infusion of 0.125% bupivacaine or greater used for maintenance). Epidural or intrathecal opioids alone will not reliably block AH.

Blood pressure and heart rate should be closely monitored throughout labor and the postpartum period. Hypertension should be taken as evidence of inadequate regional block. If any difficulties exist in measuring blood pressure via cuff, an arterial line should be strongly considered for continuous monitoring. As some patients with high levels of spinal cord injury have compromised ventilatory status, care should be taken not to overzealously raise the level of block and further restrict ventilation.

Regional anesthesia also works well for cesarean delivery. Standard dosing guidelines (as used in nonspinal cord injured patients) should apply, although careful assessment of ventilatory status before and during the procedure is necessary. Should general anesthesia be desired or necessary for cesarean delivery, as with any patient, careful preoperative assessment of the airway is indicated. Succinylcholine can be used in most patients, as succinylcholine-induced hyperkalemia should not be a problem if the injury is over 12 months old. If there is any doubt regarding the safety of succinylcholine in a given patient, a nondepolarizing muscle relaxant can be used if preoperative evaluation indicates no difficulty expected at intubation. Almost any nondepolarizer can be used, as an increased induction (intubating) dose of the relaxant will speed onset, albeit at the expense of a markedly prolonged duration of action. The very short acting nondepolarizers, rocuronium or rapacuronium, are probably the best choices in this situation (Table 13.18).

Depth of anesthesia during the maintenance phase of the anesthetic should be somewhat deeper than usually practiced during cesarean delivery in order to prevent autonomic hyperreflexia effectively. This may result in transient neonatal depression after delivery; the neonatal resuscitation team should be warned of this possibility and be prepared to support the neonate if necessary. After surgery, careful surveillance for AH should be continued for 24 to 48 hours.

13.5.4 Other problems

Seizure disorder

A preexisting seizure disorder should have little impact on the anesthetic management of a parturient; anticonvulsant medications should be continued at the discretion of the obstetrician during pregnancy when possible. The major concern is the differential diagnosis of a new seizure disorder appearing during pregnancy; first among the etiologies to be excluded is eclampsia. Other possible causes of new onset seizures during pregnancy include intracranial hemorrhage, tumor, drug or alcohol abuse or withdrawal, and trauma. When there is any doubt, early consultation with a neurologist is indicated.

Few regional anesthetic techniques or anesthetic agents are contraindicated in the parturient with a seizure disorder. Regional anesthesia may be advantageous during labor, by decreasing maternal hyperventilation and subsequent hypocarbia (which can lower threshold in some patients). Enflurane, which at higher concentrations can decrease seizure threshold, should not be a problem at the lower concentrations commonly used during cesarean delivery. Ketamine, which can cause seizure-like EEG activity in patients with seizure disorders, should generally be avoided.

Intracranial lesions

For the most part, anesthetic management of the pregnant woman with an intracranial lesion will be dictated by the type and clinical course of the lesion. With corrected vascular lesions, there should be little impact on anesthetic management. Uncorrected vascular lesions may pose problems, however. Labor and delivery must be managed to minimize the chance of the lesion bleeding or rebleeding. Generally, this means eliminating the stress and catecholamine response to labor (and resulting increased blood pressure, which increases transmural wall stress on the lesion). Solid epidural anesthesia during labor can effectively limit this response and attenuate the 'bearing down' or 'pushing' urges during the second stage (associated Valsalva maneuvers transiently increase intracranial pressure and wall stress on the vascular lesion).

At cesarean delivery, induction and maintenance dose of agents need to be increased to eliminate any hypertensive response. Solid

---

Table 13.18 Nondepolarizing relaxants for 'rapid-sequence' induction (recommended for use only when succinylcholine is contraindicated)

Agent	Dose	Minimum time to reversal
Rocuronium	1.2 mg/kg	~ 40 min
Rapacuronium	2.5 mg/kg	~ 25 min

Note: (i) Reversal times are approximate due to limited clinical experience and individual variation. (ii) Close neonatal surveillance necessary due to potential for placental transfer.

regional (epidural) anesthesia is effective in this regard; should general anesthesia become necessary, particular attention must be paid to blunting the response to laryngoscopy and intubation, using higher than usual doses of induction agents. This may increase the risk of neonatal depression, but with prior notification of the neonatal resuscitation team should not cause problems for the neonate.

With mass lesions, the primary anesthetic concern is elevated intracranial pressure (ICP). If there is any evidence of elevated ICP, dural puncture should be carefully avoided, as there is a small risk of herniation. In the absence of elevated ICP or cerebrospinal fluid pressure, regional anesthesia can be performed routinely. If intracranial compliance is reduced, even epidural injection of local anesthetics can transiently increase intracranial pressure, so small, divided doses should be used.

With evidence of markedly increased ICP, delivery will likely be via cesarean section, under general anesthesia. In this setting, a neuroanesthesia-type induction should be performed, with a slower induction using larger doses of opioids, barbiturates, and a nondepolarizing relaxant while cricoid pressure is maintained (*Table 13.19*). The parturient should be denitrogenated (preoxygenated) prior to induction, and hyperventilated before intubation. Again, the goal of this technique is to eliminate any hypertensive response to laryngoscopy and intubation, which could cause a precipitous increase in ICP in a patient with altered intracranial compliance. Careful attention to neonatal resuscitation is necessary. Ergot alkaloid and prostaglandin oxytocics should probably be avoided in these patients due to their ability to increase maternal blood pressure.

Table 13.19 Anesthetic considerations for cesarean delivery with increased intracranial pressure

Induction	Avoid 'rapid-sequence' induction
	Maintain cricoid pressure until intubated
	Induction agents:
	  Fentanyl 5–10 µg/kg
	  Thiopental 4–5 mg/kg
	  Relaxant:

Maintenance	Fentanyl/isoflurane/relaxant as necessary Oxytocin post-delivery
Emergence	Avoid hypertension; consider nitroprusside infusion
Other considerations	Possible need for neonatal resuscitation Avoid ergot alkaloids and prostaglandins (ICP)

Further reading

Baum, V.C. and Perloff, J.K. (1993) Anesthetic implications of adults with congenital heart disease. *Anesth. Analg.* **76**:1342–1358.

Brighouse, D., Whitfield, A. and Holdcroft, A. (1998) Anaesthesia for Caesarean section in patients with aortic stenosis: the case for regional anaesthesia/ the case for general anaesthesia (editorial). *Anaesthesia* **53**:107–112.

Desai, D.K., Adanlawo, M., Naidoo, D.P. *et al.* (2000) Mitral stenosis in pregnancy: a four-year esperience at King Edward VIII Hospital, Durban, South Africa. *Br. J. Obstet. Gynaecol.* **107**:953–958.

Easterling, T.R., Chadwick, H.S., Otto, C.M. and Benedetti, T.J. (1988) Aortic stenosis in pregnancy. *Obstet. Gynecol.* **72**:113–117.

George, L.M., Gatt S.P. and Lowe, S. (1997) Peripartum cardiomyopathy: four case histories and a commentary on anaesthetic management. Anaesth. *Intensive Care* **25**:292–296.

Khan, M.J. Bhatt, S.B. and Krye, J.J. (1996) Anesthetic considerations for parturients with primary pulmonary hypertension: review of the literature and clinical presentations. *Int. J. Obstet. Anesth.* **5**:36–42.

Lipscomb, K.J., Clayton Smit, J., Clarke, B. *et al.* (1997) Outcome of pregnancy in women with Marfan's syndrome. *Br. J. obstet. Gynaecol.* **104**:210–206.

Paix, B., Cyan, A., belperio, P. and Simmons, S. (1999) Epidural analgesia for labour and delivery in a parturient with congenital hypertrophic obstructive cardiomyopathy. Anaesth. *Intensive Care* **27**:59–62.

Smedstadt, K.G., Cramb, R. and Morison, D.H. (1994) Pulmonary hypertension and pregnancy: a series of eight cases. *Can. J. Anaesth.* **41**:502–512.

Chapter 14

Nonanesthetic drugs and obstetric anesthesia

Michael Paech, FANZCA

Contents

14.1 **Magnesium**

14.1.1 Physiology and pharmacology

Magnesium is an important regulator of intracellular function (*Table 14.1*). It is the second most plentiful intracellular cation (after potassium) and an antagonist and regulator of calcium activity. The body contains approximately 1000 mmol, of which half is in bone and over 20% in muscle. Only 1% is in the extracellular fluid compartment, with 0.3% in plasma, 60% as free, unionized magnesium. The normal dietary requirement (chief sources are green vegetables, cereals, meat and water) of over 300 mg day^{-1} is increased during pregnancy and lactation. Renal excretion controls plasma levels (normal range 0.7–1.0 mmol/l or 1.4–2.2 mEq/l, magnesium being a divalent ion). Magnesium deficiency is common, and the role of magnesium in the genesis of preeclampsia (PE) remains uncertain.

14.1.2 Obstetric applications

Preeclampsia and eclampsia

Eclampsia complicates 1 in 2000 pregnancies in developed countries and up to 1 in 100 in some countries (see also Chapter 9). In the Confidential Enquiries into Maternal Death in the UK it contributes to 15% of maternal deaths and worldwide has been estimated to cause 50 000 deaths per year. Mortality ranges from 2% to

Table 14.1 Physiological roles of magnesium

Activation of over 300 enzyme systems, mainly involved in energy metabolism

An essential cofactor in oxidative phosphorylation and adenosine triphosphate physiology

Essential for the synthesis of DNA, RNA, protein, and bone

Involved in hormone receptor binding and gating of calcium channels; transmembrane ion flux; and regulation of adenylate cyclase

Involved in vasomotor tone; cardiac excitability, and neuromuscular function

Regulation of neuronal activity, including the NMDA receptor in central transmission of nociceptive stimuli

5% and the prevention and control of convulsions are basic principles of management.

Magnesium therapy has been used for over 70 years in the USA to control eclamptic convulsions, although only recently have controlled clinical trials established magnesium as the agent of choice for this purpose. Many regimens have been used to establish hypermagnesemia, a popular intravenous dosing schedule being a 4 g intravenous (IV) load followed by a continuous infusion of 1–3 g/h (1 g of magnesium sulfate is equivalent to 4 mmol of elemental magnesium). The target concentration for anticonvulsant effect is 5–8 mEq/l.

Magnesium crosses the blood–brain barrier poorly, so in contrast to conventional anticonvulsant drugs its efficacy is due to alternative mechanisms. Possibilities include calcium and N-methyl-D-aspartate (NMDA) antagonism (with protection against ischemic neuronal injury) or cerebral vasodilatation (with relief of the cerebral vasospasm associated with preeclampsia and eclampsia). The most compelling evidence for magnesium as an anticonvulsant was provided by the Collaborative Eclampsia Trial (a multicenter, multinational randomized trial) which found lower rates of recurrent seizure with magnesium therapy compared with diazepam or phenytoin. Although magnesium therapy is also used in severe preeclampsia, this role is less firmly established. Magnesium may also be used to halt an established convulsion, although most centers use diazepam as first-line treatment.

Tocolysis and other applications

In the US, magnesium has been used to treat premature labor since 1959. It inhibits myometrial contractility due to calcium antagonism. The efficacy is similar to the β-sympathomimetic drugs, but side effects (flushing, nausea, and chest pain) are infrequent and postpartum hemorrhage is not significantly increased (see also Section 12.2.6).

Magnesium is safe for the fetus, although fetal heart rate variability may be reduced, making interpretation more difficult. In the

Collaborative Eclampsia Trial, Apgar scores were better than in other groups and fewer babies needed intensive care. There is an association between maternal magnesium exposure and a lower rate of cerebral palsy and increased survival among low birthweight infants, although prospective evidence is being sought to confirm its possible benefits.

Magnesium toxicity

A young woman who experienced complete paralysis after ingestion of magnesium salts in 1891 is the first recorded case of magnesium poisoning. The most important factor in the development of toxicity is impaired renal function, and caution is required should renal excretion be compromised (see also *Table 12.3*). The neuromuscular effects of magnesium may unmask respiratory muscle pathology, but in the normal patient weakness only becomes apparent as plasma levels rise above 10 mEq/l, with depression of tendon reflexes. Respiratory volumes, especially forced expiratory volumes, fall with therapeutic levels, but arterial carbon dioxide tension does not rise. Respiratory impairment may be seen at 14 mEq/l, reflecting muscle weakness rather than central depression. Magnesium competes with calcium at prejunctional sites (especially the P-channel) within skeletal muscle endplates, where it inhibits release of acetylcholine, with a less important action on the postjunctional membrane. Monitoring of patellar reflexes and respiratory rate may be used as an alternative to estimations of serum concentration.

Vasodilatation is produced by direct and indirect actions, and vascular tone may be reduced due to sympathetic block and inhibition of catecholamine release. This is relevant when postpartum hemorrhage occurs during magnesium therapy. However, reduced myocardial contractility is not significant, and although cardiac arrest has been reported (at levels approaching 25 mEq l^{-1}), during controlled ventilation magnesium levels above 15 mEq/l are tolerated. There are also modest effects on platelet adhesiveness and a small effect on the thromboelastograph, but no clinical consequences, such as increased blood loss.

14.1.3 Implications for obstetric anesthesia

Neuromuscular effects

The pre- and postjunctional effects of magnesium at the neuromuscular end plate potentiate the action of nondepolarizing muscle relaxants used during anesthesia. Reduced doses are required (the ED$_{50}$ is reduced by at least 25%) and duration may be doubled, so monitoring of neuromuscular blockade with a peripheral nerve stimulator is necessary. The technique of precurarization or 'priming' to hasten onset of neuromuscular block is not recommended, because an exaggerated effect is likely. Neuromuscular block may recur up to an hour after reversal of muscle paralysis and in an emergency, calcium administration can be used to antagonize the effects of magnesium.

The action of succinylcholine in the presence of hypermagnesemia is less clear. Prolongation has been shown experimentally, but in clinical practice the effects are inconsistent. Fasciculations are usually not seen, so when using succinylcholine for intubation, the effect should be followed with a peripheral nerve stimulator.

Regional anesthesia

Regional anesthesia can be safely used during magnesium therapy; it has no significant adverse maternal or fetal effects. In animal models, greater falls in blood pressure are seen when regional anesthesia is used in the presence of hypermagnesemia, possibly due to the sympatholytic effect of magnesium. However, while magnesium attenuates the increase in uterine vascular resistance seen with α-adrenergic agonists, ephedrine remains the vasopressor of choice.

Control of blood pressure

The vasodilator activity of magnesium contributes to control of hypertension in PE.

Likewise, magnesium aids in the control of hypertension induced by catecholamine release and sympathetic stimulation, such as at direct laryngoscopy and intubation (see Table 7.23) or during surgery of pheochromocytoma in pregnancy. An IV bolus of 40–60 mg/kg (depending on the current serum magnesium level) immediately following induction of general anesthesia in parturients with severe PE is more effective than alfentanil or lidocaine and does not produce respiratory depression, although a combination of opioid and magnesium may be optimal.

The sympatholytic action of magnesium and potential inhibition of compensatory cerebral blood flow increase should be remembered when obstetric hemorrhage occurs. Close attention must be paid to restoring adequate intravascular volume with IV fluids.

14.2 Vasopressors

14.2.1 Principles of vasopressor use in obstetrics

Uterine blood flow at term is about 700 ml/min and is proportional to the perfusion pressure (uterine arterial minus uterine venous pressure) and inversely proportional to the uterine vascular resistance. The effects of vasopressors on both these factors, secondary to cardiac and peripheral vasoconstrictor activity (see *Table 14.2*), must be balanced. The tool of Doppler recording of uteroplacental and fetoplacental flow velocity waveforms, to estimate a 'pulsatility index', provides a semiquantitative measure of vascular resistance; this can be used to assess the effects of hypotension and vasopressors. In addition, outcomes such as fetal and neonatal cord acid–base analysis and clinical parameters are used.

Hypotension usually results in a rise in the pulsatility index that is not necessarily corrected by restoration of BP with vasopressor, highlighting the importance of the early treatment of hypotension during pregnancy. Good fetal and neonatal outcome is dependent on prompt correction of sustained or profound hypotension (*Figure 14.1*), regardless of the cause.

Treatment of hypotension with a single bolus of a predominantly α-adrenergic vasopressor such as methoxamine or phenylephrine does not improve flow waveform indices, whereas treatment with ephedrine or metaraminol does so. Early administration, either as prophylaxis or in response to BP fall (see Section 7.4.5), is now common practice. This strategy is supported by the low efficacy of IV fluid loading before regional anesthesia for cesarean section (CS) and a lower incidence of severe hypotension and better neonatal acid–base status after prophylactic vasopressor (*Figure 14.2*). The choice of vasopressor is far less important for fetal health than is avoiding hypotension, and consequently in recent years there has been renewed anesthetic interest in vasopressors other than ephedrine.

Table 14.2 Relative α- and β-adrenergic effects of vasopressors		
Drug	**α$_1$ (vasoconstriction)**	**β$_1$ (cardiac inotropic and chronotropic)**
Ephedrine	+	+
Phenylephrine	++	−
Metaraminol	+++	−
Methoxamine	++	−
Dopamine <3 µg/kg/min	−	+
Dopamine >5 µg/kg/min	++	+++
Dobutamine	+	+++
Norepinephrine	+++	+
Epinephrine	+++	+++

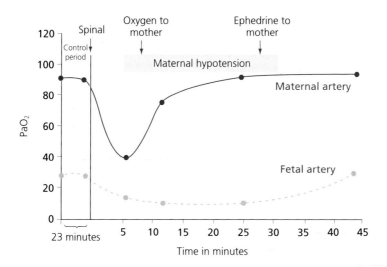

Figure 14.1 Changes in arterial oxygen tension in the fetus after spinal anesthesia-induced hypotension, hypoxia, oxygen and ephedrine administration to the mother. Reproduced with permission of Harcourt Health Sciences, Orlando from Shnider, S.M. *et al.* (1968) Vasopressors in obstetrics. I. Correction of fetal acidosis with ephedrine during spinal hypotension. *Am. J. Obstet. Gynecol.* **102**: 917.

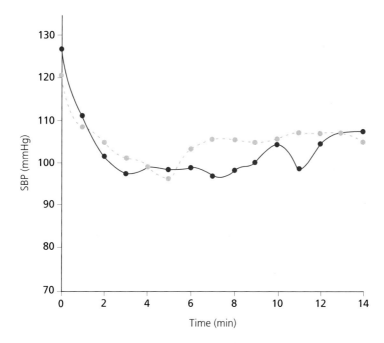

Figure 14.2 Mean systolic blood pressures for ephedrine infusion (0.25 mg/kg over 3 min) (○) versus crystalloid preload 20 ml/kg (●) during the first 14 minutes after spinal anesthesia. Reproduced with permission of Blackwell Science from Chan, W.S. *et al.* (1997) Prevention of hypotension during spinal anaesthesia for caesarean section: ephedrine infusion versus fluid preload. *Anaesthesia* **52**: 911.

14.2.2 Pharmacology

Ephedrine

Ephedrine, an active component of the Chinese plant Ma Huang, was introduced to Western culture in the 1920s and was the first vasopressor used to treat hypotension after spinal anesthesia. It has both direct and indirect actions at adrenergic nerve endings, some inhibition of monoamine oxidase, but mainly β-sympathomimetic effects. This results in an increase in heart rate and cardiac output, with little change in peripheral resistance, and an increase in systolic BP in particular. Other effects include cerebral stimulation and bronchodilation, and decreases in both cerebral and renal blood flow. Increased myocardial irritability may rarely manifest as an arrhythmia (e.g. ventricular tachycardia). Usual IV doses are 3–10 mg (duration 10 minutes) and IM or subcutaneous doses 15–50 mg, but tachyphylaxis is a prominent feature.

Ephedrine has long been considered the vasopressor of choice in obstetric anesthesia. A landmark animal study in 1974 compared large equipotent doses of several vasopressors, and found that ephedrine maintained uterine blood flow better than metaraminol and methoxamine. Ephedrine appears to have a more select vasoconstrictor action on systemic vessels, sparing the uterine artery compared with metaraminol. However, in some circumstances, the inotropic and chronotropic activity of ephedrine is best avoided (see Section 13.2). Caution is required when used with ergot derivative oxytocics to avoid hypertension, and transplacental transfer may increase fetal heart rate and beat-to-beat variability. Also, as the dose of ephedrine administered increases, the beneficial effect on arterial BP is negated possibly by an increase in uterine vascular resistance or direct fetal effects, leading to fetal acidemia (*Figure 14.3*). Thus, despite its advantage of minimal vasoconstrictor activity,

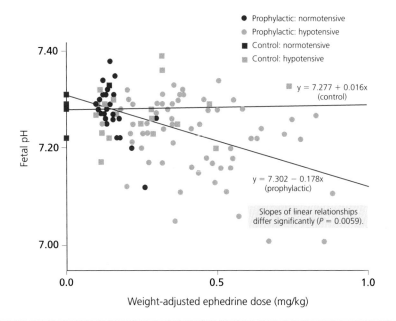

Figure 14.3 Relationship between maternal ephedrine dosage and umbilical artery blood pH. Reproduced with permission of Wiley-Liss Inc., a subsidiary of John Wiley & Sons Inc. from Shearer, V.E. *et al.* (1996) Fetal effects of prophylactic ephedrine and maternal hypotension during regional anesthesia for cesarean section. *J. Mat. Fet. Med.* **5**: 82.

most studies using effective clinical doses have found lower fetal pH when ephedrine is used prophylactically or therapeutically. The advantages of ephedrine are thus being questioned.

Metaraminol, phenylephrine and methoxamine

Metaraminol has direct and indirect α- and β-adrenergic effects and few other side effects. After IV injection it has rapid onset over 1–3 minutes and duration of up to 25 minutes, this being doubled by IM administration. Titrated infusion can also be used. In a pregnant sheep model, large doses are likely to raise BP but significantly reduce uterine blood flow, and consequently there are few data on its obstetric use. However, recent investigation suggests that metaraminol may be both safe and useful. Phenylephrine is principally a direct α₁-agonist with no effect on myocardial contractility. Vasoconstriction increases BP and may cause a reflex bradycardia. Appropriate IV doses are 50–100 µg, with larger doses likely to produce severe hypertension, despite reduced vascular responsiveness during pregnancy. The duration of action is very short (2–5 min), so titrated infusion is again suitable. Like metaraminol, phenylephrine is useful clinically, especially where tachycardia is present or best avoided, or where tachyphylaxis to ephedrine has occurred.

Methoxamine has not been used in obstetric anesthesia. It has direct α₁-activity and weak β-blockade, leading to vasoconstriction, increased systolic and diastolic BP and cardiac output, and reflex bradycardia. Despite restoration of BP, uterine blood flow may fall significantly; uterine hypertonia may result from myometrial stimulation and interaction with oxytocics can lead to severe hypertension.

Norepinephrine, dopamine, dobutamine and epinephrine

Norepinephrine (noradrenaline) has predominantly α-agonist activity and little role in obstetrics except in the intensive care unit. Dopamine has dose-dependent actions, but despite prominent α-agonist activity only at high rates (above 20 µg/kg/min), it may also reduce uterine flow; it produces adverse fetal acid-base changes compared to ephedrine and is generally avoided. Dopamine's dopaminergic receptor mediated splanchnic and coronary vasodilator action and renal effects are occasionally exploited in low urine output states in preeclampsia and in intensive care, although there is no evidence to support improved outcome. Dobutamine is a racemic mixture with mixed effects due to varying receptor activity of the two enantiomers. It has relatively greater inotropic than chronotropic cardiac effect and produces little change in peripheral vascular tone.

Epinephrine (adrenaline) is the predominant endogenous catecholamine and has potent α- and β-agonist effects. These are dose dependent, and 0.1 µg/kg IV or absorbed drug after epidural doses of 50–100 µg may produce some β-mediated vasodilatation. During regional anesthesia, local anesthetic combined with epinephrine is likely to produce greater falls in mean arterial BP and peripheral resistance and a greater increase in cardiac output. However, α-agonist properties usually predominate, and because effects are very short-lived, infusion is the most appropriate method of administration, except in acute resuscitation. Obstetric use is confined to its usual indications: resuscitation (1 mg boluses repeated as required), unresolved severe bronchospasm or severe anaphylaxis (100 µg boluses with or without continuous infusion), and inotropic support in intensive care.

Others

Ornithine-8-vasopressin (POR-8) is a synthetic derivative of vasopressin with enhanced vasoconstrictor and diminished antidiuretic activity. It is sometimes used as an alternative to epinephrine as a local vasoconstrictor. Side effects include skin pallor, nausea, increased gut motility, hypertension and reflex bradycardia, with the potential for myocardial ischemia, myometrial ischemia and pulmonary edema after overdose or accidental intravenous injection. The maximum recommended dose is 5 IU at a concentration of 1 IU/ml.

Angiotensin II causes less vasoconstriction in uterine vessels than other systemic vessels in animal models and increases blood pressure without increasing heart rate. Umbilical acid–base status is superior to that after ephedrine when given prophylactically during regional anesthesia for CS. Despite these desirable effects, it has an ultra-short half-life (15 s) and high potency. This makes clinical use difficult and it is not currently commercially available.

14.2.3 Management strategies for control of blood pressure

Prophylaxis

Despite inconsistent results, in situations where hypotension is very common, especially regional anesthesia for elective CS, prophylactic vasopressor administration is popular. Better BP stability can be achieved with ephedrine prophylaxis (from the time of spinal anesthesia) than with mere treatment of hypotension. Intramuscular ephedrine (at least 30 mg) is effective, but occasionally causes hypertension, so IV dosing is preferable. The optimum dose and regimen of ephedrine depends, in part, on the anesthetic technique, and as little as 5 mg significantly lowers the incidence of hypotension after a sequential combined spinal-epidural anesthetic using low dose subarachnoid bupivacaine and fentanyl. In contrast, after spinal anesthesia using bupivacaine 10 mg, the optimum single IV bolus may be as much as 30 mg. However, such large boluses of ephedrine will cause significant tachycardia and hypertension in some parturients, and a 10 mg bolus followed by titrated infusion at 5 mg/min, reducing to about 1 mg/min, is a more rational approach. The alternative of a 20 mg bolus, then 10 mg repeated as required, is more likely to be associated with maternal nausea (from decreased cerebral perfusion) unless BP is monitored continuously. The argument against prophylaxis is that ephedrine use is often high (above 30 mg), the incidence of hypotension remains unsatisfactory, and the proportion of umbilical artery pH values less than 7.2 increases.

Treatment

Maternal syncope, significant fetal heart-rate change (associated with decreased BP), or BP reduction by 30% or to less than 90 mmHg, are uncommon after regional analgesia during labor (approximately 5%). With combined spinal-epidural analgesia in labor, the frequency of hypotensive episodes is similar to that after epidural analgesia, but the onset is more rapid. During labor, there is no evidence that routine IV fluid loading is of benefit in preventing hemodynamic change, so early vasopressor administration is appropriate. Hemodynamic disturbance is usually transient and repeated boluses or infusions are rarely necessary.

In contrast, hypotension after anesthesia for CS is very common (50–90%), and several drugs effectively restore BP and are safe for the healthy fetus. As noted above, ephedrine has long been and remains the standard for treatment and prophylaxis of hypotension, but is under challenge.

When used in uncomplicated CS, boluses of phenylephrine 100 µg IV to maintain systolic BP >100 mmHg have no adverse effects on fetal acid–base status or outcome, and fetal hypoxia is less common than after ephedrine 5 mg. A phenylephrine infusion (*Figure 14.4*), up to a dose rate of 50–100 µg/min to avoid α-adrenergic effects on the uteroplacental circulation, is another option. Maternal heart rate after phenylephrine is lower than after ephedrine. Metaraminol is also currently undergoing re-evaluation in obstetric anesthesia and appears promising. A bolus of 0.5 mg and infusion at 0.25 mg/min effectively restores BP, and despite a higher uterine artery pulsatility index (reflecting higher vascular resistance), fetal acid–base status remains better preserved than when an ephedrine regimen of similar efficacy is used. Nevertheless, until more data are available and larger studies have been performed, these drugs are arguably best reserved for second-line treatment or special circumstances, and ephedrine 5–10 mg IV should continue to be the routine vasopressor for treatment of hypotension in healthy parturients.

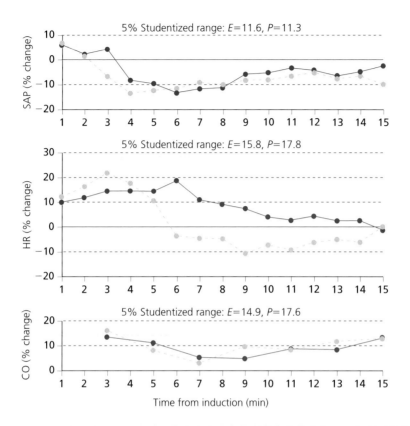

Figure 14.4 Mean percentage changes in systolic arterial pressure (SAP), heart rate (HR) and cardiac output (CO) from baseline values after induction of spinal anesthesia in the ephedrine bolus (●) and phenylephrine bolus (○) groups. Reproduced with permission of Oxford University Press from Thomas, D.G. *et al.* (1996) Randomized trial of bolus phenylephrine or ephedrine for maintenance of arterial pressure during spinal anaesthesia for caesarean section. *Br. J. Anaesth.* **76**: 63.

Further reading

Anonymous (1995) Which anticonvulsant for women with eclampsia? Evidence from the Collaborative Eclampsia Trial. *Lancet* **345**: 1455–1463.

Fawcett, W.J., Haxby, E.J. and Male, D.A. (1999) Magnesium: physiology and pharmacology. *Br. J. Anaesth.* **83**: 302–320.

Gajraj, N.M., Victory, R.A., Pace, N.A. *et al.* (1993) Comparison of an ephedrine infusion with crystalloid administration for prevention of hypotension during spinal anesthesia. *Anesth. Analg.* **76**: 1023–1026.

Higgins, J.R. and Brennecke, S.P. (1998) Preeclampsia and eclampsia: magnesium salts for all? *Med. J. Aus.* **168**: 151–152.

James, M.F.M. (1992) Clinical use of magnesium infusions in anesthesia. *Anesth. Analg.* **74**: 129–136.

James, M.F.M. (1998) Magnesium in obstetric anesthesia. *Int. J. Obstet. Anesth.* **7**: 115–123.

Morgan, P. (1994) The role of vasopressors in the management of hypotension induced by spinal and epidural anaesthesia. *Can. J. Anaesth.* **41**: 404–413.

Ralston, D.H., Shnider, S.M. and deLorimier, A.A. (1974) Effects of equipotent ephedrine, metaraminol, mephenteramine, and methoxamine on uterine blood flow in the pregnant ewe. *Anesthesiology* **40**: 354–370.

Rocke, D.A. and Rout, C.C. (1995) Volume preloading, spinal hypotension and Caesarean section. *Br. J. Anaesth.* **75**: 257–259.

Shnider, S.M. (1983) Vasopressors in obstetrics. *Reg. Anesth.* **8**: 74–80.

Chapter 15

Complications of obstetric anesthesia and analgesia

Michael Paech, FANZCA

Contents

15.1 Post-dural puncture headache

15.1.1 Incidence of post-dural puncture headache (PDPH)

Post-dural puncture headache (PDPH) may follow either deliberate breach of the dura (spinal or continuous spinal anesthesia or analgesia) or accidental dural puncture during epidural insertion. From a practical perspective, the latter is one of the most common and significant complications of an epidural technique. Post-dural puncture headache may develop acutely from pneumoencephalus if air has been injected during the loss-of-resistance technique, but usually presents 12–36 hours later. In contrast to PDPH after spinal needle puncture, onset after 48 hours is uncommon with PDPH due to an epidural needle, and the natural history of this headache and its associated symptoms differs. In general, headache severity is greater and its duration prolonged. The impact of PDPH on healthcare cost is substantial, due to the need for treatment intervention, increased length of hospital stay and, occasionally, patient complaint and litigation.

The reported incidence of accidental dural puncture during epidural insertion varies with several factors (*Table 15.1*). Unless patient follow-up is regular for several days, PDPH may be missed. In large teaching units the range of incidence of PDPH is 0.19–3.6%, usually about 0.5–1.0% (1 in 100–200 epidural attempts). The risk of accidental dural puncture correlates with experience. More punctures occur overnight, although the relative contribution of staff experience or operator fatigue is unknown. There is strong epidemiological evidence that loss-of-resistance technique with saline leads to lower rates of accidental puncture than with air. A saline-filled syringe permits continuous pressure on the plunger of the syringe as the needle advances, enhancing tactile feel to ensure minimal forward movement as the ligamentum flavum is penetrated. Injected fluid may push away the dura, which may lie in apposition to the ligament. A large personal series by a single anesthesiologist skilled with both mediums found no difference in rate between saline and air, but a lower incidence of subsequent PDPH with saline. Advocates of the needle-through-needle combined spinal-epidural technique claim this approach also lowers risk, because in cases of doubt, the spinal needle confirms the correct location. If accidental dural puncture occurs with a 16–18 gauge epidural needle, 80% of parturients develop PDPH. In two-thirds of these, headache is severe and the majority will seek intervention to relieve symptoms.

Several factors influence the rate of PDPH after spinal needle insertion, but in the obstetric population the principal determinants are the size of the dural hole and the type of needle used (*Tables 15.2* and *15.3*). Sharp-bevel 22 gauge Quincke spinal needles produce a high incidence (at least 10%) and this is greatly reduced with smaller gauge pencil-point or conical-tip needles (24–29 gauge Sprotte or Whitacre-style, see *Figure 15.1*). It appears the 'tin-lid' flap made by a cutting-edge needle is

Table 15.1 Risk factors for accidental dural puncture with an epidural needle

Experience
- Increased risk during initial learning phase

Training, especially loss-of-resistance technique
- Lower risk with saline than air

Fatigue or haste?
- Higher incidence overnight

Accuracy of audit
- Cases missed unless daily follow-up continues for several days

Table 15.2 Risk factors for post-dural puncture headache (PDPH)

Younger age

Larger needle gauge

Cutting-edge Quincke-style spinal needle

Cephalad or caudal orientation of Quincke needles

History of PDPH or migraine

Table 15.3 Influence of needle on incidence of post-dural puncture headache (PDPH)

Type of needle	Incidence of PDPH
16 gauge epidural	80%
17 or 18 gauge epidural	up to 80%
22 gauge Quincke	30–50%
25 gauge Quincke	8–10%
24 gauge Sprotte	3–5%
26 gauge Atraucan	5%
24 gauge Gertie Marx	4%
25 gauge modified Whitacre	2–3%
27 gauge modified Whitacre	0.5–1%

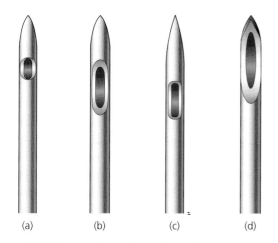

(a) (b) (c) (d)

Figure 15.1 Spinal needle tip design for (a) Gertie Marx, (b) Sprotte, (c) Whitacre, (d) Atraucan needle. These needles result in a lower incidence of postdural puncture headache than sharp-bevel (Quincke) needles of equivalent size. Reproduced from Holdcroft, A. and Thomas, T.A. (2000) Regional anaesthetic techniques. In: *Principles and Practice of Obstetric Anaesthesia and Analgesia,* p. 248. With permission from Blackwell Science Ltd, Oxford.

less likely to close, allowing persistent CSF leak, although an alternative explanation is that disruption of dural fibers is greater with pencil-point needles and the resultant intense inflammatory response aids earlier closure.

15.1.2 Etiology and differential diagnosis

Spinal headache is a consequence of low CSF pressure, secondary to acute leak of as little as 20 ml of CSF. When headache commences, pressures are about half normal. Symptoms result probably because intracranial hypotension produces traction on sensitive meningeal and vascular structures. Magnetic resonance imaging supports changes in the meningeal tissue during PDPH. It is very likely cerebral vasodilatation also contributes to headache, because migraine sufferers appear more prone, a throbbing quality is common, Doppler studies show higher flow velocities, and drugs with cerebral vasoconstrictor activity (such as the 5-hydroxytryptamine agonist, sumatriptan) reduce its severity.

There are several important reasons why PDPH needs to be diagnosed correctly. First, headache in the early postpartum period has multiple etiologies (*Table 15.4*) and is very common (up to 40% incidence), irrespective of whether or not regional analgesia was used. Second, up to 30% of accidental dural punctures are unrecognized and after dural injury, the breach of the closely apposed arachnoid membrane by the epidural catheter may occasionally be a late event. Finally, untreated PDPH may lead to chronic headache, permanent impairment or, exceptionally rarely, fatal 'coning' and brainstem death. Convulsions in association with PDPH may be due to areas of cerebral vasospasm, but other conditions (eclampsia, pneumocephalus, meningitis, hypertensive encephalopathy, subdural hematoma, other causes of raised intracranial pressure, caffeine toxicity or water intoxication, drug and alcohol withdrawal) should be excluded. The etiology of isolated seizures is sometimes never determined despite extensive investigation.

15.1.3 Features of PDPH

The signs and symptoms of PDPH may be immediate, especially if air is injected in the sitting position, but are typically of delayed onset (>50% within 24 hours and <10% more than 48 hours after dural puncture). These

Table 15.4 Causes of postpartum headache

Occurrence	Causes
Common	Tension headache
	Migraine or sinus headache
	Caffeine-withdrawal
	Pneumoencephalus after accidental air injection
	Low CSF pressure post-dural puncture headache
	Drug induced
Rare and serious	Impending eclampsia
	Cortical vein thrombosis (<1 in 5000; associated sweating, nausea and pyrexia)
	Subdural hematoma (post-trauma or PDPH)
	Subarachnoid hemorrhage
	Meningitis
	Pre-existing space-occupying lesions

Table 15.5 Characteristics of post-dural puncture headache (PDPH)

Postural
- Relieved with recumbency

Variable character
- Often throbbing

Variable distribution
- Over 50% nuchal and occipital

Relieved by abdominal compression
- Positive sitting epigastric pressure test (raised intra-abdominal pressure transmitted to cerebral venous pressure transiently relieves headache)

Other
- Auditory or visual symptoms (tinnitus, uni- or bilateral loss of low-frequency hearing, vertigo, photophobia, nausea) <1% incidence
- Cranial nerve palsy (especially diplopia – sixth nerve) <1 in 5000 (0.02%) incidence
- Epidural fluid collection visible with imaging (magnetic resonance imaging to exclude other pathology)

typically present when the parturient is erect or ambulatory. The magnitude of CSF leak is greater from a hole made by an epidural needle than a spinal needle and consequently the onset of PDPH after spinal techniques is often delayed until two or more days later. Although up to 75% of headaches following spinal techniques resolve spontaneously within a week, this is much less likely after epidural needle puncture and, if untreated, up to 10% will become chronic.

Postdural puncture headache has several diagnostic characteristics, the most characteristic being a strong postural element (*Table 15.5*). Traction on intracranial structures is referred via the trigeminal nerve (frontal) or the vagal, glossopharyngeal and upper cervical nerves (to the neck and occiput). Associated symptoms include nausea, dizziness, visual disturbance and rarely cranial nerve palsies. Severe PDPH can be extremely debilitating, preventing normal mother–infant interaction, including the establishment of breastfeeding.

15.1.4 Prevention of PDPH

Although most obstetric anesthesiologists recognize the importance of using noncutting bevel fine-gauge spinal needles, many medical practitioners continue to use inappropriate needles for anesthesia, diagnostic lumbar puncture, and radiological procedures during pregnancy. Nevertheless, PDPH cannot be completely eliminated with current spinal needles and accidental dural puncture with an epidural needle remains a low incidence complication of epidural insertion. Many strategies have been implemented to reduce the likelihood of PDPH (*Table 15.6*). Most are of modest benefit and often impractical. Forced bed rest for 24–48 hours has no effect, except to delay the presentation of headache, although recumbency is sensible advice in the presence of established PDPH. Forced oral or intravenous hydration serves only to worsen symptoms by increasing the need to mobilize to urinate. Abdominal binders are ineffective and epidural Dextran or saline injection has short-lived benefit. Epidural saline bolusing (40–60 ml) is time-consuming and infusion (20 ml/h) restricts activity, as well as being beset by practical problems such as difficulty maintaining flow and back pain. Epidural and spinal opioids, and possible adverse effects of hyperbaric local anesthetics have not been studied systematically. Opioids are probably of no prophylactic value, but provide some symptomatic relief.

There may be a reduction in the severity of PDPH associated with deliberate insertion of a catheter into the subarachnoid space, although the influence of the duration of catheterization is uncertain. Many units now opt for this approach, rather than epidural re-insertion at another interspace, because this provides the clinical advantages of continuous spinal analgesia in labor and subarachnoid anesthesia for surgery. Prophylactic epidural blood patching has been claimed to reduce PDPH by 50–75%, although clinical experience varies widely and this is only feasible if an epidural catheter has been placed following the dural puncture.

15.1.5 Treatment of PDPH

Based on its etiology, treatment aims should be to increase CSF production and epidural space pressure, reduce cerebral vasodilatation and pain, and seal the hole in the dura. In practice, based on consultation with the patient and the severity and anticipated time-course of headache, either an expectant approach awaiting resolution of the headache, or intervention in the form of an epidural blood patch, is adopted (*Table 15.7*).

Psychological support, frank discussion and regular review are mandatory, as the parturient's preference is likely to depend on her ability to cope with the headache. Bed rest and oral analgesia are recommended. Cerebral vasoconstrictors (theophylline 300 mg orally, sumatriptan, 6 mg subcutaneously or 100 mg orally, caffeine up to several hundred mg/day) may reduce mild PDPH, but are ineffective against severe PDPH. Oral or intravenous caffeine (including in beverages) is popular in the USA, but the central stimulatory effects (insomnia, palpitation and tremor) are often

Table 15.6 Evidence[a] supporting strategies to minimize the risk or severity of post-dural puncture headache (PDPH)

Strategy	
Level 1	Puncture dura with small (25 gauge or less) pencil-point style spinal needles
Level 2	Prophylactic epidural blood patch
Level 3	Avoid accidental dural puncture • training and experience • loss-of-resistance to saline Prophylactic epidural saline ± opioid injection Subarachnoid catheterization for spinal analgesia

[a]Level 1 evidence, systematic review or meta-analysis; Level 2, one or more randomized trials; Level 3, cohort data, prospective series, epidemiological data; Level 4, expert or consensus opinion

Table 15.7 Treatment of post-dural puncture headache (PDPH)

Bed rest (horizontal position)

Intravenous hydration
• ineffective

Abdominal compression/binders
• impractical/ineffective

Oral, parenteral, and epidural analgesics
• acetaminophen, nonsteroidal anti-inflammatories, codeine, opioids

Cerebral vasoconstrictors
• oral and intravenous caffeine, theophylline, sumatriptan

Adrenocorticotrophic hormone
• unproven

Epidural 'patching'
• blood
• saline
• Dextran
• Gelfoam
• fibrin glue

disruptive. Synthetic adrenocorticotrophic hormone has been suggested but not scientifically investigated.

Treatment with an epidural blood patch (EBP) is the 'gold standard', although its efficacy has been overestimated. Blood patching requires re-identification of the epidural space (risking repeat dural puncture) and injection of sterile autologous blood obtained by venipuncture. The blood clot distributes over several segments, increases epidural pressure and redistributes lumbar CSF cranially, leading to rapid relief of symptoms. The gelatinous clot then 'plugs' the dural hole to tamponade CSF leak before gradual reabsorption over many hours (*Figure 15.2*). The success rate of EBP partly depends on its timing and possibly on the volume injected (originally 2 ml, but currently 15–25 ml is recommended).

Epidural blood patch will cure 80–90% of PDPH after spinal techniques, and initially resolve a similar proportion following accidental dural puncture with an epidural needle. In the latter situation, permanent cure is more likely if blood patch is delayed at least 48 hours. When EBP is provided on demand, the recurrent headache rate (usually at 12–36 hours) is approximately 30%. A repeat blood patch may be required.

The invasive nature of EBP mandates informed consent. There is concern about introducing infected blood if bacteremia is present, so the patient should be afebrile and otherwise well (routine blood culture is not cost-effective). Patient comfort is enhanced if the lateral position is used and ideally an assistant performs venipuncture, using full aseptic technique. The success of EBP is optimized if recumbency is enforced for at least 2 hours after the procedure. The patient should be warned about back stiffness (from blood tracking back through the interspinous ligaments to the subcutaneous area), but serious complications (bradycardia, localized or radicular back pain, epidural abscess or meningitis, subdural hematoma, cranial nerve palsy, convulsion) are rare. Epidural blood patch should be recommended if complications of PDPH arise or if PDPH persists beyond a week.

Alternatives to blood for epidural injection are albumin, gelatin, Dextran 40 and fibrin glue. Only the latter two substances have been subject to more than anecdotal evaluation and preliminary histopathological evaluation in animals found no changes. The mass effect of colloid may be greater than that of saline due to slower reabsorption, and Dextran has been advocated when the safety of blood is in doubt (e.g. possible bacteremia) or blood is unacceptable (the Jehovah's Witness).

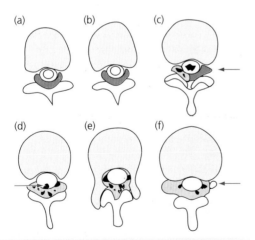

Figure 15.2 Each figure shows the distribution derived from both axial T_1 and sagittal STIR images. Images range from T_{10} (a) to L_3 (f) intervertebral level. Reproduced with permission of Oxford University Press, from Beards, S.C. *et al.* (1993) Magnetic resonance imaging of extradural blood patches: appearances from 30 min to 18 h. *Br. J. Anaesth.* **71**: 183.

15.2 Back pain

15.2.1 Back pain during pregnancy and postpartum

Backache is one of the most common symptoms experienced in adult life and tends to be more severe during pregnancy. Seventy-five percent of pregnant women describe back pain, this being new for 60%. A third find it interferes with normal activities and 10% are incapable of working. Musculoskeletal pain arises because of the exaggerated lumbar lordosis adopted to counterbalance the growing uterus and the increased mobility of sacroiliac, sacrococcygeal and pubic joints due to ligamentous relaxation under the influence of relaxin. Neural pain, such as sciatica, may arise from compression of the lumbosacral plexus by the fetal head. At times the diagnosis is apparent, but frequently the etiology of pain is uncertain and treatment difficult.

Excluding those with a past history of backache, 50% of parturients experience back pain on the first day after delivery and in 25% it persists beyond the first week. Mild postpartum backache may arise or be exacerbated by abnormal posture and strain during delivery, breastfeeding, and child-care, but if symptoms are severe more serious pathology such as disc prolapse, acute sacroiliitis or osteomyelitis, and incidental pathology (spinal tumor, septic pelvic thrombophlebitis or aortic dissection) must be excluded. Symptoms are usually lumbar or sacroiliac in distribution, but fortunately do not normally interfere with activity, prove amenable to physiotherapy and other physical therapies, and resolve with time. Risk factors for postpartum back pain are younger age and higher body mass index, but the major factor for pregnancy and postpartum backache is pre-existing back pain.

15.2.2 Back pain due to regional analgesia and anesthesia

At least a third of parturients suffer localized tenderness from soft tissue trauma after insertion of a 16 gauge epidural needle, irrespective of the insertion technique (paramedian versus midline). A lower incidence with spinal techniques suggests that needle size is relevant, although the relation to epidural needle size has not been systematically evaluated. The number of passes of a spinal needle correlates with the incidence of subsequent pain, despite MRI scans after delivery failing to find any association between soft tissue changes and the mode of analgesia, delivery, or the severity of backache. A persistent discrete tender spot at the insertion site is seen in about 1 in 2000 cases and may be due to neuroma formation.

Obstetric staff should be able to recognize and initiate investigation of the complications of regional anesthesia that present with back pain (*Table 15.8*). When the local anesthetic 2-chloroprocaine was formulated with the calcium chelator EDTA, severe back pain lasting up to 36 hours was reported, possibly due to muscle spasm from local hypocalcemia. Direct injury to a nerve root or the spinal cord is usually accompanied by severe transient local or radicular pain and paresthesia, and subsequently presents as a neurological deficit.

Epidural abscess and hematoma are the most serious complications that cause back pain (see Sections 15.3 and 15.4). A high index of suspicion is of vital importance, so that early diagnostic tests and management are instituted. Epidural abscess is often associated with skin-site infection, or subcutaneous cellulitis or abscess formation. Exquisite local tenderness is common with epidural abscess, but it may present as deep pain with or without fever and neurological symptoms. Early microbiological testing and imaging, and appropriate antibiotic treatment (before the onset of neurological signs, which may not develop for several days) may eliminate the need for decompressive laminectomy and lead to a good outcome.

Epidural hematoma may present more acutely and is usually associated with concurrent drug therapy with anticoagulant or

---

Table 15.8 Causes of back pain due to regional block

Cause

Short-term local tenderness due to tissue trauma (very common)

Short duration backache from 2-chloroprocaine with EDTA

Short-term tenderness due to epidural skin-site infection (<1%)

Long-term localized tenderness, possibly from neuroma formation (<0.1%)

Transient severe pain from neural trauma (rare)

Back pain and tenderness from epidural abscess (rare)

Back pain from epidural hematoma (very rare)

antithrombotic drugs or patient coagulopathy. In the presence of neurological signs and symptoms rapid surgical decompression is mandated, preferably within 8 hours, to optimize the chance of full neurological recovery.

15.2.3 Epidural analgesia in labor and backache

In 1990, a well-publicized retrospective survey noted an association between postpartum backache and epidural analgesia in labor, but not epidural anesthesia for cesarean section (CS). The authors concluded that backache '... is not solely a consequence of epidural anesthesia, but is probably due to a combination of muscular relaxation and postural stresses in labor'. Despite the problems inherent in the retrospective analysis (information relied on recollections from up to 9 years prior) and the significant underreporting of antenatal backache, a causal relationship was assumed by the lay press and subsequently both the general public and many antenatal educators. Consequently, for over a decade, postpartum backache has been considered 'due to the epidural' unless proven otherwise.

Several investigators have now addressed this issue. Examination of characteristics by which epidural analgesia in labor might produce backache failed to elucidate a mechanism, with no association found with difficulty of insertion, duration of analgesia, the concentration of local anesthetic given or the intensity of motor block. The first prospective study of over 1000 parturients found a 70% rate of pre-pregnancy or antenatal back pain, a 44% incidence in the postpartum period (of which 6% was severe), and no difference between those who did and did not receive epidural analgesia in labor. There are now at least four other prospective cohort studies, including almost 2000 women from several countries. All found similar rates of new backache up to 6 months postpartum (10% and 5% at 3 and 6 months, respectively), irrespective of labor analgesic technique. A cohort study with 1-year review also found no increased risk with epidural analgesia (risk

ratio 0.63, CI 0.25–1.56). Twenty-five percent of parturients with pre-pregnancy back pain have worsening of symptoms, but there is no correlation with epidural analgesia.

The most telling evidence comes from two large randomized trials involving almost 1200 nulliparous women and preliminary data from another (*Table 15.9*). These trials assigned parturients to either epidural analgesia or alternatives (continuous midwifery support, intramuscular meperidine, or intravenous opioid analgesia) during labor. Despite high cross-over rates, both intention-to-treat and per protocol analyses found identical rates of postpartum backache at 3 and 6 months. This was also true of women who had a past history of back pain or new back pain in the antenatal period. Apart from the specific causes mentioned (see *Table 15.8*), there is no causal relationship between

Table 15.9 Incidence of new low back pain after labor

Author	n	Epidural analgesia	Nonepidural analgesia
Dickinson, J. et al.	950	60%[a]	61%[a]
Loughlan, B.A. et al.	409	31%	28%
Breen, T.W. et al.	93	31%	27%
Howell, C.J. et al.	369	35%	34%

Intention-to-treat data from randomized controlled trials, 2–6 months postpartum after epidural or nonepidural methods of labor analgesia.

[a]Severe back pain 8% epidural analgesia versus 10% nonepidural analgesia.

Data reproduced with permission from Dickinson, J.E. et al. The impact of intrapartum analgesia on labour and delivery outcomes in nulliparous women. Aust. NZ. J. Obstet. Gynaecol. (accepted); Loughlan, B.A. et al. (1997) The influence of epidural analgesia on the development of new backache in primiparous women: report of a randomized controlled trial. (abstract) Int. J. Obstet. Anesth. 6: 203–204; Breen, T.W. et al. (1999) Epidural analgesia and back pain following delivery: a prospective randomized study. (abstract) Anesthesiology (Suppl.) SOAP abstracts: A7; Howell, C.J. et al. (2001) A randomised controlled trial of epidural compared with non-epidural analgesia in labour. Br. J. Obstet. Gynaecol. **108**: 27–33.

epidural analgesia in labor and either the development of postpartum backache, or a deterioration of pre-existing back pain.

15.3 Infection

15.3.1 Introduction

Infection is a major issue in obstetric anesthesia. Serious infection has been held to be rare, but case reporting provides no information about incidence and the experience of many obstetric anesthesiologists is that serious infection is becoming more prevalent. A comprehensive review of almost 11 000 obstetric epidurals between 1989 and 1994 from the author's unit found no serious infections. Since then, six cases of either meningitis or epidural abscess have occurred among a similar number of epidural techniques. Data from general surgical populations also suggest that serious infection is more common than previously thought, the incidence of epidural abscess being about 1 in 2000.

Infection can follow direct introduction of bacteria into the vertebral canal (at insertion or within injected solution), spread from the skin insertion site, or hematogenous spread. There are few systematic data on infection control, but extrapolating from venous catheterization, factors of relevance include asepsis during insertion (*Table 15.10*), minimization of 'breaks' into the catheter connections, sterile technique during drug injection, dressing care, and regular inspection of the catheter site. Rare mechanisms are direct contamination of the epidural site via oropharyngeal droplet spread from the anesthesiologist and 'seeding' of the epidural space during bacteremia. In the presence of a distant focus of infection, the risk of intraspinal infection remains low. Indeed, it is likely that many parturients have an epidural catheter placed while bacteremic due to chorioamnionitis or other infection. The most common source of bacterial infection is the patient's skin flora, and both skin-site and deep infection are predominantly due to staphylococcal species, especially *S. aureus*. Bacteriophage typing may be useful in determining the source of infection.

Table 15.10 Aseptic insertion technique for regional block

1. Operator performs thorough hand-washing; wears mask and gloves (sterile gown?)
2. Skin prepared with antiseptic such as chlorhexidine 0.5–2% (with or without alcohol 70%) by thorough scrubbing and two separate applications after drying
3. Sterile field maintained and sterile solutions injected
4. Needle(s) and catheter inserted with 'no-touch' technique
5. Transparent moisture-permeable dressing applied
6. Skin site inspected for fluid collection or inflammation and regular review organized

15.3.2 Epidural skin site infection

Prospective series indicate that 2–5% of skin sites become inflamed once epidural catheters have been in place longer than 24 hours. The colonization rate of the catheter tip rises dramatically in the presence of inflammation, mandating catheter removal. Purulence or surrounding cellulitis is an indication for empiric antibiotic therapy with an agent such as flucloxacillin, on the basis of likely *S. aureus* infection, until a definitive microbiological diagnosis is made. Higher catheter tip colonization rates are associated with more than one skin puncture within an interspace, catheterization beyond 48 hours and morbid obesity. The onset of severe back pain or headache, signs of meningeal irritation, or neurological disturbance merits immediate further investigation and neurological consultation.

15.3.3 Epidural abscess

Epidural abscess can develop spontaneously or after surgery, particularly in immunosuppressed patients, but in the obstetric population is usually associated with epidural techniques. About 50% of reported cases had an epidural catheter for more than 2 days and blood cultures usually prove negative. Depending on the segmental distribution of the abscess, compromise of the vascular supply to the spinal cord or cord compression may cause bowel and bladder dysfunction, leg weakness, or paraplegia (*Table 15.11*). Imaging is best achieved with a gadolinium-enhanced magnetic resonance image (MRI; *Figure 15.3*). In the absence of a neurological deficit, prolonged conservative therapy with intravenous antibiotics is appropriate therapy. However, a large abscess or signs of neurological dysfunction mandate decompression within 6–12 hours if recovery is to occur. Surgical laminectomy is normally performed, although percutaneous drainage by irrigation of epidural catheters located on either side of the abscess has also been described.

15.3.4 Meningitis

Meningitis has complicated spinal, epidural or combined spinal-epidural techniques, and epidural blood patch. The overall incidence, and the relative risk in each situation, is unknown. Despite concern that meningitis might increase because of the introduction of combined techniques for labor analgesia, extensive clinical experience with tens of thousands of cases since the early 1990s has been reassuring.

The etiology of meningitis (bacterial, viral, aseptic) is sometimes uncertain, although chemical irritation by contaminants is now rare and the diagnosis of viral meningitis is usually evident after history and laboratory investigation. Bacterial meningitis is probably most common and may be associated with skin-site infection. Unfortunately, CSF culture

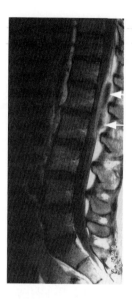

Figure 15.3 Sagittal T$_1$ weighted magnetic resonance image of a posterior epidural abscess (arrowed) in a parturient. The abscess was predominantly on the left and is shown compressing the spinal cord anteriorly. Reproduced with permission of the Journal of the Australian Society of Anaesthetists, Sydney from Collier, C.B.and Gatt, S.P. (1999) Epidural abscess in an obstetric patient. *Anaesth. Intens. Care* **27**: 663.

often proves negative, due to preceding antibiotic therapy (for prophylaxis against wound infection or for treatment of skin-site inflammation). CSF features indicative of bacterial etiology include increased leukocyte count, decreased glucose, increased protein, and positive Gram stain. Unlike community-acquired meningitis and epidural abscess, the prognosis is good, with full recovery likely if therapy is instituted early. Nevertheless, prolonged central venous access for antibiotic therapy and community nursing after control of the acute phase in hospital is costly.

15.4 **Epidural and subdural hematoma**

In contrast to other surgical populations, epidural and subdural hematoma are exceptionally rare complications in parturients.

Table 15.11 Presentation of epidural abscess

Severe back pain
- worse with flexion; sometimes with radiation in the involved nerve root distribution

Severe local tenderness

Fever, malaise, meningitis-like headache with neck stiffness

Laboratory changes
- elevated white blood cell count, raised erythrocyte sedimentation rate, and positive blood culture

Progression over hours to days to neurological deficit or osteomyelitis

There are only a handful of published cases and the incidence is unknown, although apparently one in several hundred thousand. Hematoma occurring either spontaneously or after regional block is usually associated with a hematological abnormality, especially coagulopathy or anticoagulant therapy. The rarity of this complication is partly explained by the widespread interest in 'safe' platelet numbers for regional block in thrombocytopenic parturients and adherence to traditional dogma that such techniques are contraindicated when the platelet count is <100 000 or a bleeding or clotting disorder is present. Nevertheless, these criteria have long been challenged and currently the majority of obstetric anesthesiologists support epidural catheterization provided the platelet count is greater than 75–80 000 with no other risk factors present. Laboratory evidence, including thromboelastography, supports the safety of this more pragmatic approach, based on an individual risk-benefit assessment. In the absence of clinical bleeding, significant coagulopathy, or severe thrombocytopenia (count less than 50 000), regional techniques (especially single-shot SA) may well retain a favorable cost–benefit assessment.

Major risk factors for hematoma after regional block appear to be fibrinolytic drug administration or full anticoagulation. Concurrent administration of low molecular-weight heparin, which is antithrombotic because of both anti-factor Xa and weak fibrinolytic activity, also warrants caution and adherence to consensus guidelines (*Table 15.12*). An important message from examination of case reports is that epidural catheter removal carries some risk, and coagulation status at that time should be optimized.

The presentation of intraspinal hematoma is similar to that of epidural abscess, with the exception of more rapid progression and less local tenderness. Cranial and spinal subdural hematoma may present acutely, but are often more chronic lesions, and may be associated with pathology such as ependymoma and shearing of dural vessels because of low CSF pressure after accidental dural puncture.

Table 15.12 Recommendations for regional block in association with low molecular-weight heparin (LMWH)

Avoid regional block for at least 24 hours if therapeutically anticoagulated with LMWH (e.g. enoxaparin 1 mg/kg)

Discuss the timing of prophylactic LMWH and regional block with the obstetrician

Avoid regional block for at least 12 hours after prophylactic LMWH

If not high risk or insertion is traumatic, begin prophylactic LMWH at least 12 (preferably 24 h) postoperatively

Remove epidural catheters when activity is low, for example at least 12 hours after the last dose

To avoid clot disruption and fibrinolysis, do not administer LMWH until 2–4 hours after regional block or catheter removal

Avoid concurrent administration of nonsteroidal anti-inflammatory drugs, other antiplatelet drugs including aspirin and Dextran; and other anticoagulants

Consider adjusting dosage and monitoring anti-Xa activity in selected patients

15.5 Neurological deficit

15.5.1 Introduction

Neurological dysfunction has multiple etiologies (*Table 15.13*), including a complication of regional block (see Sections 15.3 and 15.4 above and *Table 15.14*). However, the most common cause of major neurological dysfunction during pregnancy and after delivery is compressive neuropathy or 'obstetric palsy'. Obstetric palsies were first described in 1838. Subclinical sensory changes can be detected in up to 20% of parturients and often involve the femoral and obturator nerves after difficult labor. This high incidence of minor and major neurological deficit from nerve compression during childbirth contrasts with an incidence of 1 in 5–10 000 for needle- or catheter-related nerve injury after central neuraxial block. The propensity to blame epidural analgesia for all such events highlights the important role anesthesiologists can play in the assessment and diagnosis of obstetric neurological injury.

Table 15.13 Causes of postpartum neurological dysfunction

Type	Causes
Spontaneous or incidental	Epidural abscess; epidural hematoma; anterior spinal artery syndrome Disc prolapse, undiagnosed central nervous system disease Diabetic or viral neuropathy
Pregnancy-related neuropraxia	Meralgia parasthetica, carpal tunnel syndrome
Delivery-related neuropraxia	Lumbosacral plexus neuropathy; femoral or obturator nerve palsy
Posture-induced neuropraxia	Sciatic, femoral or lateral popliteal nerve compression Compression of cutaneous branches of posterior rami of spinal nerves
Surgery-related neuropraxia or transection	Femoral nerve palsy Injury to cutaneous branches of anterior thoracic nerves
Regional anesthesia- or analgesia-related	

Table 15.14 Causes of neurological dysfunction due to regional block

Cause

Direct needle or catheter trauma
- to spinal cord or nerve root

Neurotoxicity
- local anesthetic
- accidental injection of other neurotoxic drugs
- cauda equina syndrome associated with lidocaine and spinal microcatheters

Infection
- epidural abscess or meningitis; arachnoiditis

Hematoma
- epidural or subdural; spinal or intracranial

Low CSF pressure-related
- cranial nerve palsy or subdural hematoma after dural puncture

High pressure or ischemia-induced injury
- spinal canal stenosis, pre-existing pathology such as bleeding arteriovenous malformation, edema of spinal cord tumor

Other causes of nerve compression injury are surgical (intraoperative retraction or stretching) and position-related (especially lateral cutaneous nerve of the thigh or femoral nerve compression with hip flexion; lateral popliteal nerve or sciatic compression while sensation is diminished by epidural analgesia; and peroneal nerve compression from squatting).

15.5.2 Assessment and management

Neurological injury after delivery is a serious complication and common cause of litigation. All neurological dysfunction requires early appraisal. An adequate history, prompt neurological examination, and sometimes further investigation are of paramount importance to accurate diagnosis and management. Consultation with a neurologist or neurosurgeon is not necessary for minor and transient deficits, but early expert opinion can facilitate the opportunity for recovery from neurological deficit due to epidural abscess or hematoma. Hospital policies and processes should be directed to staff awareness and vigilance, and monitoring of postpartum and postoperative lower limb motor function, so that possible compressive pathology is identified and notified, rather than symptoms being ascribed to persisting regional block.

Some sensory deficits are easily diagnosed from their onset and dermatomal distribution. The dysfunction may involve single or multiple nerve roots, a specific peripheral nerve, or a nonanatomical mechanism. Entrapment syndromes such as meralgia paresthetica (outer thigh dysesthesia from inguinal ligament entrapment of the lateral cutaneous nerve of the thigh from L_2–L_3) are common. Other cases require specialist diagnostic expertise, imaging of spinal canal anatomy, and occasionally electrophysiological testing. Nerve conduction velocity studies and electromyography may indicate a pre-existing abnormality, a delivery injury, or the location of injury peripherally. Other investigations include late-response studies, somatosensory evoked potentials and motor evoked potentials.

Axonotmesis (axon degeneration within an intact sheath due to ischemia or compression) and neurotmesis (cutting or shearing of the axon and sheath) have a poor prognosis compared with neuropraxia, which leaves the nerve and its axonal sheath intact. Localized damage with loss of myelin is more likely to repair and recover within several weeks or months. Depending on the extent of damage, paresthesia, dysesthesia, hypoesthesia, and motor deficit may persist for months or become permanent.

Management of persisting dysfunction, especially muscle weakness, often involves physical therapy, physiotherapy, occupational therapy and orthotics. Occasionally, steroids are used to reduce swelling (e.g. facial nerve palsy), but an expectant approach, awaiting resolution, is typical.

15.5.3 Specific neurological injuries

Transient mild paresthesias are common (10–25%) during epidural insertion and probably represent passage of the catheter near a nerve root, because the incidence is markedly reduced (<5%) with soft, flexible tip catheters. Direct contact with the spinal cord or a nerve root is usually associated with immediate, severe lancinating pain. This serves as a warning to withdraw the needle or catheter or to stop injection and may avoid intraneural or intracord injection and permanent injury. Due to variability in the point of termination of the spinal cord (about L_2), spinal needles must never be inserted above the $L_{2/3}$ interspace. The surface landmark of Tuffier's line across the iliac crests approximates the $L_{4/5}$ disc level. However, the unreliability of palpation or visualization in determining the intervertebral level (the correct interspace is only identified in 25–40% of cases, see *Figure 15.4*) suggests it is wise to aim below the supracristal line, hopefully at $L_{3/4}$ or $L_{4/5}$.

Lumbosacral plexus injury, especially of the lower roots, results from fetal head or forceps compression within the pelvis and presents as sensory change, foot-drop, and pain. This deficit must be distinguished from common peroneal nerve injury at the head of the fibula, due to stretch or compression (e.g. prolonged squatting). The incidence of femoral nerve (L_{2-4}) injury has fallen due to earlier surgical intervention for arrest of labor, but nerve compression at the inguinal ligament occurs in the lithotomy position and follows abdominal surgical retraction injuries. Characteristic features are loss of quadriceps power, diminished knee jerk, and loss of sensation over the L_{2-4} dermatomes. The obturator nerve (also L_{2-4}) may be compressed near the obturator foramen, presenting with mild inner thigh hypoesthesia and weakness of hip adduction; and sciatic nerve compression injury during labor has also been described. A number of other neurological deficits (radial, ulnar and cranial nerves) and syndromes (carpal tunnel, Bell's palsy) are associated with pregnancy.

15.6 High regional block

15.6.1 Total spinal block

Clinical presentation

Total spinal anesthesia was once an accepted method of anesthesia, so while not without risk, every obstetric anesthesiologist should be capable of managing this complication of SA or EA with a high likelihood of excellent maternal and fetal outcome. The Confidential Enquiries into Maternal Death in England and Wales once regularly noted substandard care associated with deaths from this complication. Rising standards, including better resuscitation training and better levels of supervision, may have contributed to an absence of such deaths between 1985 and 1993, and one (the only maternal death directly attributable to anesthesia) in the 1994–1996 report.

Occasionally, total spinal block manifests as rapidly ascending sensory change and rising paralysis, followed by apnea, hypotension, and unconsciousness. More often, the first

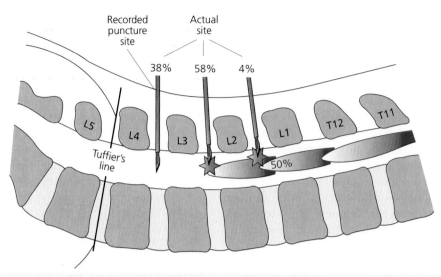

Figure 15.4 Hazard to the spinal cord from spinal needle insertion due to error in estimating the correct intervertebral level (because of variations in anatomical level of the supracristal or Tuffier's line) and due to variability in the level of termination of the spinal cord. Planned insertion at $L_{3/4}$ was radiologically demonstrated as incorrect in 62% of cases. Reproduced from Bromage, P.R. (1999) Neurologic complications of labor, delivery, and regional anesthesia. In: *Obstetric Anesthesia* (ed. Chestnut, D.H.), 2nd edn, p. 651. With permission from Mosby, Inc. St. Louis, MO.

indication is sudden loss of consciousness and apnea shortly after accidental injection of epidural local anesthetic (LA) into the subarachnoid space. High spread of subarachnoid or epidural LA, whether after deliberate spinal anesthesia or intended epidural injection, is usually immediate or within several minutes, but occasionally presents up to 30–45 minutes later, especially following a change of patient position.

High spinal (or indeed epidural or subdural) block that compromises swallowing, phonation, or respiration also gives rise to concern, and may require intervention to prevent aspiration or hypoxia. The consequences of accidental subarachnoid injection of LA are partly dose-dependent, and bupivacaine 12.5–15 mg, even in a high volume of diluent, is unlikely to produce clinical collapse. This supports the philosophy of incremental injection of small volumes of epidural LA, and the use of low-dose epidural LA and opioid combinations during labor.

Mechanisms of high block

Several scenarios may lead to high or total central neuraxial block (*Table 15.15*). Life-threatening high block may be due to accidental subarachnoid injection of epidural solution, but unrecognized subarachnoid placement of an epidural needle or catheter is uncommon (about 1 in 5000). Even less common is late subarachnoid migration of a well-functioning epidural catheter. Differential flow from a multi-holed epidural catheter, straddling the dura, favors fluid exit from the distal (subarachnoid space) orifice with more forceful injection. After accidental dural puncture and replacement of an epidural catheter, epidural drugs may pass to the subdural or subarachnoid space, with the size of the dural hole an important determinant of the proportion transferred. All drug doses should be given incrementally, looking for abnormal or excessive spread. The incidence of total spinal block associated with replaced epidural catheters after dural puncture may be as high 1 in 10.

Many obstetric anesthesiologists thus prefer deliberate subarachnoid placement of the epidural catheter for continuous spinal analgesia or anesthesia.

Excessive spread of spinal LA, especially after failed epidural block (due to compression of the lumbar intrathecal sac and reduced CSF volume) is possible, although the incidence varies widely. When cephalad spread is inadequate despite large volumes of epidural LA, an alternative to SA is injection of a small volume of LA through a second low thoracic epidural catheter. Irrespective of the reason for the failure of EA, a further option is conversion to sequential CSE anesthesia (see Section 7.6.3). Nevertheless, even single-shot SA may be safely performed if meticulous attention is paid to patient positioning, such that the thoracic curve is accentuated, limiting the spread of hyperbaric solution to mid-thoracic segments.

Detection of subarachnoid catheter location

Prior to epidural injection, aspiration looking for CSF is a simple safety measure. A variety of tests to distinguish CSF from saline or LA have been used, including measuring fluid temperature; glucose, pH, and protein content analysis; or testing with sodium pentothal for precipitation (acidic LA precipitates in alkaline sodium pentothal up to a dilution of 1 in 4). Test-dosing with LA is controversial, and many case reports document a false negative test-dose prior to the total spinal block. When accidental subarachnoid injection is recognized immediately, aspiration of 20–30 ml of LA-contaminated CSF may recover up to 50% of the drug, although the effectiveness of this strategy has not been tested in a clinical setting.

Management of high block

Management (*Table 15.16*) involves basic resuscitation principles (airway, breathing, circulation), plus avoidance of aortocaval compression, early protection of the airway, aggressive vasopressor support to maintain cardiac output, and intensive maternal and fetal monitoring. Opioid-induced respiratory depression may contribute to hypoventilation or apnea when intraspinal opioids have also been administered, and intravenous naloxone is recommended. Early resuscitation, ventilation, and circulatory support should result in a normal maternal outcome and the prognosis for the fetus remains excellent, provided oxygenation is maintained and sustained hypotension avoided. Urgent cesarean section is by no means

Table 15.15 Mechanisms of high central neuraxial block

Mechanism

Epidural catheter initially inserted into subarachnoid space but not recognized

Epidural catheter in multicompartment (epidural, subdural, subarachnoid) location

Multicompartment (epidural, subdural) epidural catheter previously functioning normally penetrates arachnoid mater

Epidural catheter adjacent to dural puncture hole

Spinal or epidural– exaggerated spread of anesthetic drugs

Spinal after epidural analgesia or failed epidural anesthesia

Table 15.16 Management of total spinal block

Basic resuscitation
- airway, breathing, circulation
- avoid aortocaval compression; elevate lower limbs
- early protection of the airway
- aggressive vasopressor support and intravenous fluid

Naloxone
- for previous intraspinal opioid

Intensive maternal monitoring

Intensive fetal monitoring

Maintain maternal sedation

Cerebrospinal fluid withdrawal?
- 20–30 ml from subarachnoid catheter

mandatory and should be based on fetal assessment after maternal stabilization. Anesthesia or sedation until the block regresses to safe levels, as judged by clinical evaluation, is usually required for 1–3 hours.

15.6.2 Subdural block
Anatomy and diagnosis
The precise anatomy of the subdural space is controversial, but it is classically described as lying between the dura and arachnoid mater, with a small intracranial extension. Deliberate identification of the subdural space is difficult, although cervical subdural block and endoscopy are possible, and accidental injection of contrast during myelography is not infrequent. Many clinical reports of accidental subdural catheterization or drug injection involve parturients, although the incidence is unclear. One in 1400 (from a prospective series of almost 11 000 obstetric epidurals) is probably an underestimate, as subdural injection is sometimes unrecognized and most clinically evident cases are not reported. Diagnosis is based on clinical grounds, but atypical presentation or multicompartment block (a multi-holed catheter traversing two or more of the epidural, subdural or subarachnoid spaces) create confusion. Definitive diagnosis using imaging (radiographic contrast) is seldom performed, but typically shows a 'rail-road track' appearance, without spread into intervertebral foramina as seen with an epidurogram (*Figure 15.5*).

Clinical characteristics and management
Subdural injection of LA has a number of potential consequences. Clinical presentation varies widely (*Table 15.17*), from early or delayed high sensory block with minimal systemic disturbance through to immediate life-threatening apnea, hypotension, and loss of consciousness. Most commonly, high cephalad spread occurs, even after small LA volumes (2–10 ml). Sensory changes may involve cervical roots or cranial nerves, including trigeminal nerve block and Horner's syndrome. Asymmetry of sensory block, usually with sacral sparing, is common. The onset and recovery are similar

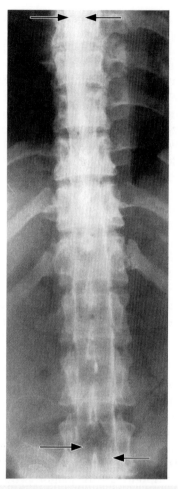

Figure 15.5 Typical appearance of subdural spread on anteroposterior epidurogram after injection of radiographic contrast through the epidural catheter. Arrows indicate 'railroad track' bilateral distribution of subdural contrast from the mid-lumbar to the mid-thoracic region. Reproduced from Collier, C.B. (1998). *An Atlas of Epidurograms. Epidural Blocks Investigated.* With permission from Taylor and Francis

to epidural injection (rather than subarachnoid), although the duration of effect of subdural opioid may be prolonged. Hypotension tends to be moderate unless an extremely high block occurs, and motor block variable in density, but often minimal. These characteristics reflect pooling of solution in the wider subdural space around the dorsal nerve roots and variable distention of the subdural space.

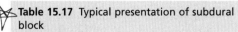

Table 15.17 Typical presentation of subdural block

Presentation

Uneventful epidural identification and catheter insertion

Sensory change over 10–20 minutes

Excessive spread for volume injected

High cephalad spread with poor caudal spread and sacral sparing

Asymmetric distribution

Minimal or moderate motor block

Minimal or easily controlled hypotension

Subdural block usually requires reinsertion of the catheter into the epidural space, although occasionally analgesia or anesthesia is satisfactory. Deliberate dosing of a subdural catheter for anesthesia or postoperative analgesia is unwise, because results are unpredictable. Rarely, high subdural block requires intervention, including ventilation and intubation.

15.7 Intravenous injection of local anesthetic

15.7.1 Background and prevention

Cannulation of an epidural vein (incidence 3–15%) is more likely in pregnancy, probably because of engorgement of the epidural venous plexus and the relatively low venous pressure. Venous trauma is lower when at least 10 ml of normal saline is injected through the epidural needle, and if soft, flexible-tipped catheters are used. In the 1980s, severe LA toxicity (seizures, respiratory and/or cardiac arrest) from IV bupivacaine was a prominent cause of maternal death from regional anesthesia, especially in the USA. This complication now appears to have declined significantly, perhaps due to greater awareness and better prevention of accidental IV injection (routine aspiration of the catheter, slow injection of incremental boluses; the reduction of therapeutic doses for epidural analgesia in labor; and test dosing). The decline of caudal epidural anesthesia (which carries a much

greater risk than lumbar injection), the use of local anesthetics with higher therapeutic indices (for example, lidocaine with epinephrine, chloroprocaine, and ropivacaine), and the increased use of SA are other possible reasons. The incidence of LA-induced convulsions in tertiary obstetric units is less than 1 in 10 000.

A tenet of safe practice is to prevent intravascular injection of epidural LA (*Table 15.18*). Intravenous placement of about 70% of uniport catheters and almost 100% of multiholed, closed-tip catheters can be detected at the time of insertion by simple aspiration. The strategy of incremental dosing (with individual boluses of no more than 20–25 mg of bupivacaine or ropivacaine and 100 mg of lidocaine) has not been validated and may fail to detect about 25% of intravascular catheters, but is nevertheless sensible. Slower injection is likely to reduce peak LA levels and allow detection of toxicity prior to a convulsion or arrhythmia. All test doses designed to detect intravenous injection have limitations; the most sensitive

Table 15.18 Prevention of accidental intravenous injection of local anesthetic

Method

Epidural technique
- Use loss-of-resistance to saline and inject 10 ml through epidural needle before threading catheter
- Avoid injection through epidural needle
- Use soft-tip flexible epidural catheter

Appropriate regional technique and choice of local anesthetic

Aspiration
- Needle and catheter
- Before attaching to connector and filter look for efflux of blood with catheter end dependent and open to air

Slow incremental bolus

Test dose
- Air
- Epinephrine-containing local anesthetic
- Other

Maintain a high index of suspicion

and specific, the injection of 1–2 ml of air using Doppler monitoring for cardiac emboli, is somewhat impractical. Small doses of intravenous LA may produce premonitory symptoms. Although LA with epinephrine 15 μg in the presence of heart rate and BP monitoring is useful in some circumstances, its reliability in the presence of labor pain is reduced and its value as a routine debatable. Sensitivity to chronotropes is reduced in pregnancy, the criteria for a positive response (normally >20 beats per minute) needs modification in the presence of contraction pain, and epinephrine has potentially adverse effects in preeclampsia, cardiac disease and the compromised fetus.

There is no single strategy that can eliminate the possibility of LA toxicity. A low rate requires multiple preventive strategies, including appropriate selection of regional technique, drug and dose; awareness of factors that may modify patient response to accidental IV injection; and tests to exclude intravascular placement.

15.7.2 Clinical presentation and management

The pathophysiology of central nervous and cardiovascular system LA toxicity is complex. Toxicity occurs within a wide range of plasma concentrations, specific for each individual drug. In obstetric anesthesia, toxicity from excessive doses (from a rise in concentration with repeated injection or continuous infusion) is rare. The response to accidental IV administration of epidural LA is only partly dose related, also being dependent on other pharmacological (e.g., rate of rise of plasma level) and patient (e.g., level of sedation) factors. Symptoms, when present, are mild, transient and nonspecific, classically involving the central nervous system (e.g., tinnitus, visual disturbance, perioral tingling and numbness, metallic taste, drowsiness, agitation, jitteriness, and slurring of speech). However, severe toxicity may present with the sudden onset of convulsions or a cardiac arrest.

Table 15.19 Management of local anesthetic toxicity

Get help and prevent patient injury while convulsing

Airway
- Ensure a clear airway, especially when seizure terminates
- Maintain safe patient positioning – avoid aortocaval compression

Breathing
- Watch for and treat hypoventilation (oxygen, bag and mask ventilation or tracheal tube ventilation) in the post-ictal phase

Circulation
- Assess clinically looking for hypotension, arrhythmia or cardiac arrest
- Establish ECG monitoring for ventricular arrhythmias

Terminate convulsions
- Benzodiazepine (diazepam, midazolam) preferable to sodium pentothal if not self-terminating
- Second-line anticonvulsants (e.g. phenytoin) seldom required

Treat arrhythmias and myocardial depression
- Best combination not determined, but for profound collapse use large doses of epinephrine, consider bretylium and magnesium for arrhythmias; clonidine and dobutamine
- Manage cardiac arrest with external cardiac massage, defibrillation, appropriate pharmacological therapy, prevention of aortocaval compression and immediate delivery if feasible

All obstetric medical and nursing staff should be capable of diagnosing and managing LA toxicity. Fortunately, convulsions are usually self-limiting and cardiac arrest rare. Management principles include immediate summoning of help, clearing the airway, protecting the parturient from injury, terminating convulsions (preferably with IV benzodiazepine), prevention of seizure-related hypoxemia and hypercarbia (including early intubation and hyperventilation if required), support of the circulation and fetal monitoring (*Table 15.19*).

15.8 **Complications of general anesthesia**

15.8.1 Introduction

All complications of general anesthesia (GA) are relevant to obstetric anesthesia during pregnancy and for cesarean section (CS), but those that feature prominently in the obstetric population are failed intubation, aspiration of gastric content, awareness, hypotension and hypertension (see Chapters 7 and 14) and adverse neonatal effects (see Chapter 7).

The pharmacological prevention of gastric aspiration and steps taken during GA have been addressed earlier (see Sections 7.3.1, 7.9.2 and *Figure 15.6*). However, the pregnant woman is at risk of aspiration-induced upper airway obstruction or subsequent pneumonitis not only at the induction of GA, but also at extubation, during emesis in the recovery room and after normal delivery, in the postpartum period for up to 48 hours, after convulsions, during high regional block and during cardiopulmonary resuscitation. When aspiration is suspected, immediate management is to suction the hypopharynx, to consider turning the patient to the lateral head-down position, and to secure the airway with a tracheal tube. Close observation thereafter is mandatory. This includes monitoring of clinical signs and symptoms (especially respiratory vital signs, bronchospasm and atelectasis; cardiovascular status); oximetry and arterial blood gas analysis; and chest radiography. In the absence of obvious changes within a couple of hours, serious aspiration is unlikely. However, if aspiration is significant, supportive respiratory care must be arranged, including oxygen therapy, physiotherapy, and ventilation in intensive care if severe. Steroids are contraindicated and antibiotic therapy used only for specific indications.

15.8.2 Failed intubation

Failed intubation is probably the most common cause of anesthetic-related maternal death in developed countries. The incidence of failed intubation in obstetrics is about 1 in

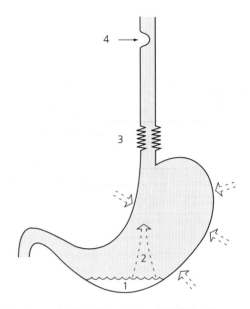

Figure 15.6 Measures directed at preventing aspiration pneumonitis associated with obstetric anesthesia. (1) Emptying of solids from the stomach and reduction of gastric fluid volume and acidity. (2) Prevention of sudden increases in intragastric pressure. (3) Prevention of fall in lower esophageal sphincter pressure and reflux. (4) Cricoid pressure to prevent regurgitation into the pharynx; and maintenance of active upper airway and laryngeal reflexes to prevent aspiration into the trachea. Reproduced with permission of Canadian Anaesthesiologists Society, Toronto from Davies, J.M. *et al.* (1990) The stomach: factors of importance to the anaesthetist. *Can. J. Anaesth.* **37**: 902.

300–500, compared with that of the general surgical population of 1 in 2500, in part due to the anatomical changes of pregnancy (see Section 2.3). The upper airway may be compromised by fat deposition in the head and neck, mucosal edema of the tongue, oral and nasopharyngeal mucosa. Deterioration in Mallampati score may occur as labor progresses.

Airway assessment is a crucial component of safe practice (see Section 7.3.1), although most measures to identify women at greater risk and to predict the success of tracheal intubation show poor sensitivity and specificity. With GA, the airway must be rapidly secured, to avoid a rapid fall in oxygen tension associated with the respiratory changes in pregnancy and increased oxygen consumption.

If difficult intubation is anticipated, early insertion of an epidural catheter during labor is sensible and regional anesthesia advisable for CS. Awake fiberoptic intubation, avoiding the nasal route because of a high risk of severe epistaxis, may be warranted if GA is indicated. Whenever GA is induced and difficulty is suspected, it is prudent to confirm that ventilation is possible with a face mask before neuromuscular block with succinylcholine.

In all obstetric units and operating rooms, a set of specialized airway management equipment is recommended (see *Table 9.4*) and patient position should be optimized before induction (see *Figure 7.11*). Poorly applied cricoid pressure with distortion of laryngeal anatomy is a common cause of inadequate direct laryngoscopic view. Attempts to pass the tracheal tube prematurely in an inadequately paralyzed patient may predispose to regurgitation of gastric content.

The obstetric anesthesiologist must be well trained and well prepared. This includes a management plan and skills should intubation fail (*Figures 15.7* and *15.8*). Many management algorithms have been devised as guidelines, all based on the principles of establishing oxygenation and ventilation while preventing regurgitation and aspiration, and on decision-making guided by the perceived best interests of the mother and fetus. In most cases, having decided to abandon attempts to intubate, cricoid pressure is maintained while oxygenation and ventilation are achieved using a bag and face mask with oral airway initially, or a laryngeal mask airway subsequently. It is often appropriate to waken the mother and postpone surgery, converting to regional anesthesia or awake intubation prior to GA. Rarely, in the interests of fetal survival and provided a clear airway can be maintained, GA with cricoid pressure is continued without intubation. The need to proceed to cricothyroidotomy or similar transtracheal ventilation is, fortunately, exceptionally rare.

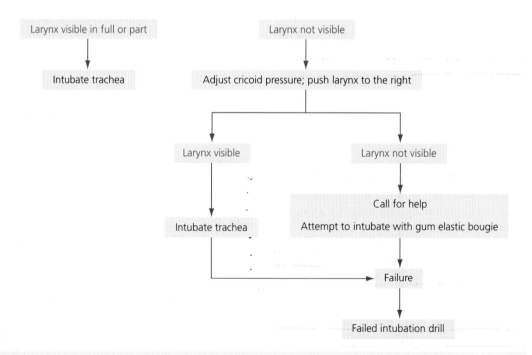

Figure 15.7 Management of difficult intubation based on view at direct laryngoscopy.

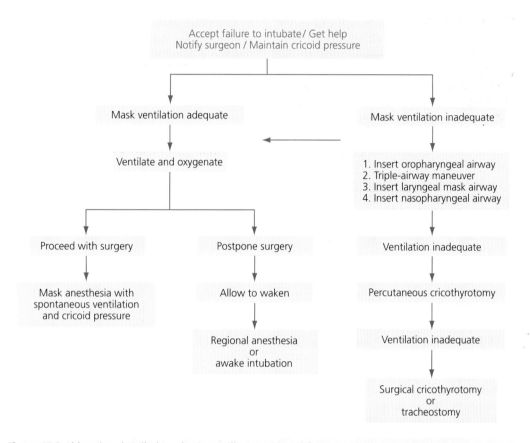

Figure 15.8 Abbreviated 'Failed Intubation Drill'. Reproduced from Paech, M.J. (1997) Obstetric airway management. In: *Airway Management*. (eds Hanowell, L.H. and Waldron, R.J.), p. 351. With permission from Lippincott-Raven Publishers, Philadelphia, PA.

15.8.2 Awareness (conscious recall)

During GA, obstetric patients are at high risk for both intraoperative responsiveness, and more importantly, recall of sounds, events, or experiences postoperatively (to which the term 'explicit recall', or 'awareness', is commonly applied). Despite the reduced minimum alveolar concentration (MAC) of inhalational anesthetics in pregnancy, major contributing factors to this increased risk are the desire to limit fetal drug exposure and the tocolytic effect of volatile anesthetics, and to allow rapid return of airway reflexes after anesthesia. The common practices of avoiding sedative premedication, using reduced doses of induction drug, restricting inhalational volatile anesthetic to 0.5 MAC with high inspired oxygen concentration, and stopping inhalational anesthetic shortly after delivery all contribute. Consequently, awareness has been a frequent complication that may involve auditory perception, feelings of paralysis, anxiety and panic, recall of intubation, and pain. Such events occur mainly during the period of 'light' anesthesia, between induction and transition to adequate anesthetic depth with inhalational anesthetics, but also at delivery and final suturing. Although ketamine induction is less likely to result in intraoperative responsiveness (without recall), the risk associated with propofol is uncertain and sodium pentothal has remained the induction drug of choice. Recently reported rates of explicit recall (0.2–0.5%, with nonspecific 'dreaming'

1–6%) have been attained as a result of appreciation that inadequate anesthesia is likely to be of detriment to the fetus and that a more liberal approach to general anesthetic drug dosing is safe. A modified technique permits larger sodium pentothal doses (5 mg/kg); overpressure with high fresh gas flows and temporarily up to 2 MAC inspired inhalational anesthetic (using agent monitoring to rapidly attain adequate depth); pre-delivery opioid dosing when appropriate; and maintenance of inhalational agent until near the completion of surgery.

Awareness is now most likely to be a consequence of equipment problems or errors (e.g., an unfilled vaporizer) or drug errors (such as incorrect induction drugs or drug sequence). However, patients with a history of awareness may have decreased susceptibility to anesthetic drugs and meticulous attention must be paid to drug dosing and technique. The development of new monitoring technologies such as the bispectral index, respiratory sinus arrhythmia or auditory evoked cortical potential monitors, may prove further aids to reducing this complication.

In the event of conscious recall, sympathetic patient counseling is important, including acknowledgement of the parturient's experience and provision of reasonable explanations. This should be in the presence of a witness and be followed by thorough documentation. The anesthesiologist must prepare for the possible medicolegal consequences, irrespective of whether or not the cause of awareness was apparent.

15.8.3 Neonatal effects
Information about the effects of GA on neonatal condition, both at birth and during the following 24 hours, comes from small prospective series. Most comparisons with regional anesthesia are retrospective cohort or epidemiological studies and are subject to selection bias. Additionally, changes in both GA technique (more liberal use of volatile anesthetics) and regional anesthesia management (more aggressive control of hypotension) make it difficult to generalize from older data. Anesthetic technique does not correlate with neonatal mortality, but GA is associated with an increased need for neonatal resuscitation (lower Apgar scores at birth, oxygen and intubation) and possibly with poorer reflex tone and alertness (lower neurobehavioral scores) in the first few hours of life. In urgent CS due to fetal hypoxemia and acidosis, the acid–base status of the infant improves with either method of anesthesia.

In recent years, the dogma that opioids should not be given before delivery has been challenged. Many anesthesiologists believe that pre-induction opioid administration (alfentanil 15–30 µg/kg; fentanyl 5–10 µg/kg) has some little neonatal consequence, but of considerable maternal benefit in certain circumstances (principally to obtund adverse hemodynamic responses to intubation in severe preeclampsia, cardiac and neurological disease). Although neonatal respiration may be affected, provided the neonatologist, pediatrician or doctor is aware of opioid exposure and naloxone is available as an antagonist, clinical outcome is usually good.

15.9 Medicolegal considerations

15.9.1 Introduction
Obstetric anesthesiologists are frequently faced with situations of crisis when the parturient is particularly vulnerable. Irrespective of the standard of care, inevitably, when a good outcome is not achieved, some parents will seek compensation through legal recourse. This has extended to lawsuits for inadequate pain relief during labor and failure to address intraoperative pain during CS under regional anesthesia.

In some countries, medical litigation over obstetric practice is rising at over 25% per year. This appears to have been fuelled by high (and some might say unrealistic) consumer expectations, prolonged periods of liability, and huge settlement claims. Obstetric anesthesiologists have inevitably become involved in this litigious climate, either as co-defendants with obstetricians, or in independent cases of negligence. There can be nothing more damaging to our professional and emotional well-being than appearing in court to defend one's practice, so it is perhaps not surprising that many anesthesiologists avoid obstetrics, finding little appeal in dealing with patients at stressful and emotionally vulnerable times, often at unsociable hours. In contrast, others are devotees who are prepared to face such personal and professional challenges and find obstetric anesthesia a richly rewarding subspecialty.

The legal definition of medical negligence or malpractice varies across legal systems, but, in general, a plaintiff must prove a breach of duty (the anesthesiologist failed to meet a standard of care) and that damages were caused by that violation of the standard. How the standard of care is defined also varies. The Bolam principle of 'in accordance with the practice accepted as proper by a reasonable body of medical men skilled in that particular art' has now been replaced in some countries by a standard largely determined by the court rather than the defendant's medical peers. The question of consent (see Section 7.3.1) is often critical, as is the level of communication and rapport established in the doctor–patient relationship. The onus is on the anesthesiologist to inform the parturient about both complications that are minor but common, and those that are rare but that might influence the decision of 'a reasonable person'. As a group, prospective parents are usually keen to receive high levels of disclosure about interventions and procedures. Even during painful labor, retention of relevant information is high, especially when antenatal or other education classes have been attended previously. Other areas of medicolegal involvement of anesthesiologists are preparation of reports for legal firms, insurers or regulatory authorities, and acting as an expert witness.

15.9.2 Avoiding medical litigation

Informed consent is clearly critical, but debate continues about the process (verbal, written, or both), the validity (in a parturient in great pain and distress and influenced by potent sedative and analgesic drugs during labor), and the detail of documentation. From a legal perspective, comprehensive legible documentation with accurate notation of timing is of great importance. It may be impossible to prove something was discussed or done several years after the event when the plaintiff's and defendant's memories are at odds. Contemporaneous notes act as an *aide memoir*, even though in emergency settings and in labor, a brief explanation of a procedure and acknowledgement of the limitations of the circumstances may be the best that can be done. Consent to continue should be sought if the patient is distressed or the procedure is proving difficult.

Poor doctor–patient communication is the factor most likely to lead to future difficulties and, thus, the art of establishing rapport is a paramount skill in avoiding litigation. An honest and empathetic approach is advocated (*Table 15.20*).

Table 15.20 Suggestions for avoiding medicolegal claims
Suggestions
Develop communication skills and establish rapport
See elective patients in advance
Provide parturients and partners with realistic information about benefits, disadvantages, complications and options
Answer questions honestly and thoroughly; do not accept or assign blame
Consult with specialist colleagues
Document details of management, monitoring, and the timing of events
Document discussions with parturient and partner
Make detailed notes after an event or crisis, date and sign them
Never attempt to alter, delete, or surreptitiously add to previous documentation
Contact your insurer, medical board or other relevant legal representation

15.9.3 Specific situations

Although accurate data are not available, information such as that in the American Society of Anesthesiologists Closed Claims Study provides an indication of claim patterns. Many examples can be cited, but the most common claims for negligence probably involve pain experienced during regional anesthesia for cesarean section (see Section 7.8.2), neurological dysfunction and post-dural puncture headache after regional block, and awareness during GA (see Sections 15.1, 15.5, 15.6, 15.8). Ethical dilemmas include management of the obstetric Jehovah's Witness experiencing major obstetric hemorrhage, termination of pregnancy and human embryo donation.

Further reading

Aitkenhead, A.R. (1990) Awareness during anaesthesia: what should the patient be told? (editorial). *Anaesthesia* **45**: 351–352.

Bogod, D. (2000) Medicolegal implications. In: *Regional Analgesia in Obstetrics. A Millennium Update* (ed. Reynolds, F.), pp. 371–380. Springer-Verlag, London.

Collier, C.B. (1992) Accidental subdural block: four more cases and a radiological review. *Anaesth. Intensive Care* **20**: 215–232.

Duffy, P.J. and Crosby, E.T. (1999) The epidural blood patch. Resolving the controversies. *Can. J. Anaesth.* **46**: 878–886.

Harmer, M. (1997) Difficult and failed intubation in obstetrics. *Int. J. Obstet. Anesth.* **6**: 25–31.

Hogan, Q. (1996) Local anesthetic toxicity: an update. *Reg. Anesth.* **21**(6S): 43–50.

Holdcroft, A., Gibberd, F.B., Hargrove, R.L. *et al.* (1995) Neurological complications associated with pregnancy. *Br. J. Anaesth.* **75**: 522–526.

Hull, C.J. and Thorburn, J. (1997) Proposer. Opposer. Awareness is due to negligence during general anaesthesia for caesarean section. *Int. J. Obstet. Anesth.* **6**: 178–181.

Kindler, C.H., Seeberger, M.D. and Staender, S.E. (1998) Epidural abscess complicating epidural anaesthesia and analgesia. An analysis of the literature. *Acta Anaesthesiol. Scand.* **42**: 614–620.

Loo, C.C., Dahlgren, G. and Irestedt, L. (2000) Neurological complications in obstetric regional anaesthesia. *Int. J. Obstet. Anesth.* **9**: 99–124.

Moore, D.C. (1986) Toxicity of local anaesthetics in obstetrics IV: management. *Clin. Anaesthesiol.* **4**: 113–124.

Morgan, B. (1990) Unexpectedly extensive conduction blocks in obstetric epidural analgesia. *Anaesthesia* **45**: 148–152.

Newman, L.M. (1999) Legal and ethical issues in obstetric anesthesia. In: *Obstetric Anesthesia,* 2nd edn (ed. Norris, M.C.), pp. 765–778. Lippincott, Williams and Wilkins, Philadelphia, PA.

Paech, M.J. (1996) Obstetric airway management. In: *Airway Management.* (eds Hanowell, L.H. and Waldron, R.J.), pp. 343–355. Lippincott-Raven Publishers, Philadelphia, PA.

Paech, M. (2001) Regional anaesthesia, anticoagulation and antithrombosis. In: *Anaesth. Intensive Care Med.* Issue 2:6, pp. 216–218. The Medicine Publishing Company, Abingdon, UK.

Reynolds, F. (2000) Dural puncture and headache. In: *Regional Analgesia in Obstetrics. A Millennium Update* (ed. Reynolds, F.), pp. 307–319. Springer-Verlag, London.

Reynolds, F. (2001) Damage to the conus medullaris following spinal anaesthesia. *Anaesthesia* **56**: 235–247.

Reynolds, F. and Speedy, H.M. (1990) The subdural space: the third place to go astray. *Anaesthesia* **45**: 120–123.

Robinson, P.N., Salmon, P. and Yentis, S.M. (1998) Maternal satisfaction. *Int. J. Obstet. Anesth.* **7**: 32–37.

Russell, I.F. (1997) Postpartum neurological problems. In: *Clinical Problems in Obstetric Anaesthesia* (eds Russell, I.F., Lyons, G.), pp. 149–160. Chapman and Hall, London.

Russell, R. (2000) Long term sequelae of childbirth: backache. In: *Regional Analgesia in Obstetrics. A Millennium Update* (ed. Reynolds, F.), pp. 321–332. Springer-Verlag, London.

Vandermeulen, E.P., Van Aken, H. and Vermylen, J. (1994) Anticoagulants and spinal-epidural anesthesia. *Anesth. Analg.* **79**: 1165–1177.

Chapter 16

Neonatal resuscitation

Valerie A. Arkoosh, MD

Contents

16.1 Introduction

At birth, numerous physiological changes must occur for a fetus to successfully make the transition to a neonate. Despite the complexity of this process, only 6% of newborns born in the United States require life support in the delivery room. This percentage rises quickly among newborns who weigh less than 1500 g. Delivery room personnel must understand the neonatal adaptations to extrauterine life, make provision for resuscitation, understand the predictors of need for resuscitation and respond appropriately.

16.2 Neonatal adaptation to extrauterine life

The fetus depends on placental blood flow for gas exchange. Pulmonary vascular resistance (PVR) is high, with 90% of right ventricular output shunting across the ductus arteriosus (*Figure 16.1*). Systemic vascular resistance (SVR) is low: 40% of cardiac output flows to the low-resistance placenta. During vaginal delivery, compression of the infant thorax expels fluid from the mouth and upper airways. With crying, the lungs fill with air, surfactant is released, and oxygenation increased. These changes greatly decrease PVR. Simultaneously, clamping of the umbilical cord removes the low-resistance placental bed from the circulation, increasing SVR. Within minutes, the right-to-left shunt across the foramen ovale and ductus arteriosus is substantially reduced (*Figure 16.2*).

Transient hypoxemia or acidosis is well tolerated by a normal newborn and prompt intervention usually prevents any permanent sequelae. Prolonged neonatal hypoxemia or acidosis impedes the transition from fetal to neonatal physiology. The fetus/neonate initially responds to hypoxemia by redistributing blood flow to the heart, brain and adrenal glands. Tissue oxygen extraction increases. Eventually, myocardial contractility and cardiac output decrease. Hypoxemia and acidosis promote patency of the ductus arteriosus,

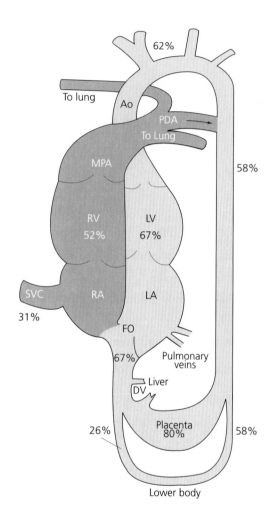

Figure 16.1 Diagrammatic representation of the fetal circulation. *In utero*, pulmonary vascular resistance is high and 90% of right ventricular output flows across the ductus arteriosus. Numbers represent SaO$_2$ in vessels or chambers.

counteracting the normal neonatal increase in pulmonary artery blood flow. Ventilatory drive is reduced by both indirect central nervous system depression and direct diaphragmatic depression. The net result of these physiological responses is a neonate with persistent pulmonary hypertension and little or no ventilatory drive. Prompt intervention is necessary in these neonates.

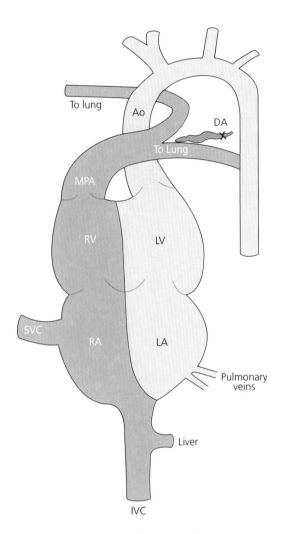

To lung

Ao

DA

To Lung

MPA

RV

LV

SVC

RA

LA

Pulmonary veins

Liver

IVC

Figure 16.2 Diagram of adult (post-birth) circulation. At birth, pulmonary vascular resistance drops dramatically, and the ductus arteriosus constricts; right ventricular output now flows primarily through the lungs. Changes in vascular resistance markedly decrease the shunt across the foramen ovale.

16.3 Requirements for effective neonatal resuscitation

Preparation for neonatal resuscitation encompasses a number of activities including acquisition and maintenance of the proper equipment; identification, education, and training of responding personnel; and development of contingency plans for additional personnel if needed. Equipment and medications should be organized together in one location in the delivery room, checked frequently for proper functioning and expiration date, and replenished immediately after use (*Table 16.1*).

At least one person skilled in newborn resuscitation should attend every delivery. Additional personnel should be available if a high-risk delivery is anticipated. The importance of trained personnel following protocol-driven maneuvers is critical. In one hospital in China, neonatal mortality was reduced from 9.9% to 3.4% after the introduction of Neonatal Resuscitation Program Guidelines. In the United States, an obstetric anesthesia workforce survey conducted by Hawkins *et al.*, in 1992, found that anesthesiologists performed neonatal resuscitation in fewer than 10% of cesarean deliveries. This percentage has decreased from 23% when a similar survey was administered in 1981. Pediatricians, obstetricians, nurse specialists, family practitioners, respiratory therapists or CRNAs not medically directed by an anesthesiologist performed the remainder of the resuscitations. In a 1991 survey of Midwestern community hospitals, routine involvement of anesthesia personnel in neonatal resuscitation was noted by 31% of respondents. Looking forward, the need for anesthesia personnel to participate in neonatal resuscitation may increase as pediatric residents spend more time in primary care training and less in neonatology.

In determining need for personnel trained in neonatal resuscitation, practitioners in the United States can refer to Guideline VII of the American Society of Anesthesiology, Guidelines for Regional Anesthesia in Obstetrics (see *Table 5.2*). The guideline states:

'Qualified personnel, other than the anesthesiologist attending the mother, should be immediately available to assume responsibility for resuscitation of the newborn. The primary responsibility of the anesthesiologist is to provide care to the mother. If the anesthe-

Table 16.1 Equipment and medications for neonatal resuscitation

Suction equipment	Bag and mask equipment
Bulb syringe	Neonatal resuscitation bag with pressure relief valve
Mechanical suction	Face masks – newborn and premature sizes
Suction catheters 5F–10F	Oral airways
Meconium aspirator	Oxygen with flowmeter and tubing
Intubation equipment	**Medications**
Laryngoscope	Epinephrine 1:10 000
Straight blades #0 and #1	Naloxone hydrochloride 0.4 mg/ml or 1.0 mg/ml
Extra bulbs and batteries	Volume expander
Endotracheal tubes 2.5–4.0 mm	Sodium bicarbonate 4.2% (5 mEq/10 ml)
Stylet	Dextrose 10%
Scissors and gloves	Sterile water and normal saline
Miscellaneous	
Radiant warmer	Umbilical artery catheterization tray
Stethoscope	Umbilical tape
ECG	Umbilical catheters 3.5F, 5F
Adhesive tape	Three-way stopcocks
Syringes and needles	Feeding tube, 5F
Alcohol sponges	

siologist is also requested to provide brief assistance in the care of the newborn, the benefit to the child must be compared to the risk to the mother.'

16.4 Antepartum assessment of risk

With careful ante- and intrapartum fetal assessment, the need for neonatal resuscitation can be predicted in about 80% of cases. Antepartum assessment includes evaluation for major fetal anomalies and identification of maternal factors that may influence fetal wellbeing (*Table 16.2*). Intrapartum events often predict the need for neonatal resuscitation (*Table 16.3*). Assessment must continue throughout labor as the clinical situation can change rapidly. Intrapartum evaluation includes fetal heart rate monitoring with, when indicated, fetal scalp stimulation or fetal scalp blood sampling for pH determination. Even in the presence of a reassuring fetal heart rate trace nearly 50% of babies born by cesarean section will require some active form of resuscitation as will virtually all of those with nonreassuring fetal heart rate tracings.

Intrapartum fetal heart rate (FHR) monitoring is the first line of fetal assessment (see Section 3.6). FHR monitoring is most reliable in confirming fetal wellbeing and is more than 90% accurate in predicting a 5 minute Apgar score greater than 7. In predicting fetal compromise, however, FHR monitoring has a false positive rate of 35–50%. A recent study examined fetal heart rate monitoring strips of singleton infants with birth weights of at least 2500 g and moderate to severe cerebral palsy and compared them with fetal heart rate strips from control children. The 21 children with cerebral palsy who had multiple late decelerations, or decreased heart rate variability represented 0.19% of the infants who had these fetal heart rate monitor findings. Thus, the false positive rate in this patient population was 99.8%. Nonetheless, practitioners have little else with which to judge fetal wellbeing and clinical decisions regarding delivery are often based on a careful evaluation of the FHR trace.

In the presence of a nonreassuring fetal heart rate trace, the practitioner may wish confirmatory studies of fetal wellbeing or lack thereof. Digital stimulation of the fetal scalp or

Table 16.2 Maternal and fetal factors associated with need for resuscitation

Maternal diabetes	Post-term gestation
Pregnancy-induced hypertension	Pre-term gestation
Chronic hypertension	Multiple gestation
Previous Rh sensitization	Size-dates discrepancy
Previous stillbirth	Polyhydramnios
Bleeding in the second or third trimester	Oligohydramnios
Maternal infection	Maternal drug therapy including
Lack of prenatal care	• Reserpine, lithium carbonate
Maternal substance abuse	• Magnesium, adrenergic-blockers
Known fetal anomalies	

Table 16.3 Intrapartum events associated with need for resuscitation

Cesarean delivery	General anesthesia
Abnormal fetal presentation	Uterine tetany
Premature labor	Meconium-stained amniotic fluid
Rupture of membranes > 24 hours	Prolapsed cord
Chorioamnionitis	Abruptio placentae
Precipitous labor	Uterine rupture
Prolonged labor > 24 hours	Difficult instrumental delivery
Prolonged second stage > 3–4 hours	Maternal systemic narcotics within 4 hours of delivery
Nonreassuring fetal heart rate patterns	

vibroacoustic stimulation through the maternal abdomen will result in fetal heart rate accelerations in a healthy, nonacidotic fetus. Fetal scalp pH determination can confirm or exclude fetal acidosis. A pH of less than 7.2 is considered abnormal and if confirmed by a second measurement may indicate the need for delivery.

Predictors of need for endotracheal intubation include administration of general anesthesia to the mother and low infant weight. In growth-restricted infants, factors predicting low uterine artery pH and/or 5 minute Apgar score <7 include: preeclampsia, fetal distress, breech delivery, forceps use, older maternal age, amnioinfusion, general anesthesia, and nalbuphine use during labor.

16.5 **Essentials of neonatal resuscitation**

16.5.1 Intrapartum management

Intrapartum resuscitation should be attempted once fetal compromise is identified (see also Section 3.7). Maternal factors that may impair oxygen delivery to the fetus must be identified and corrected if possible. These include maternal hypotension or decreased cardiac output secondary to aortocaval compression, sympathectomy, hemorrhage or cardiac disease. Disease states that may interfere with maternal oxygenation such as asthma, pneumonia, or pulmonary edema should be considered and if present, treated appropriately.

Attention must also be directed to the uterus where hyperstimulation, tetany, abruption, or rupture may interfere with blood flow to the fetus. Stopping oxytocin infusion or administering a tocolytic agent will reduce uterine tone. Delivery will be required if abruption or rupture are severe.

Umbilical cord prolapse should always be considered if fetal heart rate changes are sudden, severe and prolonged. Oligohydramnios is a risk factor for umbilical cord compression and variable decelerations. Obstetricians frequently use saline amnioinfusion to attempt to alleviate cord compression. Saline amnioinfusion is performed by infusing saline into the uterus via an intrauterine pressure catheter. Amnioinfusion is also being used in cases of thick meconium in an attempt to dilute the meconium, hopefully decreasing the severity of meconium aspiration syndrome.

16.5.2 Delivery

The American Heart Association/American Academy of Pediatrics recommends the neonatal resuscitation protocol that follows. New protocol recommendations were released in 2000. The initial steps in neonatal resuscitation include an assessment of the overall condition of the neonate and steps to minimize heat loss (*Figure 16.3*). Depressed, asphyxiated infants often have an unstable thermal regulatory system. Additionally, cold stress leads to hypoxemia, hypercarbia, and metabolic acidosis, all of which will promote persistence of the fetal circulation and hinder resuscitation. Within the first 20 seconds of birth, the newborn should be dried, placed under a radiant warmer, and undergo suctioning of mouth and nose.

In the presence of meconium, routine endotracheal intubation and suctioning is no longer recommended. Tracheal suctioning is only recommended if there is meconium-stained fluid *and* the baby is not vigorous (*Figure 16.4*).

The second step (within 30 seconds of birth) is assessment of neonatal respiration. If gasping or apneic, positive-pressure ventilation (PPV) should be instituted at a rate of 40–60 breaths per minute with 100% oxygen. Peak inspiratory pressures of 30–40 cmH$_2$O or higher are necessary for initial lung expansion. The large majority of infants requiring any resuscitation will respond to these first two steps. Indications for endotracheal intubation include ineffective bag and mask ventilation, an anticipated need for prolonged mechanical ventilation, or to establish a route for administration of medicine (*Table 16.4*). With prolonged bag and mask ventilation, a nasal or oro-gastric tube should be inserted to decompress the stomach.

The third step is assessment of neonatal heart rate (within 1 minute of birth). Chest compressions are required in only 0.03% of deliveries. Neonatal cardiac arrest is generally secondary to respiratory failure producing hypoxemia and tissue acidosis. The result of these metabolic changes is bradycardia, decreased cardiac contractility and, eventually, cardiac arrest. Chest compressions should be instituted at a rate of 90 per minute when after 30 seconds of PPV the heart rate is below 60. Chest compressions should be stopped when the heart rate is greater than 60. Chest compressions can be performed using either the thumb method or the two-finger method. The depth of compressions should be approximately one-third of the anterior-posterior diameter of the chest. Pressure should be applied to the lower third of the sternum that lies between the nipple line and the xyphoid process. The ratio between chest compressions and ventilations should be 3:1, producing 90 compressions and 30 ventilations each minute. In practice, this equals 30, 2-second cycles per minute. A 2-second cycle consists of three chest compressions in 1.5 s, leaving 0.5 s for ventilation. In most neonates with adequate ventilation, cardiac function normalizes quickly.

The above three steps should all occur within the first 90 seconds of birth. Although 1- and 5-minute Apgar scores (*Table 16.5*) are recorded as one way of assessing neonatal response to resuscitation, the practitioner

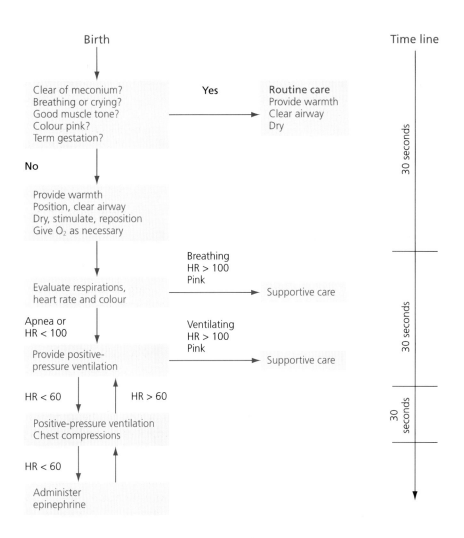

Figure 16.3 Time-flow diagram of neonatal resuscitation.

should not wait for the 1-minute score to begin resuscitation. If the 5-minute score is less than 7, additional scores should be obtained every 5 minutes until 20 minutes have passed or until two successive scores are greater than or equal to 7. In a study of stillborn infants, 66.6% were resuscitated and left the delivery room alive. Of these, 39% survived beyond the neonatal period. Survival is unlikely if the Apgar score is 0 at 10 minutes of age.

Medications are indicated if, after adequate ventilation with 100% oxygen and chest compressions for 30 s, heart rate remains below 60 beats per minute. Medications, doses and routes of administration are given in *Table 16.6*. Naloxone hydrochloride is indicated specifically for neonatal respiratory depression due to maternal opioid administration, but should not be given to a neonate born of a narcotic addicted mother as this can precipitate acute withdrawal in the neonate. Sodium bicarbonate should only be used when ventilation is adequate (or respiratory acidosis will replace metabolic acidosis) AND metabolic acidosis is documented or presumed, or all other measures have been unsuccessful. The use of blood volume expanders is rarely indicated and may be detrimental. Their use should be

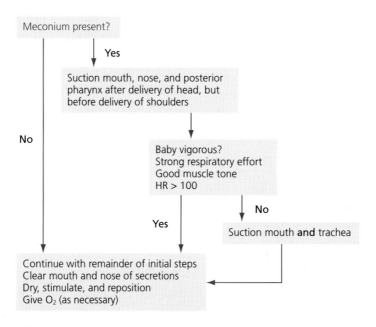

Meconium present?

Yes

Suction mouth, nose, and posterior pharynx after delivery of head, but before delivery of shoulders

No

Baby vigorous?
Strong respiratory effort
Good muscle tone
HR > 100

No

Yes

Suction mouth **and** trachea

Continue with remainder of initial steps
Clear mouth and nose of secretions
Dry, stimulate, and reposition
Give O₂ (as necessary)

Figure 16.4 Appropriate response to the presence of meconium.

Table 16.4 Suggested endotracheal tube size

Gestational age (weeks)	Weight (kg)	ET tube size (ID, mm)	Depth insertion (cm from upper lip)
<28	<1.0	2.5	6–7
28–34	1.0–2.0	3.0	7–8
34–38	2.0–3.0	3.5	8–9
>38	>3.0	3.5–4.0	9–10

Table 16.5 Determination of APGAR score

Sign	0	1	2
Heart rate	Absent	< 100 bpm	> 100 bpm
Respiratory effort	Absent	Slow, irregular	Crying
Muscle tone	Flaccid	Some flexion of extremities	Active motion
Reflex irritabililty	No response	Grimace	Vigorous cry
Color	Blue, pale	Blue extremities	Completely pink

* Infants are assigned a value of 0, 1, or 2 for each of the five signs. These are totaled to determine the Apgar score, which can range from 0–10.

restricted to situations in which there is evidence of acute blood loss, such as feto-maternal hemorrhage, accompanied by clear signs of shock. Atropine is not indicated in neonatal resuscitation because vagal stimulation is rarely the cause of bradycardia in a newborn requiring resuscitation. Direct laryngoscopy, however, may cause a transient decrease in heart rate.

Once the need for medications is established, there are three possible routes of administration: umbilical vein, peripheral veins, or endotracheal instillation. Endotracheal epinephrine effects are delayed up to one minute compared to intravenous administration. Although increasing the dose of endotracheally administered epinephrine may be recommended in pediatric resuscitation, a change in dose is not recommended in neonatal resuscitation. The larger dose of endotracheally administered epinephrine is associated with prolonged hypertension in an animal model. Given the association between intraventricular hemorrhage and hypertension, the current recommendation is to administer the same dose of epinephrine (0.01–0.03 mg/kg) intravenously or endotracheally. If there is no response after endotracheal administration of epinephrine, intravenous access should be established as quickly as possible. Naloxone can also be instilled into the trachea.

16.5.3 Neonatal airway management
Laryngeal mask airway (LMA)
Recently, the size-1 LMA has been used successfully to resuscitate newborns of both normal and low birthweight requiring PPV at birth. In a descriptive study by Paterson *et al.*, eligible newborns weighed at least 2.5 kg and were of 35 weeks gestation or greater. Twenty of 21 neonates were successfully resuscitated with the LMA. One neonate underwent tracheal intubation to facilitate administration of epinephrine. Time for LMA insertion averaged 8.6 s, circuit pressure at audible leak averaged 22 cmH$_2$O and peak circuit pressure obtained averaged 37 cmH$_2$O. Gastric distention was not observed during the resuscitation procedure. The successful use of the LMA has also been described in neonates with Pierre-Robin syndrome in whom both bag and mask ventilation and endotracheal intubation had failed. Further studies are needed to assess the reliability of this technique of airway management in the neonate requiring resuscitation.

16.5.4 Practical issues
Neonatal hypoglycemia
Approximately 10% of healthy term neonates have transient hypoglycemia. Other neonates at risk include those born of diabetic mothers or mothers who received a large amount of

Table 16.6 Medications for neonatal resuscitation

Medication	Concentration	Dosage / Route	Rate
Epinephrine	1:10 000	0.01–0.03 mg/kg ET or IV	(0.1–0.3 ml/kg) Give rapidly. Flush catheter/ET tube with saline.
Volume expanders	Normal saline	O negative blood IV (umbilical vein)	10 ml/kg Give over 5–10 minutes.
Sodium Bicarbonate	0.5 mEq/mL	(4.2% solution) IV (umbilical vein)	2 mEq/kg (4 ml/kg) Give slowly, over at least 2 minutes.
Naloxone hydrochloride	0.4 mg/ml	0.1 mg/kg IV or ET	Give rapidly
Dopamine	2–20 µg/kg/min	IV	

ET = endotracheal, IV = intravenous

intravenous dextrose during labor. Macrosomic, pre- or postmature neonates also are prone to hypoglycemia. A dextrose strip blood glucose test is easily obtained on any infant at risk and should also be obtained from neonates who appear lethargic at birth without obvious cause. If the glucose level is <40 to 45 mg/dl, the neonate should be treated either with oral feedings (2–3 cc/kg D10% in water) or by intravenous infusion (8 mg/kg min).

16.6 Summary

Successful neonatal resuscitation requires an understanding of neonatal physiology and adequate preparation of personnel and supplies. Good ante- and intrapartum assessment will identify the majority of infants who will require resuscitation. Those who frequent the delivery room, even when not designated as primary responders to neonatal resuscitations, should understand how to initiate neonatal resuscitation.

Further reading

American Heart Association, American Academy of Pediatrics (2000) *Textbook of Neonatal Resuscitation*. American Heart Association, Dallas, TX.

American Heart Association (1992) Standards and guidelines for cardiopulmonary resuscitation and emergency care. *JAMA* **268**: 2276.

Denny, N.M., Desilva, K.D. and Webber, P.A. (1990) Laryngeal mask airway for emergency tracheostomy in a neonate. *Anaesthesia* **45**: 895–900.

Fanaroff, A.A. and Marrin, R.J. (eds) (1992) Neonatal-perinatal medicine. In: *Diseases of the Fetus and Infant*, 5th edn. Mosby Year Book, St. Louis, MO.

Frand, M.N., Honig, K.L. and Hageman, J.R. (1998) Neonatal cardiopulmonary resuscitation: The good news and the bad. *Pediatr. Clin. N. Am.* **45**: 587–598.

Friedlich, P.R., Chan, L. and Miller, D. (2000) Relationship between fetal monitoring and resuscitative needs: fetal distress versus routine cesarean deliveries. *J. Perinatol.* **20**: 101–104.

Gandini, D. and Brimacombe, J.R. (1999) Neonatal resuscitation with the laryngeal mask airway in normal and low birth weight infants. *Anesth. Analg.* **89**: 642–643.

Guay, J. (1991) Fetal monitoring and neonatal resuscitation: what the anaesthetist should know. *Can. J. Anaesth.* **38**: R83–R88.

Hawkins, J.L., Gibbs, C.P., Orleans, M., Martin-Salvaj, G. and Beaty, B. (1997) Obstetric anesthesia workforce survey – 1981 versus 1992. *Anesthesiology* **87**: 135–143.

Hein, H.A. (1993) The use of sodium bicarbonate in neonatal resuscitation: Help or harm? (letter). *Pediatrics* **91**: 496–497.

Jain, L. and Vidyasagar, D. (1995) Controversies in neonatal resuscitation. *Pediatr. Ann.* **24**: 540–545.

Jain, L., Ferre, C., Vidyasagar, D., Nath, S. and Sheftel, D. (1991) Cardiopulmonary resuscitation of apparently stillborn infants: Survival and long-term outcome. *J. Pediatr.* **118**: 778–782.

Krebs, H.B., Petres, R.E., Dunn, L.J., Jordan, H.V.F. and Segreti, A. (1979) Intrapartum fetal heart rate monitoring I. Classification and prognosis of fetal heart rate patterns. *Am. J. Obstet. Gynecol.* **133**: 762–772.

Leuthner, S.R., Jansen, R.D. and Hageman, J.R. (1994) Cardiopulmonary resuscitation of the newborn. *Pediatr. Clin. N. Am.* **41**: 893–907.

Levy, B.T., Dawson, J.D., Toth, P.P. and Bowdler, N. (1998) Predictors of neonatal resuscitation, low Apgar scores, and umbilical artery pH among growth-restricted neonates. *Obstet. Gynecol.* **91**: 909–916.

Nelson, K.B., Dambrosia, J.M., Ting, T.Y. and Grether, J.K. (1996) Uncertain value of electronic fetal monitoring in predicting cerebral palsy. *New Engl. J. Med.* **334**: 613–618.

Ostheimer, G.W. (1993) Anaesthetists' role in neonatal resuscitation and care of the newborn. *Can. J. Anaesth.* **40**: R50–R56.

Paterson, S.J., Byrne, P.J., Molesky, M.G., Seal, R.F. and Finucane, B.T. (1994) Neonatal resuscitation using the laryngeal mask airway. *Anesthesiology* **80**: 1248–1253.

Saugstad, O.D. (1998) Practical aspects of resuscitating asphyxiated newborn infants. *Eur. J. Pediatr.* **157**: S11–S15.

Tejani, N., Mann, L.I. and Bhakthavathsalan, A. (1976) Correlation of fetal heart rate patterns and fetal pH with neonatal outcome. *Obstet. Gynecol.* **48**: 460–463.

Wimmer, J.E. (1994) Neonatal resuscitation. *Pediatrics in Review* **15**: 255–265.

Zhu, X.Y., Fang, H.Q., Zeng, S.P., Li, Y.M., Lin, H.L. and Shi, S.Z. (1997) The impact of the neonatal resuscitation program guidelines (NRPG) on the neonatal mortality in a hospital in Zhuhai, China. *Singapore Med. J.* **38**: 485–487.

Chapter 17

Obstetric anesthesia in the developing world

Paul M. Fenton, MD

Contents

17.1 Introduction to the developing world

The purpose of this final section is to educate, as a matter of general information, the western-trained anesthesiologist in the different types of practice in the poorer parts of the world. In addition, it will serve as a practical guide for anesthesiologists who have the opportunity to go to developing countries to provide anesthesia services. This author's experience has been in Africa and most of the information presented refers to this area.

The descriptive term 'developing countries' may be misleading to residents of countries that are considered 'developed'. It contains an implied consensus on where those countries are and also a uniformity of medical practice that has no basis in fact. The great variety in anesthesia practice worldwide means it is impossible to adequately describe obstetric anesthesia in all developing countries in a few pages, as this chapter purports to do. Further, the term itself ('developing countries') is a misnomer in large parts of the globe today: many countries are not actually *developing* but are doing the reverse and, after a few advances in health care in recent decades, they are returning to the baseline from which their development began.

Little research is carried out, and still fewer publications emanate from most developing countries. In current practice, where publication and communication are increasingly important, this silence from developing countries is troubling. No news is not good news, and development (as the term is usually understood), has probably stopped in many places. A poster presented at the *1st All Africa Anaesthetic Congress* (Harare, Zimbabwe) in 1997 demonstrated graphically the dearth of facts available with the title *'Terra Anaesthetica Incognita'*. A Medline search of the National Library of Medicine in Bethesda, Maryland using the subject headings 'cesarean section', 'Africa', and 'anesthesia', returns just one article published in the last decade.

No new term has been devised for this phenomenon of *'nondeveloping'*. This chapter uses the old terminology, but provides insight into the less technological practice of anesthesia in Africa (from personal experience in Malawi) and in other countries (from published reports) in the poorer parts of the world. The latter reports are usually from the heads of departments in larger cities of their respective countries; they tend to be optimistic and conspicuously fail to include reports of maternal outcome.

Sub-Saharan Africa is pre-eminent among areas considered 'developing' in health care, but other areas that must be considered include India, China, Central Asia, South East Asia, Eastern Europe, and Central and South America; this list comprises most of the world. A major problem is that the contrasts within even small areas of these regions (especially in the cities) are as great as between the poorest parts of rural Africa and the richest parts of the industrialized North.

The cost of anesthesia plays an important part in the quality of the service, but should not be overemphasized. The basic cost of anesthesia for a cesarean section in Malawi in 1999 was $8–$10 (US) for the small equipment and drugs, and $1 for the services of the anesthetist. A good service with acceptable morbidity and mortality can be provided in Africa for a tiny fraction of its cost in the West. Government money for health care is spread very thinly, however, and dictates the quality of care. For example, the ratio of the annual per capita expenditure on health in Malawi to the estimated maternal mortality rate is surprisingly similar to the opposite ratio in The Netherlands (*Table 17.1*). The result of these realities is that many – perhaps the majority – of mothers in Africa cannot afford the surgery necessary to either survive or completely recover from the mechanical trauma of childbirth, and these injuries are ultimately fatal.

Childbirth is a growth industry in many developing countries. In Africa, with fertility rates (lifetime number of births per female of child-bearing age) of 6 or 7, obstetric operations comprise an average of 75% (up to 95% in some hospitals) of all major surgical proce-

Table 17.1 Public sector health care expenditures and maternal mortality

Country	Annual per capita health expenditure (US dollars)	Estimated maternal mortality rate (deaths/100 000 births)
Sierra Leone	?	2000
Malawi	$5	1000
Zimbabwe	$14	400
Developed countries (average)	$1000	17
Netherlands (Europe)	$2000	7

dures. All these procedures require anesthesia, but anesthesiology as a medical specialty has not received the emphasis in developing countries that it has in the West. In the developing world, unfortunately, whether in medical or paramedical categories, anesthesia has few career attractions; to a great extent anesthesiologists themselves are to blame for this situation.

17.2 Manpower

The obstetric anesthesiologist does not exist as a specialist in most of the developing world: all anesthesiologists and anesthetists in Africa spend much of their time with female patients dealing with the complications of childbirth, 95% of which present as emergencies.

The status and training of anesthetists varies widely throughout the world (*Table 17.2*): in Africa, not less than 95% of personnel are nonphysicians, usually called clinical officers. Some of these have formal training as anesthetists, some not. In rural China, nurse anesthetists comprise 50–90% of anesthesia manpower (according to different reports),

while in Chinese cities, anesthesiologists predominate. In Central Asia, even in poorer countries like Mongolia, anesthesiologists are the norm and paramedical anesthetists are almost unknown.

Including India in this chapter is perhaps questionable, because it is so vast and diverse. Liver transplants are conducted a few kilometers up the road from where cesarean sections are given ketamine or open drop ether because halothane is too expensive. Personnel are equally diverse, but very little information exists on the ratio of physician to nonphysician anesthesia personnel in India.

Indonesia, although also having a huge population, has a more uniform spectrum of anesthetic practice, more like Africa. Nurses administer 80% of anesthetics. This practice is consistent throughout the rest of the poorer countries of South East Asia such as Cambodia, Laos and Vietnam.

Developing countries with all-physician anesthesia services (like many former Soviet block countries) always emphasize the importance of this position, clearly regarding

Table 17.2 Anesthesia providers by region

Region	Physician	Clinical officer/ paramedical	Nurse
Southern Africa	++	−	++
East Africa	+	+++	−
Central/West Africa	+	−	+++
SE Asia	+	−	+++
China – urban	++	−	++
China – rural	+	−	+++
South America	++	++	−
Central Asia	+++	−	−

the use of the nurse anesthetist as a backward step. South America also tends to scorn the nonphysician anesthetist; while paramedical anesthetists exist (*'technicos'*), they are excluded from joining national associations of anesthetists. Guyana, however, is the exception and actively trains them, especially for rural practice.

The overall picture is bewildering and raises three significant questions: why are there physicians in one place and paramedics in another? What is the difference between anesthesiologists, nurse anesthetists and anesthetic clinical officers? How does one measure their relative merits and cost-effectiveness?

On the first question, there seems little logic: in Bangladesh and Nepal, two of the poorest countries in the world, all anesthetics are performed by physicians, whereas in the relatively more affluent Thailand there are twice as many nurses as physicians practicing anesthesia. Politics does play a major role: governments may perceive nurse anesthetists as a cheap form of labor compared to physicians. Surgeons, who often have a disproportionately strong voice in ministries of health, generally favor nurse anesthetists as they are less troublesome: when malpractice occurs in the management of surgical patients, the nurse anesthetist can be blamed for both surgical *and* anesthetic mishaps! The general public, in the interest of its own safety, favors more physicians in anesthesia, but is unfortunately not well informed about the importance of the specialty. It is in the interest of many surgeons to keep it that way.

In terms of patient outcome, it is almost impossible to compare the merits of physicians with nonphysicians in anesthesia; where both personnel are available, the physician will always be called upon to care for difficult cases which, by their very nature, have a higher rate of complication. For cesarean section in Mozambique, near-equivalence in postoperative outcome for physician and nonphysician surgery has been reported.

In summary, it is logical to assume a trained anesthesiologist will perform better than a paramedical anesthetist where both are working in a similar environment. The leadership necessary to make progress in the specialty of anesthesia within a developing country can only come from the physician anesthetist. In order to provide services to the bulk of a scattered rural population, however, the paramedical anesthetist is essential.

17.3 Equipment

The variety of anesthetic equipment in developing countries is as great as the variety of anesthetic providers. A thorough understanding of gas flow, pressures, pipelines, types of vaporizers, ventilators, and system function is far more important to the anesthetist in the developing world than it is in the West. The reason is simple: the technical support that the Western anesthesiologist expects in buying, installing and servicing equipment is usually completely absent in the developing world. Of necessity, the physician becomes a 'jack-of-all-trades'. A lack of familiarity with basic principles of anesthesia apparatus is often evident when developed world anesthesiologists visit developing countries.

In terms of equipment, one can define four broad categories. The first is the urban private hospital, almost identical to western practice. The second is the larger urban hospital (usually government-run) that was created along a western model some decades ago, but where management, finance and expertise have not been sustained. In these, there are older style continuous flow machines in use, often giving 100% oxygen because nitrous oxide is no longer available. Leaking or defunct pipeline systems may be in evidence, or oxygen may come from cylinders located in the operating room. General anesthesia with halothane is the norm and regional techniques are rare. The third category is the smaller government or mission hospital in rural areas where assorted apparatus is found, sometimes based on draw-over vaporizers or other free-standing device, but more often based on old, adapted continuous flow anesthesia machines. Unfortunately, draw-over anesthesia has long been abandoned in most of the West, and anesthesiologists from the developed world are rarely familiar with its principles. Spinal anesthesia and solo-ketamine general anesthesia are widely used. Oxygen may come from oxygen concentrators. The last category is the rural hospital where some resuscitation items exist (possibly oxygen, but not in the operating theatre) and ketamine is the only anesthetic drug available.

It is remarkable that in the year 2001, there has been no anesthesia machine developed that is suitable for the developing countries where most of the population of the planet live.

17.4 Obstetric practice and obstetric anesthesia

Obstetric practice and obstetric anesthesia differ drastically from western practice, and it is essential to recognize the differences. Obstetrics in developing countries is largely a matter of dealing with emergencies. No mother is prepared and the presenting condition of the mother is unpredictable. Obstetric shock, hemorrhage, anemia, and sepsis are everyday events and rates of morbidity and mortality are very high. The anesthesiologist must match his expertise and services to the prevailing circumstances (which can rarely be changed) and not try to do the reverse. The welfare of the mother is considered far more important than that of the baby and anesthesia decisions must reflect that.

17.4.1 Labor analgesia.

Labor analgesia (i.e., regional analgesia) as discussed in most of this text is not available in the developing world. Opiates such as meperidine are given to the lucky few, and nothing to the rest. A few countries in the developing world will provide Entonox (a premixed container of 50% nitrous oxide and 50% oxygen, delivered through a negative pressure valve and face mask) and fewer still an epidural service. A number of obstacles stand between the laboring mother and analgesia: she does not know about it or does not make any noise during contractions; the midwives may feel she 'needs' the pain of childbirth for her own good or they are too busy; the drug is located elsewhere and needs to be signed out; or she comes late to hospital and is too close to delivery. In the largest hospital in Malawi, about 3% of laboring mothers receive a single dose of pethidine. In rural areas, analgesia is rarely given. The majority of deliveries take place in the village or township, some supervised by traditional birth attendants.

Even should an enthusiastic practitioner be available, a labor epidural analgesia service is not usually a viable option. Epidural sets are expensive, sterility is doubtful, and conditions on most labor wards generally unsuitable. The midwives probably do not understand the function of the catheter, so the physician will be spending his entire time supervising epidurals instead of resuscitating emergencies elsewhere. Likewise, Entonox is not a realistic option: the gas is expensive, may be misused, or the apparatus is inoperable. For these reasons, labor analgesia is not even within the job description of public sector anesthetists in most developing countries.

17.4.2 Cesarean section

Background
Cesarean section (CS) is the most common major operation in many areas of the developing world. Management of CS is the everyday activity of the average anesthetist in Africa, whether physician or clinical officer. Much of the following section is based on a study of over 8000 cesarean deliveries carried out in Malawi between 1998 and 2000.

In the West, CS is performed largely for fetal indications during a well-monitored labor. A different situation exists in Africa: mothers present *in extremis*, usually in arrested labor due to cephalopelvic disproportion (CPD), or with a ruptured uterus of several days duration. Cesarean delivery is therefore performed most commonly to save the mother's life, not produce a baby. Opinion on the merits or demerits of CS in the West cannot, therefore, be applied in Africa.

The role of CS in reducing maternal mortality is one of the major controversies in obstetrics today. In rural Africa, CS rates are around 1%, in urban areas about 10–25%. The great difference between rural and urban areas does not have a clear correlation with known maternal mortality due to CPD, and it is not clear what happens to those mothers in rural areas whose labor arrests but who are not delivered by CS.

There are other risks associated with CS in Africa that further limit the indications: a mortality of 1–5% is associated with the operation itself, including the postoperative period. There is a high rate of serious wound infection due to poor surgical technique and HIV-seroprevalence; postoperative wound care may be poor and effective antibiotics unavailable. Puerperal sepsis is probably the largest single cause of maternal mortality in most African hospitals after delivery, and post-cesarean patients are at greatest risk. While this mortality rate seems high by Western standards, the mortality rate without cesarean delivery in this population is between 50 and 100%.

Anesthetic practice

The focus on regional anesthesia for CS that has occurred in recent years in the West has not been seen in Africa; both general and spinal anesthesia are used more-or-less equally. Epidural anesthesia is much less common due to the time, expense, and expertise required with the technique. A recent survey of maternal preferences showed spinal anesthesia to be the most popular method; the first reason given was fear of death under general anesthesia, while bonding with the baby was a distant second.

Spinal anesthesia

Methods do not differ greatly from those in developed countries. Hyperbaric lidocaine 5% with 7.5% dextrose is commonly used, as it is inexpensive. Unfortunately, with a duration of only 45–60 minutes the surgeon must be experienced and the CS uncomplicated. Meperidine or ketamine may be required towards the end of the procedure if the mother is experiencing pain. Hypotension and respiratory difficulty are remarkably common, and therefore a generous intravenous pre-load (over 1 l) should be given, and oxygen and resuscitation equipment should always be available. Ephedrine is often necessary, but if not available, 1 mg epinephrine diluted in 20 ml water and given 0.5 ml (25 µg) at a time is effective for pressure support, though rather abrupt in onset and offset.

The small stature of most women in developing countries should be remembered: 60–75 mg of hyperbaric lidocaine is usually sufficient. In urban areas, however, large women with multiple previous cesarean deliveries are found and 10–12 mg 0.5% isobaric or hyperbaric bupivacaine is preferable.

The lack of post-dural puncture headache (PDPH) is a controversial issue in Africa. Use of the 22–gauge needle (or even 20–gauge) is widespread, but PDPH is rare. Whether this is due to cultural, anatomical (i.e. racial), socioeconomic, or other reasons is unknown.

General anesthesia

Apart from lower operative blood loss with spinal anesthesia (*Table 17.3*), there is little reason to choose spinal over general anesthesia in terms of maternal safety in Africa. This is for two reasons: the risk of regurgitation and aspiration is lower in Africa and difficult intubations are rare.

In rural areas, intravenous ketamine with spontaneous ventilation is widely used without any safeguards of the airway. Practitioners of this method claim it serves the requirements of economy and safety in the hands of the untrained, unequipped people providing anesthesia, who should not be attempting intubation or spinal anesthesia. It cannot be recommended as a safe method, however.

Halothane in oxygen and air with spontaneous ventilation is also widely used. Among the methods of general anesthesia, this is the least satisfactory due to uterine relaxation

Table 17.3 Blood loss at cesarean delivery and anesthetic technique

Technique	Drug	Number	Percent	Mean blood loss (ml)
General anesthetic	**Total**	4891	60.6%	
	Ether	1629	33.3%	420
	Halothane	3124	63.9%	405
	Ketamine	138	2.8%	N/A
Spinal	**Total**	3135	38.8%	296
	Lidocaine 5%	2478	79.0%	N/A
	Bupivacaine 0.5%	657	21.0%	N/A

from high halothane concentrations and the poor analgesia. Though operative blood loss using halothane is no worse than with ether, postoperative hemorrhage after halothane anesthesia is a particular hazard. If general anesthesia is used, ether is the safest method, given that postoperative care is usually inadequate. Ether does contribute to postoperative nausea and vomiting, and electrocautery cannot be used, but is not necessary for the performance of a CS.

Ether technique
Diethyl ether may be given using a draw-over system or a continuous flow apparatus. If using draw-over vaporizers, note should be taken that the performance of vaporizers varies considerably, with some delivering reduced concentrations at high flows.

After the usual rapid-sequence induction with pentothal and succinylcholine, the patient is intubated and ether started at 10–15% in oxygen and air using moderate hyperventilation by hand. Scavenging is necessary to reduce irritation to staff by the vapor. Surgery starts as soon as successful intubation is confirmed. If, after about 10 minutes the baby is still not out, reducing the ether concentration to 4% and giving small increments of succinylcholine is satisfactory and does not produce awareness. The baby often smells of ether but is not usually depressed by it. It is important to switch off ether as soon as possible, well before the end of surgery. This may produce a rather bumpy closure for the sur-

geon, but it is safer for the patient to be as awake as possible on extubation.

Cricoid pressure does not appear to be as important in Africa as it is in the West. In 4918 CSs performed under general anesthesia, cricoid pressure was reported applied in 61% and not applied in the remainder. There were 139 cases of regurgitation (2.8%) reported, mostly seen at extubation, with the same incidence in the cricoid and no-cricoid groups (*Table 17.4*).

17.5 **Common obstetric problems and procedures**

17.5.1 Evacuation of uterus; retained products of conception
This is a surprisingly common procedure in Africa, especially when you include dilation and curettage (D&C) for septic or induced abortions. Neglected retained products are an important cause of puerperal sepsis (and therefore death), hence uterine evacuations must be treated as urgent.

Methods of anesthesia vary: inhalation induction and maintenance of anesthesia with halothane is widespread. The general rule of avoiding high concentrations of volatile agents for fear of causing uterine relaxation and hemorrhage is sound, but without nitrous oxide or muscle relaxants it is difficult to keep a patient from moving at less than 2–3% halothane. Trichloroethylene from a vaporizer mounted in series with halothane is sometimes used to reduce the halothane dose.

Table 17.4 General anesthesia, cricoid pressure, and risk of regurgitation

	Cricoid pressure applied (n)	Percentage	No cricoid pressure applied (n)	Percentage
Total cases (n = 4918)	2985	61	1933	39
Regurgitation (n = 139)	78	2.6	61	3.2
Time of occurrence:				
At intubation (n = 36)	24	31	12	20
At extubation (n = 76)	45	58	31	51
In recovery, including vomiting (n = 27)	9	11	18	30

Good clinical judgment is important: late presenting or septic evacuations with pre-existing anemia have a high risk of hemorrhage with halothane above 1%. Intravenous ketamine 1–2 mg/kg is preferable for both the cardiovascular system and the uterus due to its oxytocic effects.

Another technique used when an anesthetist is not available is meperidine and diazepam. This is rarely satisfactory because analgesia is poor, and patient movement can interfere with completion of the procedure.

17.5.2 Preeclampsia

Preeclampsia and eclampsia are more common in Africa than in the West. The rate is about 3% in all mothers at term and 4.5% in those undergoing cesarean section. Eclampsia is common since the prodromal state is often unrecognized and proceeds untreated until the mother seizes. Anecdotal evidence from Africa suggests the onset of eclampsia is less related to maternal blood pressure than is observed in the West. The dangers of eclampsia are still significant: in a study in Malawi of 328 women undergoing cesarean section with preeclampsia or eclampsia, 46% had one or more seizures, with four deaths among the eclamptics and three deaths in the preeclamptics who had not seized. Two of the four deaths among

the eclamptics were reported due to uncontrollable eclampsia, while in the other two the cause of death was unknown. In the preeclamptics, all three died of avoidable surgical or anesthetic complications (*Table 17.5*).

Preeclampsia is generally poorly managed in Africa. Although primarily a cardiovascular disease, the mainstay of treatment is often limited to diazepam given by obstetricians. Hydralazine is used, but most often in inadequate doses; magnesium sulfate is not generally available. Renal failure is a common and often fatal complication. Furosemide is widely used and may produce diuresis, but it is not clear that this offers any benefit without correcting the hypovolemic state. Considering the generally poor management, the disease seems to follow a slightly more benign course than in the West, and high blood pressures seem to be well tolerated by the mother. Syn-

Table 17.5 Maternal survival in preeclampsia and eclampsia

	Died n (%)	Survived n (%)	Total
Eclamptics	4 (2.6)	148 (97.4)	152
Preeclamptics	3 (1.7)	173 (98.3)	176
Total	7 (2.1)	321 (97.9)	328

dromes such as HELLP would not be diagnosed even if they did occur. Renal failure may be the most common cause of death in preeclampsia in developing countries.

The optimal method of cesarean anesthesia in preeclampsia is debatable: general anesthesia with halothane is traditional. Ether releases catecholamines that should exacerbate the condition, but ether 8–10% with spontaneous ventilation has been used without exacerbating blood pressure. As ether is generally preferable to halothane for CS, it also seems a reasonable choice for general anesthesia in preeclampsia. Spinal anesthesia is preferable to general anesthesia for hemodynamic reasons, as well as avoiding the hypertensive response to intubation and avoiding airway management problems. Clotting studies are rarely available, but a carefully executed spinal anesthetic using a 25 gauge needle would be very unlikely to cause problems, and is the method of choice in a cooperative, conscious patient.

17.5.3 Obstetric shock

The management of hypovolemic shock is not different from the West; management problems will arise because of the shortage of blood and colloid plasma expanders, however. Obtaining more than 2 units of blood in most African countries is difficult, and plasma expanders may be unavailable. However, recent data have shown that volume expansion with clear fluids, whether colloid or crystalloid, can markedly improve outcome. When blood is in short supply it should be given after hemorrhage is controlled.

Table 17.6 presents a useful algorithm for determining the clinical necessity for transfusion.

17.5.4 Ruptured uterus

This is a surprisingly common condition in Africa, seen much less frequently in the West. Forty-one percent of all deaths in mothers undergoing CS in Malawi (see 17.4.2) were due to ruptured uterus, mainly in those who had had no previous CS. 'Local medicine' probably plays a large role: there are many types of these herbal medicines used in Africa, but one increases uterine contractions and appears to be very effective for this purpose. In a region where the small pelvis is a common female characteristic, this natural oxytocic is believed to be responsible for many cases of ruptured uterus. Another factor contributing to uterine rupture is neglect of CPD in labor (a 2–month history of 'labor' is the record known to this author). Regurgitation of stomach contents on induction of general anesthesia is also widely blamed on local medicine ingestion during labor.

Uterine rupture can present at any time after the onset of labor. Initially, there is internal hemorrhage and hypovolemic shock and the abdomen assumes a characteristic shape that is both visible and palpable. The parturient usually presents very anemic and soon becomes septic. Fetal demise is the rule, though occasionally at operation the baby survives. In the modern poverty of the developing world, ruptured uterus can present at urban hospitals in similar numbers as at rural hospitals (*Table 17.7*).

Management of the patient with a ruptured uterus is the same as for any hypovolemic patient undergoing surgery. Emphasis should be on speed of anesthetic induction and immediate surgery, rather than prolonged volume resuscitation. An internal jugular line is recommended in addition to a large peripheral catheter, not to measure CVP, but because of ease of placement and the ability to rapidly infuse volume and resuscitation drugs if required, especially in the postoperative period. Induction is performed with ketamine 50 mg and succinylcholine 50 mg, conveniently mixed together in the same syringe and given into the central line. Ether anesthesia or further doses of ketamine are used for maintenance. Total hysterectomy may be carried out, or repair.

17.5.5 Obstetric sepsis

As mentioned above, obstetric sepsis is probably the largest single cause of maternal mortality in Africa today. Septic abortions,

Table 17.6 An algorithm for determining the necessity for transfusion

1. Begin with the patient's current hemoglobin (mg/dl) and subtract 4.[a, b]

2. Subtract more numbers as follows:

(a) Surgery planned	subtract 1
OR	
Surgery with likely blood loss	subtract 2
(b) Uncertain intra-abdominal pathology	subtract 1
(c) Inexperienced surgeon	
OR	
History of large blood loss	subtract 1
(d) Significant medical problems	subtract 1
OR	
Significant respiratory or cardiac disease	subtract 2
(e) Age >50	subtract 1
OR	
Age >70	subtract 2
(f) Recent hemoglobin loss[b], surgery or intra-vascular volume shift	subtract 1
(g) Obesity	subtract 1
(h) Other significant adverse factors (age <1, long surgery, high altitude, etc.)	subtract 1

3. Add more numbers as follows:

(a) Units of blood available	add (no. of units – max 3)
(b) Urgent case	add 1
(c) Emergent case	add 2
(d) System failure (i.e., patient may not get chance for operation again)	add 1
Total:	———

If result is 0 or greater:
- surgical case – proceed with surgery and anesthesia
- medical case – no need to transfuse

If result is less than 0:
- reduce negative factors, or transfuse patient

[a]Why 4? In areas with high HIV seroprevalence and/or blood scarcity, this is the minimum hemoglobin reserve at which an 'otherwise healthy' patient should not need a blood transfusion. In the US or Europe, current practice may support a higher minimum reserve (i.e. a hemoglobin of 6 g dl^{-1}).

[b]Hemoglobin loss here covers occurrence of malaria.

ectopic pregnancies and normal deliveries (or, more commonly, cesarean sections) may develop pelvic or abdominal sepsis any time up to the 10th day post-delivery. HIV seropositivity is usual. Lack of adequate antibiotics or antiseptics, and poor operative techniques are among the reasons for the high infection rate after cesarean section. Operative drainage is usually necessary, requiring laparotomy. In severe sepsis, the argument often becomes whether to do the case at all: is the patient moribund? Predicting patient outcomes with and without operation is one of the more difficult judgments in medical practice in Africa today.

Problems faced by the anesthetist include when to give blood, how to maintain the

Table 17.7 Presenting complications, rural versus urban hospitals, Malawi, Africa, 1998–2000.

	Hemorrhagic shock	%	Anemia	%	Ruptured uterus	%
District hospital (rural) (n = 5236)	454	8.7	371	7.1	233	4.5
Central hospital (urban) (n = 2834)	156	5.5	128	4.5	100	3.5

blood pressure, how much fluid to give, what drugs to use, and whether to protect the airway. Anemia is invariable but volume replacement with crystalloid or colloid is more important in the operative stage, saving scarce blood transfusion for recovery. Intravenous ketamine is used to maintain blood pressure. Intubation is recommended, although a minimalist approach with ketamine and oxygen by mask is sometimes used. Small exploratory operations often turn into full-scale laparotomies. During lysis of adhesions, endotoxemia is maximal and sudden death in asystole may occur. Epinephrine should be ready. The patient's life is often hanging by a thread, and intubation can be seen as the last straw that kills, or a life-saving maneuver to improve oxygenation. The latter is usually the best course followed by ventilation in an ICU. Inotropic support is usually needed postoperatively.

17.6 Morbidity and mortality in obstetric anesthesia

Of all healthcare providers, anesthesiologists and anesthetists can probably make the greatest contribution to a favorable outcome in patients admitted to a hospital with complications of labor. This contribution is not in choice of technique, however, but in knowledge of, and therapy for hemodynamic complications. The majority of obstetric deaths are secondary to hemodynamic problems in parturients neglected post-operatively, who were admitted in very poor condition before delivery.

In a survey of 8070 cesarean deliveries performed in Malawi, there were 85 deaths within 72 hours of surgery (mortality rate 1.05%). A total of 139 patients were observed to regurgitate during general anesthesia; 11 died (one intraoperatively, 10 post-operatively). Aspiration of stomach contents contributed to the deaths of six parturients (five in whom cricoid pressure was applied on induction) and may have contributed to deaths of two more. All these deaths were in parturients who also had preoperative anemia, shock, and sepsis. In uncomplicated parturients, there were 94 cases of regurgitation observed, resulting in only one post-operative aspiration pneumonia and no deaths. Thus, regurgitation and aspiration appear to be an important cause of death only in parturients with other preoperative complications. Cricoid pressure did not appear to prevent it or was not properly applied.

In the same survey, 15 patients died on the operating table, of whom 13 had preoperative hemodynamic complications; two were uncomplicated, apart from cephalopelvic disproportion. Seventy other deaths occurred post-operatively. These deaths were largely unwitnessed, and no resuscitation attempts were reported. The causes were a combination of anemia, sepsis, and hypovolemic shock. Simple measures such as post-operative follow up, volume infusion, blood transfusion, and blood pressure and urine output monitoring can make a significant difference to hospital maternal mortality.

These data indicate that the practice of obstetric anesthesia in Africa, and likely in other developing countries, is complicated by anemia, sepsis, and hypovolemic shock. Anesthetists working in these countries should be aware that these conditions may be some 10 times as important as aspiration of stomach contents as a cause of maternal death.

17.7 Summary and conclusions

While cesarean delivery is the commonest major operation in the developing world, outcomes differ markedly from accepted norms in Western practice due to the differences in severity of preoperative complications, indications for delivery, and anesthetic techniques. The mortality rate associated with cesarean delivery is 1 to 5% in Africa, the major determinant of outcome being the severity of preoperative complications and the quality of postoperative care. Labor and delivery are commonly complicated by preeclampsia, uterine rupture, sepsis, and HIV seropositivity.

Despite the dominance of emergency cases in obstetric anesthetic practice in these countries with high birth rates, anesthesiology as a specialty has not been accorded its due status. While tremendous strides in medical knowledge have been made in recent decades, the chasm between the quality of health care practiced in developed and developing countries continues to widen. The contrasts are greatest in the areas of childbirth and maternal mortality. In anesthetic practice, equipment and manpower show great variation, both between and within countries, due largely to financial constraints. Unfortunately, in poor countries, an acceptable low-cost anesthesia service has not been attainable.

The management of the common complications of shock, sepsis, and hemorrhage in developing countries is no different from the rest of the world, nor is it dependent on advanced technology. It requires primarily skilled anesthetic care in the perioperative period, both before and after delivery. The provision of these skills could reduce the rate of maternal morbidity and mortality in developing countries to a very significant extent.

Further reading

Fenton, P.M. (1997) The epidemiology of district surgery in Malawi. *East Cent. Af. J. Surg.* **3**: 33–41.

Fenton, P.M. (1999) A tale from the far side. *Int. J. Obstet. Anaesth.* **8**: 145.

Fenton, P.M. (1999) Blood transfusion for caesarean section in Malawi. A study of requirements, amount given and effect on mortality. *Anaesthesia* **54**: 1055–1058.

Fenton, P.M. (2000) The pharmacology of volatile agents. *Update in Anaesthesia* **11**: 78–82.

Fenton, P.M. and Tadesse, E. (2000) Reducing perinatal and maternal mortality in the world. *Br. J. Obstet. Gynaecol.* **107**: 831–832.

Fenton, P.M., Reynolds, F. and Whitty, C. (2001) Deaths and perioperative complications of caesarean section in Malawi. *Lancet* (in press). Q2

Hardy, J-F. and Fenton, P.M. (2000) Effectiveness of blood transfusion in Malawi. *Anaesthesia* **55**: 613–614.

Iliff, P. (1995) *Health for whom? Mother and Child Care in Times of AIDS, Poverty and ESAP.* Mambo Press/Silveira House, Harare, Zimbabwe.

Lackritz, E.M., Campbell, C.C., Ruebush, T.K. et al. (1992) Effect of blood transfusion on survival of children in a Kenyan hospital. *Lancet* **340**: 524–528.

Liljestrand, J. (1999) Reducing perinatal and maternal mortality in the world: major challenges. *Br. J. Obstet. Gynaecol.* **106**: 877–880.

Liu, J. (1997) Anaesthesia in the People's Republic of China. *World Anaesthesia* **1**: 42.

Macfarlane, A. and Chamberlain, G. (1993) What is happening to caesarean section rates? *Lancet* **342**: 1005–1006.

Matthai, M., Sanghvi, H. and Guidotti, R. (2001) *Management of Complications in Pregnancy and Childbirth.* World Health Organization, Geneva, Switzerland.

Mbizvo, M.T., Fawcus, S., Lindmark, G. and Nystrom, L. (1994) *Maternal Mortality in Zimbabwe.* Uppsala University/University of Zimbabwe, Harare, Zimbabwe.

Onsrud, L. and Onsrud, M. (1996) Increasing use of caesarean sections, even in developing countries. *Tidsskrift for Den Norske Laegeforening* **116**: 67–71.

Pereira, C., Bughalho, A., Bergstrom, S. et al. (1996) Comparative study of caesarean deliveries by assistant medical officers and obstetricians in Mozambique. *Br. J. Obstet. Gynaecol.* **103**: 508–512.

Schuitmaker, N., van Roosmalen, J., Dekker G., et al. (1996) Maternal mortality after cesarean section in The Netherlands. *Acta Obstet. Gynecol. Scand.* **75**: 332–334.

Steyn, P.S., Odendaal, H.J. and Steyn, D.W. (1998) Trends in caesarean sections at Tygerberg Hospital, South Africa: a 20 year experience. *Cent. Af. J. Med.* **44**: 219–223.

Sun, D. (1993) Letter from Shanghai. *World Anaesthesia Newsletter* **10**: 2.

Thompson, K. (2000) Maternal mortality in Africa. *Anaesthesia* **55**: 191–192.

World Bank (1994) *Better Health in Africa: Experience and Lessons Learned*. World Bank, Washington DC

Index